PRACTICAL MANAGEMENT OF
EMOTIONAL PROBLEMS IN MEDICINE

Practical Management of Emotional Problems in Medicine

Revised and Expanded Edition

Hugh James Lurie, M.D.
Clinical Professor of Psychiatry and Behavioral Sciences
University of Washington School of Medicine
Seattle, Washington

Raven Press ■ New York

Raven Press, 1140 Avenue of the Americas, New York, New York 10036

© 1982 by Raven Press Books, Ltd. All rights reserved. This book is protected by copyright. No part of it may be reproduced, stored in a retrieval system, or transmitted, in any form or by any means, electronic, mechanical, photocopying, recording, or otherwise, without the prior written permission of the publisher.

Library of Congress Cataloging in Publication Data

Lurie, Hugh James.
 Practical Management of Emotional Problems in Medicine.
 Includes bibliographical references and index.
 1. Psychiatry.   I. Title.   [DNLM: 1. Family practice.
2. Mental disorders—Therapy. 3. Physician-patient
relations. 4. Primary health care. WM 100 L967c]
RC454.L87 1982   616.89   81-40019
ISBN 0-89004-707-3

Great care has been taken to maintain the accuracy of the information contained in the volume. However, Raven Press cannot be held responsible for errors or for any consequences arising from the use of the information contained herein.

To my family and friends

Preface

This book describes features and facets of a physician's practice that can make both the doctor and the patient more comfortable with each other and with the medical or psychological situation that brings the patients to the physician. Selected techniques—both ancient and contemporary—are described, touching briefly on various psychological aspects of the practice of medicine, in an attempt to provide new insights and strategies for dealing with old problems.

The present book is an extensive revision of an earlier one (published by Roche Laboratories in 1976); revisions have come from readers' comments, from my own awareness of new perspectives, attitudes, and information on old issues, and where, in my opinion, a different or new point of view might illuminate a murky or obscure issue. Some chapters are totally new, for example, Children's Issues. Other chapters have been expanded significantly. New areas of the primary physician's role—to aid the patient in expanding his own knowledge and attitudes, to serve as a scientific and educational resource person, and to be an "instructor and model," for patients and their families—are emphasized.

The areas of life planning and the physician's mental health are areas of increasing importance, in my opinion, in the lives of patients and physicians. Discussion of these topics is considerably broader and more extensive in scope than in the first publication.

Much psychiatric material had to be excluded or extensively simplified. In a monograph of this size, designed to be of practical use to the primary physician on the "firing line" but also helpful to the resident or even inquisitive medical student, my goal was conciseness, readability, and relevance to office practice. A major challenge remains for physicians: to ensure the compassionate, but effective care of patients with emotional problems or emotional reactions to their physical problems. This book is written with the intent of furthering the efforts of meeting that challenge.

Acknowledgments

Thanks go to Professor William Barger for permission to reprint parts of "The Relationship Contraption" and to reproduce Table 4-1; Ms. Victoria Campbell for permission to reprint parts of "Word Games" and "Personal Sexual History"; Ms. Alene Moris of the Individual Development Center of Seattle for permission to reprint "Life Planning Skills"; Drs. Robert Sack and James Shore and *The Western Journal of Medicine* for permission to reprint three tables from *Psychopharmacology in Medical Practice*; *Medical Aspects of Human Sexuality* for permission to reprint portions of *Sexual Complaints in Family Practice*; Ms. Doris Stevens and the Sexual Assault Center of Harborview Medical Center, Seattle, for permission to reprint *Interviewing Child Victims*, originally prepared with support of grant 77-DF-10-0016 from the Law Enforcement Assistance Administration of the U.S. Department of Justice; Dr. Herbert Benson and William Morrow, Publishers, New York, for permission to reprint "Guidelines for eliciting the relaxation response," from *The Relaxation Response*, © William Morrow, Publishers; Professor Judd Marmor, for permission to reprint the Foreword to the first edition of the book.

Special thanks to Edythe Lurie, Jeanne Longyear, Professor Eric Trupin, Dr. Regina Puryear, and Dr. Nicholas Ward, all of whom read and made helpful suggestions about portions or the whole of the manuscript. Special thanks also to Marg Anderson, who typed the manuscript.

Special appreciation to Dr. B. V. Pisha, whose support of the first and second editions of this book has been crucial in its development.

Much of the material used in the previous edition of this book was originally acquired or developed as a by-product of participanting and teaching in a program of continuing education for primary physicians in Washington State, a project financially supported by the Department of Health, Education, and Welfare, for the U.S. Public Health Service.

Foreword

The primary care physician plays a critical role in the recognition and management of emotional disorders. Nonetheless, a psychiatric diagnosis is often missed or entertained only as a "last resort" and after much time and expense. This book is designed to increase the practitioner's awareness of the patients' psychological development, coping and adaptation, and responses to illness. While of necessity limited in descriptions of psychiatric disorders, Dr. Lurie has managed to distill a great deal of complex information and psychological concepts into a practical approach to understanding patient behavior.

The life cycle from infancy through old age is discussed in detail, giving the practitioner an outline against which to measure patients' growth and ability to cope. The manifestations of psychopathology are described in sufficient detail that the practitioner can begin to identify the major psychiatric disorders as well as the personality patterns of patients and their impact on health care and patient compliance. The substantial inclusion of clinical vignettes describing problems and interactions likely to occur in a physician's office adds both spice and practicality.

This practicality extends to the presentations of different therapeutic approaches, including the roles of psychotherapy and counseling. Other therapeutic approaches are presented in detail. A summary of psychopharmacotherapeutic approaches contains good, basic information for the practitioner, while the extensive list of side effects of drugs commonly prescribed in medical practice will be an invaluable resource.

This book is unique in that it pays considerable attention to the special needs of the physician. The chapter on office milieu includes practical approaches to office management designed to assist the physician in his/her practice. The extensive discussions of values clarification, life planning, stress reduction, and prevention or early detection of stress and impairment touch on often neglected aspects of the physicians' life and work. Spouses may benefit from reviewing these chapters, and they may form the basis for some important family discussion and actions.

While no book can replace the give and take of discussion or the skill development that comes with opportunities to practice, Dr. Lurie has provided numerous ways to apply the cognitive information to help doctors be more comfortable, skilled and successful in recognizing and managing the emotional aspects of physical illness, diagnosing, treating and/or referring patients with psychiatric disorders, as well as providing for their own emotional and intellectual needs. This book taken p.r.n. will be stimulating, useful and enjoyable.

> Carolyn B. Robinowitz, M.D.
> *Deputy Medical Director*
> *Director, Office of Education*
> *American Psychiatric Association*

Foreword to the First Edition

Although there are illnesses in our midst carrying a higher mortality rate, there is none whose morbidity is greater than that of disorders of mental and emotional origin. More than 20 million people in this nation are afflicted with a psychiatric illness of sufficient severity to require some form of treatment. It is manifestly impossible for the 25,000 psychiatrists in this country to meet this overwhelming need, and as a result, other professionals—psychologists, social workers, and psychiatric nurses—even nonprofessionals or "paraprofessionals," have been called on more and more in recent years to assist in providing these urgently needed mental health services.

No one, however, carries a more important responsibility in dealing with this herculean task than those physicians who carry the primary responsibility for the general care of patients and their families. It is well known that anywhere from 50 to 75% of all persons who consult physicians for physical symptomatology have complicating or contributing mental or emotional problems. Thus, it is the primary physician who constitutes the first line of defense, so to speak, in the mental health care of most people. Anything that will enable him to do this more effectively is a matter of extreme importance not only to the quality of his practice, but also to the health of the American people.

It was clearly with the above goal in mind that the author of this volume undertook the difficult but important challenge of attempting to reduce the complex and voluminous material that is encompassed in contemporary psychiatric knowledge to terms that are readable, understandable, and useful to primary physicians and other nonpsychiatric professionals. Such a massive compression inevitably carries with it certain dangers, particularly that of making some problems or processes appear simpler than they actually are. Nevertheless, considering the difficulties involved, Dr. Lurie has succeeded admirably and the result is a volume rich in clinical wisdom and in helpful and practical approaches to the major psychiatric problems that physicians encounter in their daily practices.

Especially helpful is the delineation of the varied therapeutic approaches that can be used in dealing with these problems. Physicians reading this volume may find some approaches more compatible with their own personal styles than others. This is to be expected. We have learned in psychiatry that one of the most important instruments in the psychotherapeutic process is the personality of the therapist himself. It is essential, therefore, that the physician learn to apply his or her own personality, but always within the framework of understanding such as this volume endeavors to provide. The reader must be cautioned, moreover, that the process of psychotherapy, like that of true love, does not always run smoothly. Faith and patience are no less important for the physician than they are for his appropriately named "patient." Equally important is an awareness of the limitations imposed both by the conditions of his practice and the boundaries of his psychiatric knowledge. When those limitations are exceeded he must have both the wisdom and the humility to refer the patient for appropriate psychiatric consultation. Nonetheless, primary physicians and nonpsychiatric professionals will be gratified by how often they are able to help much more than they may be expected, by being willing to set aside enough time to listen to the patients' emotional problems and applying one or another of the techniques described in this volume, as indicated.

Dr. Lurie has performed a particularly valuable service in extending the content of his material beyond the customary psychiatric nosology taught in most medical school curricula. Thus, he deals in highly practical ways with such troublesome behavioral problems as the dependent patient, the seductive one, the hostile one, and the dying one, as well as with strategies such as crisis intervention, medical—psychiatric emergencies, and marital and sexual counseling.

The chapter on the mental health of the physician himself is one that is too often neglected, and Dr. Lurie offers a number of wise and practical suggestions that will enable the physician to tolerate better the sometimes inordinate pressures of his professional life. These pressures can indeed be great, but the rewards of learning to cope with them are even greater. In a world in which so many people are compelled to labor at relatively meaningless tasks simply to make a living, those of us who are physicians are twice blessed; we are not only involved in work that is intrinsically fascinating and challenging, but we are so often able to bring comfort and relief of suffering to those who seek our help. I know of no nobler profession than ours; and although it is true that we are often distressed by the futility of some of our efforts, to the extent that we strive constantly to broaden the horizons of our still inadequate knowledge, we can add to our sense of mastery and so lessen the stressfulness of our responsibilities. This volume offers a meaningful step in that direction.

Judd Marmor, M.D.
Franz Alexander Professor of Psychiatry Emeritus
University of Southern California

Contents

1. The Office Team 1
2. The Milieu 5
3. Holistic Medicine in the Office 8
4. Strategies of Interviewing/Primary Care Counseling .. 10
5. Social Factors and Symptoms 25
6. The Difficult/Problem Patient 28
7. Children's and Adolescents' Issues 42
8. Adult Development and Its Implications For Primary Care ... 72
9. The Aging Patient and Primary Care 80
10. The Doctor and the Dying Patient 92
11. The Depressed Patient 99
12. The Anxious Patient 131
13. Psychiatric Emergencies: The Physician's Role 139
14. Psychiatric Complications of Medical Drugs 148
15. Systems Strategy: Crisis Intervention in Office Practice ... 152
16. Adult Psychotic Illness 156
17. Posttraumatic Stress Disorder in Vietnam Veterans .. 172
18. The Alcoholic Patient 175
19. Psychological Testing 184
20. Behavioral Approaches in Office Practice 191
21. Life Planning 202
22. Marital and Family Counseling 208
23. Sexual Counseling Roles of the Physician 217
24. Mental Health of the Physician 237

Subject Index 245

1

The Office Team

Why do people come to doctors? Some come just to have prescriptions filled, leaving as quickly as possible after seeing the doctor. Others are sufficiently anxious, depressed, or worried about their psychological or physical pain to seek and welcome comfort from anyone at hand. Often such patients talk with other patients, and they would undoubtedly like to talk with the office staff and nursing personnel if these personnel were accessible and forthcoming. When patients are in emotional turmoil, they usually are seeking someone who can sense their distress and take time to be caring and supportive.

Many physicians are aware that their patients have special rapport with certain of the people who work in their offices. It is rare, however, for a doctor to realize that his office and nursing personnel are seen by his patients as an extension of his own lifestyle and style of medical practice. Often a physician's staff project his ability to offer emotional support, to intervene in crisis, and to be seen as a psychotherapeutic force in the lives of his patients.

Nurses, office personnel, and laboratory technicians are usually chosen for their efficiency, personal attractiveness, and apparent skillfulness in performing their particular "official" functions. Unfortunately, office procedures which help the doctor be the most scientific, efficient, and frugal with his time are the very procedures which, by themselves, may prevent a patient in emotional distress from feeling welcome in the doctor's office, from feeling that anyone there cares about him, and, ultimately, from feeling that he really wants to spend time in this particular doctor's office. Insight into his patient's needs allows the physician to use his personnel in a variety of innovative and imaginative ways designed to provide greater comfort to patients as well as to save his valuable time.

To structure or change an office practice so that it provides a broader network of supportive physical and mental health services requires that the physician construct, educate, and supervise his "medical team" in a way that is somewhat different from traditional models of office practice. The doctor interested in building such a team might consider implementing some of the following procedures:

1. Regular meetings of the doctor and his staff may be held to discuss how each member of the team can have a dual role: making the patient feel more comfortable as well as gathering diagnostic data to alleviate the patient's distress. For example, a female patient often confides intimate or "embarrassing" information to a female nurse that she would be reluctant to tell the male doctor.

2. The physician might encourage and support his office staff to acquire and develop the particular skills, attitudes, and self-confidence that contribute to patient care. The staff can then relate effectively with patients, rather than avoiding direct patient contact or feeling more comfortable with an "ask your doctor."

3. The physician can encourage his staff to increase their knowledge about both physical and emotional aspects of clinical medicine, so that the entire team may help "educate" the patient about ways to improve and maintain health.

4. Although the doctor remains "the captain," it makes sense for everyone on the team to feel free to contribute ideas and suggestions about how to approach a difficult patient or a clinical problem. Solving problems with a team may depend as much on a "fresh look at the data" as it does on the professional credentials of the person making the suggestion.

5. Each organization, including a private medical office, may be viewed as having both a vertical (chain-of-command) and a horizontal (colleageal) structure. The more the doctor (who is the head of the vertical structure) can treat his nurses and office personnel as colleagues and maintain an atmosphere of informality and mutual respect, the more the treatment team will seem to function as a team in the patient's eyes. The fussy patient will no longer insist on talking to the "doctor" about minor concerns and may actually be more deeply satisfied by a good chat with a sympathetic nurse.

Doctors who have constructed office support teams have utilized themselves, their personnel, and the office atmosphere in the following ways: (a) there is often a coffee pot available for waiting patients; (b) although reading materials are available for those patients who wish to sit quietly with their own thoughts, the chairs in the waiting room are arranged so that the patients face each other and are close enough to talk in small groups; (c) office personnel not only pull charts but are encouraged to act as facilitators of conversation among the patients and to offer as much support to conversations as seems appropriate.

Some patients have been able to capitalize on this welcoming and relaxed atmosphere. For example, all geriatric patients are scheduled for one afternoon, and the nurse and office personnel circulate among the patients in the waiting room, offering coffee and conversation, very much in the style of a good stewardess or steward in the first class lounge of a "747" or a *maitre d'* in an elegant hotel. A doctor who uses these ideas reports that patients often develop a strong and positive relationship with a particular nurse or staff member (1). This interchange of communication between patients and staff and the feelings of support it engenders often reduces the need of patients to spend a great deal of time with the doctor discussing small physical complaints, as much of the care they feel they receive comes from the physician's alter ego—the staff in the outer office. Other doctors report that having a young staff person or nurse as part of the team often enables teenagers to relate more easily to the office situation and alleviates some of their initial anxiety before they see the doctor. Older nurses or office personnel, with whom the elderly population can more easily feel comfortable, serve the same function for the older crowd.

Supportive psychotherapeutic groups have been established in some offices. The co-leaders are the office nurse (who may have received special training in counseling) and the physician (who is particularly able to clarify the medical issues involved). For example, in the office practice of one physician in Oregon, supportive groups are held prior to the monthly prenatal visits of a group of primiparous women (2). After one-half hour of group discussion (often stimulated by a movie about some aspect of pregnancy or child-rearing), the physician leaves to examine each woman in the group separately. While the examinations are being performed, the group continues to discuss therapeutic issues, helped along by the nurse. All sorts of topics arise, ranging from concern about loss of looks and the feeling that their husbands find them undesirable, to expressions of anxiety and depression. Many of the women develop strong positive relationships with each other through this group experience. These may continue outside the office during their shared pregnancies, constituting a "supportive network" for them. A primary physician who led one of these groups reported that such a supportive system appears to reduce significantly the morbidity of his patients as well as the number of times the patients call on him between scheduled visits.

In another family physician's office, the doctor and his nurse, who has developed skills in counseling, offer supportive psychotherapeutic counseling to individual patients, couples, or families (3). In still another primary care group practice, where many of the patients are Hispanic and speak Spanish exclusively, a Spanish-speaking licensed practical nurse plays a key role in the office, acting as translator, supportive psychotherapist, and "hostess" of the office (4). A family physician in eastern Washington state utilizes his office nurses very much like community health nurses: They make home visits to particular patients about whom he is especially concerned, and serve as "brief therapists" in the office; in the latter case, depressed or dependent patients might be "assigned" to visit the nurse every day and discuss their progress.

Similarly, if nursing personnel have sufficient time, willingness, and rapport to offer counseling and support to the families of dying patients, they may ease much of the grieving process.

The office nurse's more traditional roles, of course, continue to be important in an outpatient practice. There is an increasingly expanding role for nursing personnel to educate the patient within the primary care office setting. This may include "traditional" educational roles, such as explaining, demonstrating, or reinforcing medical or surgical techniques (e.g., insulin injections) or instructing new mothers about infant care; they may also include newer roles, such as establishing behavioral programs for diet and weight control or establishing behavioral programs for mildly confused patients to ensure that they take their medications as prescribed.

Many physicians, as they become aware of the increasing needs and demands of patients for education and information on health maintenance, and the need for informed consent for whatever treatment or medication regimen on which they might embark, have found it useful to add to their group allied health personnel, e.g., physician assistants or nurse practitioners. These persons, working under the supervision of the physician, have been trained to work with considerable independence in both diagnostic and management areas, particularly when the medical problem is reasonably straightforward. If one is adding such a new practitioner to an existing office staff, it is very important to define roles, responsibility, and procedures with the entire staff. To mix metaphors, the flexible office team, working as an extension of the physician, is both the backbone of existing primary care and the wave of the future.

REFERENCES

1. Daugherty, R. (1981): Personal communication.
2. Tozer, E. (1971): Family doctor—but with a difference. *Family Health*, 3:20.
3. De Alva, W., and Peterson, R. (1981): Personal communication.
4. Lurie, H. J., and Lawrence, G. L. (1972): Communication problems between rural Mexican-American patients and their physicians: description of a solution. *Am. J. Orthopsychiatry*, 42:777.

2

The Milieu

The lifestyle of a doctor, personally and professionally, is often a reflection of the beliefs the doctor acquired during his childhood, beliefs which were reinforced in his medical training. Thus those doctors who believe that man was placed on earth to suffer reflect this in their professional lives: They work long hours in unattractive surroundings, making their patients uncomfortable in other ways while curing them of their complaints. A doctor who believes that he is "purely a scientist"—precise, professional, efficient—may whisk his patients through a maze of well-programmed business personnel, past gleaming and antiseptic steel machinery, into starkly clean and cold examination rooms, where the patient may have the dubious pleasure of seeing himself as a laboratory specimen under the critical eye of the scientific observer.

More enlightened doctors who can separate their own spartan needs from those of their less ascetic patients have put into practice the belief that outpatient primary medical care can incorporate attractive surroundings designed for treating people with dignity and courtesy as well as efficiency. The patients of such physicians find themselves in cheerful offices surrounded by personnel who enjoy talking with them. These doctors feel that their offices meet not only their own professional need for cleanliness and efficiency but their patients' needs for comfort and restoration. Turning the doctor's "house" into a "home" where the patient feels support and a warm welcome is highly therapeutic.

When a customer walks into a bank, the experience may be exhilarating. A new bank building, particularly, often has soothing or stimulating arrangements of office furniture, bright carpets, green plants, and interesting pictures on the wall. When one walks into some doctors' offices, on the other hand, the sense of well-being produced by the sunlight and blue sky outside may vanish instantly. One side of the office may have a drab counter, behind which sits a "pawnbroker." Unattractive signs may assault the patient: "Doctor Is In," "No Smoking Please," "Please Show Your Blue Cross Card." The chairs—and this is true even in a new office—look uncomfortable and uninviting, and usually turn out to be as uncomfortable as they look. The lighting is often poor, the magazines often ancient and tattered, and the nurse in her pristine white uniform icy and unapproachable.

Although the contrast drawn here between the welcoming bank and the forbidding doctor's office may be an exaggeration, often these contrasts exist. In the lean years of the Depression, banks and medical offices looked spartan because of both the economic conditions of the day and the furnishing style of the period. Since those days, however, bankers, lawyers, airlines, and stockbrokers have caught up with the twentieth century. They use modern interior decorating techniques to help put the client at ease and make the time spent in their offices as pleasant as possible.

Physicians seem to be the last ones to catch up and catch on. Their lack of awareness and sensitivity to those things in the environment which might increase a patient's comfort has contributed to the tarnished image of medicine and physicians, and reinforced the notion that doctors are a group of cynical businessmen who care only about acquiring money and big cars and who do not give a hoot about patients as people. However, if a patient waiting in the doctor's office can feel comfortable and cared for, he is more likely to think the doctor is concerned about him. Here are some specific suggestions (all tax deductible) which might be of use in creating an atmosphere of warmth and comfort:

1. Choose a room which has enough light—either artificial or natural—so that patients do not feel they are being shut off in a clothes closet. Ideally, the most restful waiting room would be one in which the patients could look out the window onto live trees and shrubs. If windows are not possible, much the same effect can be achieved with pictures of "sympathetic" faces or exciting scenery, or with bright and interesting wallpaper. As decorators have known for years, the more light, the "brighter" the colors (e.g., red or orange), and the higher the ceilings, the greater is the intensity of emotional response to space. To cheer and excite people (and, unfortunately, make hyperactive children more "hyper"), one might consider all of the ingredients mentioned above. To produce a "restful" atmosphere, one uses soft blues and greens and less light. Unfortunately, the latter color schemes may emerge as impersonal, institutional, and cold. Each doctor must ultimately decide which decorating scheme is right for him and his practice; hopefully, the decision will be responsive to his own as well as his patients' needs.

2. Use a rug on the floor, the thicker the better. Children and adults are both attracted by thick rugs, which imply welcome. You may want to have a rug in a neutral color so the dirt does not show, but any color rug can make a difference.

3. Choose comfortable chairs, the kind you would be willing to sit in for several hours if you had to wait, as your patients have to occasionally. If possible, group the chairs in threes or fours around tables. This facilitates communication between patients and dispels the impersonal "train station" atmosphere of many waiting rooms.

4. Anything "living" (fish, green plants) is a sign of hope to patients: Live things imply that the person they are going to see is interested in health and not just illness.

Fish, particularly, are a wonderful distraction for those patients who are too fidgety or worried to be able to read.

5. If you anticipate having children in your office, play materials (e.g., blocks, a blackboard on the wall, goldfish, children's books, and low tables on which one may color) can make the child feel that this is a friendly atmosphere.

6. If coffee or tea is available for patients while they wait, it implies an atmosphere of hospitality and concern. The coffee or tea can also serve as a focus for informal, educational, supportive group experiences, facilitated by nursing or office staff (Chapter 1).

7. Choose pictures carefully. These might be simple posters of landscapes, sporting activities, or anything which appeals to the physician, but the more they suggest the world of the living (sunshine, activity, mountains, etc.) the more hopeful they seem. Diplomas or certificates on the wall may establish the credentials of the physician, but they also convey an authoritarian, distant atmosphere to a person who is already anticipating a lack of receptivity. Especially with adolescent patients, diplomas may actually undermine credibility and convince the patient that the doctor is on an "ego trip."

8. Magazines in the waiting or reception rooms should be up to date, even though their range of subject matter may be general. A 3-month-old issue of *Time* will both fail to distract the patient from his personal problems and convey the impression that the doctor is not sufficiently concerned about the patients to keep his "library" up to date.

The way in which an office is decorated conveys to a patient, rightly or wrongly, how much the doctor respects him and is likely to care for him. To paraphrase what Eliza Doolittle says in *My Fair Lady*: "What makes a lady is not what she says but how she is treated."

3

Holistic Medicine in the Office

The way in which the office is structured can promote the awareness and maintenance of health as well as the elimination of disease. In contrasting sickness with health promotion, a major shift of focus is on the increased participation of the patient in his own health care and maintenance, rather than on that care being determined exclusively or primarily by the physician or another medical authority. For this process to work in any reasonable way, of course, the patient must be informed and educated about options and implementations also must occur in a timely and efficient manner, which still permits the physician to treat a reasonable volume of patients. Information-giving must then be delegated to other people or resources in the primary care system. This can be done in the following ways:

1. Questionnaires can be used to collect data about habits, health maintenance, and lifestyle, instead of spending a great deal of personal interviewing time. Some patients resent forms, of course, so this would have to be highly individualized. Standardized data forms have been found helpful by many physicians (1).

2. Media can be used for educational purposes. This media can be films for specific groups of patients, or prerecorded videocassette programs on Beta or VHS formats, which can be shown on a television monitor in the reception area while patients are waiting to see a physician. The focus of the program may be on health maintenance (regular blood pressure checks, immunizations, diet, exercise, stress reduction techniques), or on techniques of early detection of illness (manual self-examination of the breast). Information about the effects of certain habits (cigarettes, alcohol), may also be included, but such informational approaches are rarely successful in decreasing such habits. A media presentation of information important to patients, but extremely tedious for the physician to continually explain, may increase patient awareness and save time.

3. Other educational materials can be made available. Many pediatrically oriented practitioners have for many years had informational booklets about a variety of pediatric concerns available in their waiting rooms. Increasingly, other physicians in primary care settings are making similar information available, either free or for sale or loan. Manuals, pamphlets, books, and audiotapes exist on a wide variety of topics related to health maintenance and promotion (e.g., relaxation training, parent effectiveness training, couples communication), and most patients welcome these, if they have the endorsement of their physician. They save the physician's time, and can often expand the awareness of the patient from his exclusive disease orientation to a wellness and health orientation (2).

4. Educational experiences and techniques may be used as a prescribed procedure. Many health maintenance and health-oriented organizations (e.g., health department clinics) have offered group-led, educationally-based experiences for their patients on a variety of topics, such as nutrition, communication, normal development, available community resources, etc. (3). Innovative physicians in primary care settings are doing the same thing: assigning patients to attend assertiveness, weight management, and parent effectiveness classes, etc., which either they, or one of their staff or associates runs (or referring to an appropriate resource in the community). Using available community resources to present such courses is feasible, both in terms of time and monetary constraints, and a patient is frequently pleased to discover he can become much more effective in the management of his own health life, and does not always need "experts."

REFERENCES

1. For example, the Cornell Medical Index.
2. For example, *I am Joe's heart*, a videotape developed and distributed by Medcom, Inc., of New York.
3. For example, groups developed and run by the Health Education Department of Group Health Cooperative, Seattle, Washington.

4

Strategies of Interviewing/Primary Care Counseling

Many practicing physicians have acquired their interviewing and communications skills in a rather haphazard way. In medical school, the acquisition of surgical skills is approached in a systematic fashion, with emphasis on a variety of surgical techniques and the applications of such techniques to varying situations. The acquisition of counseling and interviewing skills appears to depend much more on the personal biases of the instructor, the acuteness with which the trainee observes his supervisors, or the prevalence and strength of a particular "school" of psychological thinking within the medical school faculty, including the Department of Psychiatry.

Often there is a marked disagreement among the medical faculty about the value and need for psychological intervention. This, too, plays a role in the extent to which students imitate, try out, and become proficient in using interviewing and counseling skills in their interventions with patients in training, and subsequently, in their professional lives. For example, a psychoanalytically oriented psychiatrist in a department of psychiatry may emphasize that interviews should last for 50 min, should involve active listening and open-ended questions, and should rely on the free associations and ideas of the patient for much of the interview's direction. The professor of medicine, on the other hand, may disparage the value of psychiatry and imply that "crocks" and "goomers" aren't worth the expenditure of much of a physician's time. Patients should be told they have no organic disease ("It's in your head") and they should "get hold of themselves." Behaviorists, conversely, may suggest to medical students that students (and later, medical practitioners) can most profitably spend their time with patients who have emotional problems by teaching patients to record and observe their own behavior and to practice techniques to modify this behavior (such as relaxation techniques). Pharmacologists and biochemically minded psychiatrists may stress a purely biochemical basis for certain behavior, and suggest that students and medical practitioners would best use their time learning about distinctions in medications and how to use chemical agents more precisely and effectively for the amelioration of symptoms.

Faced with all these seemingly conflicting suggestions and attitudes, it is no wonder that some medical students become confused. It becomes easy to acquire the notion that psychological interventions are, at best, somewhat haphazard, lack much precision, and thus, require little study to determine how best and when to apply these skills in specific clinical situations. Fortunately, at the present time, some residency programs in family medicine, as well as some refresher courses focused on emotional problems in primary care, have begun to look critically at these issues. The conclusion is that different approaches to interviewing and specific strategies and approaches to patients with emotional problems may lead to fairly predictable outcomes. Interviewing, like surgical procedures, can become a matter of diagnosing the problem, choosing the appropriate interventions, and considering the advantages and shortcomings of that intervention or approach with a particular patient.

This chapter will describe a few different kinds of interviewing styles and strategies for patients, some pros and cons of these approaches, and the situations in which they seem to be most useful. Later in the chapter, guidelines about building an open relationship will be addressed, as will specific considerations for changing "interviewing" into "counseling." These descriptions of interviewing approaches are not exhaustive. Like any other kind of medical intervention, use of a particular technique requires clinical judgment and an accurate assessment of the total situation in order to be appropriate and effective. There are, of course, oversimplifications. Most seasoned interviewers use a combination of approaches with the same patient, and even in the same interview. For clarity, however, it is useful to separate the various approaches. The following assumptions apply to all of the interviewing approaches:

1. All persons sincerely seeking help are experiencing real psychological pain. Sometimes this pain may express itself as defensiveness, anger, and hostility; at other times as depression, sadness, or dependency.

2. Many people, even when they need and are driven to seek help, are uncomfortable about receiving it. They worry about whether the physician will be understanding or critical. They worry about whether the physician will push them around, not take their complaint seriously, or apply a label of "crock," "malingerer," or "silly." Patients also worry about cost. Will asking a doctor about a marital problem, during a visit for the flu, result in a higher bill? Sometimes a patient associates being ill or seeking help with feelings he had as a child. Any conflict or concerns about being dependent and relying on an authority figure may again be reactivated. If the physician is to help this patient, he must be aware that such feelings might exist, and be able to adopt a strategy to overcome such obstacles.

This strategy might initially take the form of spending sufficient time with the patient to clarify his expectations and his previous experience in seeking help. In the formidable office of the physician, and talking with a person who often may seem to be a formidable "authority," many patients feel inadequate, foolish, and embarrassed to take up the time of "The Busy Doctor." Understanding, accepting, and reassuring such a patient ("But I wish you would tell me about your concerns; that's what I'm here for. They're not trivial, if you're worried about them") are often critical factors to work with in such a patient. The physician needs to gain a clear understanding of how the patient views his relationship with the doctor, regardless of the patient's presenting problem.

3. The doctor's own level of comfort in dealing with emotionally charged issues is an extremely important variable in the success of treatment. Some kinds of problems are innately more frustrating and engender in any physician more anxiety, despair, and feelings of futility than do others. Among such difficult problems are the dying patient, certain kinds of alcoholic patients, hostile patients, etc. If the physician is going to help such patients, he must be able to acknowledge, but not be overwhelmed by, his own reactions to these individuals. Every doctor probably has some patients whom he prefers and others with whom he has more difficulty. When a patient feels inadequate (in or out of the physician's office), he may present himself nervously, demandingly, hostilely, stupidly. Understanding and empathizing with the patient's discomfort are strong ingredients in being therapeutic. The ability to maintain his objectivity and handle the situation in a "professional" and accepting manner—even if at times he would prefer to kick the patient out of the office—may be critical to the physician's success in choosing and implementing a treatment plan.

4. In most medical situations, the physician is the supreme authority, which is certainly appropriate for some medical situations and for some patients. On the other hand, the ability to respond to the variety of emotional problems which patients may present requires that the physician be able to assess objectively his role, and to change it when necessary. This role may vary from being the medical and psychological authority with some patients, to acting as a facilitator and collaborator in mutual problem-solving with other patients who would like to solve their own problems, but need fresh opinions and ideas.

5. The inclination to condemn ourselves and our patients for foibles, indiscretions, and errors of discernment and action is very strong. As an intervention technique in any kind of counseling, being judgmental is usually quite unproductive, particularly when the judgment takes the form of criticism, condemnation, or rejection. Rather than judging, clarifying over time with the patient your view and his view of his situation will both build trust and be more helpful to facilitate change.

TECHNIQUES AND STRATEGIES

The Empathic Style

Empathic interviewing is the cornerstone of supportive interactions in primary care: it conveys acceptance, understanding, and warmth to the patient, and the sense that although in trouble, one is not totally alone. Because patients with emotional problems often experience pain, isolation, low self-esteem, and the sense that no one cares, this approach, through the use and reflection of genuine feelings, can provide immediate comfort.

Guidelines

a. Establish an atmosphere of friendliness and trust.

b. Listen attentively and try to accept both the person seeking help and his problem.

c. Empathize with the patient, rather than "sympathize." Sympathy implies the kind of solace that an adult might give a child—"You poor thing, mother will make your cut all right,"—whereas empathy implies the ability of one adult to really get into another adult's shoes—"I can really feel what you're going through." Sympathy, therefore, has a slight touch of condescension and distance; empathy means that the other person is right there, suffering along with you.

d. Try to clarify issues and assist the person seeking help to diagnose his own problems.

e. Paraphrase the problem (restate in your own words what the person is saying), to let the person know that you are really listening. Identify and try to understand the patient's predominant feelings. Investigate the context of the problem.

f. Summarize.

g. Help the patient to look at alternatives, but *do not give advice*.

Advantages

a. Through this technique, the patient can uncover, understand, and begin to work through the feelings associated with his emotional problem.

b. Because this technique emphasizes that the patient is responsible for his own decisions without the interviewer giving advice, both are relieved of a burden: the interviewer of the responsibility of making a decision for someone else; the patient of the resentment he might feel at someone telling him what to do.

Disadvantages

a. This method requires enough time to be effective. One rarely feels understood or emotionally satisfied if there is an extreme time pressure to disclose and discuss too quickly a personal problem, so that the interviewer can finish up and rush out of the office to help other people.

b. If the patient is not able to clarify what the problem is and the interviewer does not offer suggestions or insist on clarification, there may be no closure or resolution by the end of the interview. At times, patients need specific advice and suggestions, as well as understanding.

c. In some emergencies in which the anxiety level of the patient may be massive, a calm and empathic approach may be misconstrued by the patient to imply that neither he nor his problem is being taken seriously. Empathy and labeling of feelings may be experienced as a rebuff.

Excited Patient: And when the kid ran into my car, I wondered if I was going to be killed.

Soothing Doc: I can see it must have been very upsetting.

Excited Patient: Of course, it was upsetting. I was scared out of my mind. What do you think I'm talking about?

d. For some patients who must and should make real decisions, a sense of being understood may prevent the necessary and desirable process of decision making.

Application

a. With dependent patients, where there is both the desire and fear that the interviewer should make the decisions for the patient.

b. With patients who are experiencing a problem in expressing, dealing with, or resolving feelings such as guilt, sorrow, anger, or self-doubt. This kind of problem is in contrast with problems where feelings are less prominent: "Should I sell the car to buy a piece of land in the country?"

c. As an exploratory technique, in which the physician may have the sense that the presenting complaint is not the "real" problem.

d. With patients in whom the physician recognizes the need and wish to ventilate and be heard, rather than be given advice, i.e., many "normal" adolescents and elderly people, and the majority of people who are grieving over a recent loss, ranging from the death of a friend to the oldest child going off to college.

THE CLARIFYING STYLE

In many psychological or emotional matters, pinning down and clarifying the problem are major steps toward solving the problem and may often, in themselves, be the major therapeutic maneuver. As with all other interviewing styles, this technique should be used with tact, and efforts to clarify must be made in a supportive and concerned manner, so that such efforts will not be seen as a rebuff, but as a further "diagnostic procedure." The purpose is to pinpoint the problem as well as expand the patient's view of it, so that he can reach his own solution.

Guidelines

a. Listen attentively to the presentation of the problem.

b. Ask questions designed to help the person diagnose his own difficulty. Some of these questions should attempt to clarify what the person means or how he feels ("Do you mean you feel angry at your wife when she says that?"). Other kinds of questions might be: Do other people see the problem differently? Has the person developed any alternative ways to solve the problem? Do some choices or options seem more relevant than others?

c. Do not give advice.

Advantages

Many patients are sufficiently upset by their emotional or psychological distress that each of their problems becomes jumbled with every other problem, thereby making a focus on specific problem solving very difficult. The clarifying approach helps (and, at times, forces) a patient to separate out one problem from another, and begin the process of identifying the separate solutions or approaches applicable to each discrete problem. The method is analogous to developing a specific problem list for a problem-oriented record, and developing priorities for which problems to approach first.

Disadvantages

a. Since the interviewer asks questions, this technique may be seen as excessively intrusive, unsympathetic, or "too scientific."

b. Even when specific problems are clarified and identified, their solution may require advice, suggestions, or support. This technique, therefore, is probably applicable in "pure form" only with those patients who have a fair degree of psychological strength and self-reliance themselves.

Application

a. With patients who are chronically confused, because of histrionic traits or personalities ("hysterics").

b. With patients overwhelmed by a number of simultaneous problems (multiple-problem families), and where the patient's concerns with "bare survival" have made any clear decisions about priorities or planning almost impossible.

c. In a serious and acute life crisis where focused thinking is difficult (a death in the family, a prospective divorce, loss of a job, a child running away).

THE CONFRONTIVE STYLE

Being able to confront a patient is a useful skill for a primary physician to have in his repertory: for example, with patients who seem unmotivated for treatment, or for those patients who appear to be wasting their time and yours in a struggle over "who's the boss." Sometimes patients contend with physicians to show that they can still be assertive; such struggles may be a way for a patient to show that he continues to be in charge of his life and that he is not totally dependent on the doctor. Struggles with a doctor may also be a way for a patient to deal with unpleasant feelings, such as depression or helplessness. Sometimes such struggles should be consciously tolerated by the physician, particularly when the doctor decides that this level of functioning is adaptive and should remain unchallenged for the moment. On the other hand, allowing patients to manipulate their treatment may not be useful for them, and may be destructive and exhausting for everyone. Using some of the confrontation techniques described below will begin to allow a clarification of what the physician and patient expect from each other, and may help bring into focus those elements interfering with their mutual collaboration. Confrontation may range from a raised eyebrow, a questioning look, or a statement pointing out a marked inconsistency in the patient's story, to a head-on collision between doctor and patient. How much, what style, and the timing of the confrontation are critical factors. The goal is to help the patient, rather than punish him.

Guidelines

a. Listen attentively to the presentation of the problem.

b. Offer concrete suggestions that might be useful. If the patient repeatedly disputes, disagrees, and argues with these proposals, point this out, and ask the patient if he is aware of this behavior.

c. When the person seeking help repeatedly blames others and "fate" for his difficulties, tactfully point this out.

> "I wonder if you notice that you keep blaming your wife for your difficulties in keeping a job."

d. Whenever there is a marked discrepancy between the *words* and the feelings (affect) expressed, point out this discrepancy.

> "You keep agreeing with me that you want to stop drinking and that you will go along with the program, but when you say it you sound sarcastic and there is a smile on your face."

e. When the person seeking help often meanders into unimportant and irrelevant details which you feel are evasions or attempts to change the subject, try to get him back on the subject and ask him about the behavior you have observed.

> "I wonder why you keep talking about things like being stranded in New York with $1.25, whenever we start getting into your relationship with your wife and children."

f. When the patient projects extreme belligerence, defiance, or an excessively ingratiating manner, you should reflect this back.

> When a patient says, "Oh, doctor, I know that only you can help me, and that you know everything about family problems, but I've tried all of those things you've suggested, and I'm sure they won't work with my family. . . ." reflect back to the person your impression that perhaps he doesn't want to change his behavior and maybe doesn't have as much confidence in you as he says.

g. Share your personal reactions to the statements being made by the patient.

> When an adolescent patient grunts, looks angry, and says, "I don't know," to every question, the doctor might comment, "It looks to me like you really don't

want to be here. I get the impression that you see me as some sort of policeman, rather than as someone who might be able to help you."

Advantages

a. The method is particularly good for cutting through the resistances and roadblocks certain patients set up to interfere with treatment and the possibility of change.

b. If a patient really does not want any help, it is nice to know it.

c. Confrontation forces a patient to decide if he really can work with the doctor trying to help him, and may help the patient decide to finally "get into treatment."

d. Confrontation sometimes works like seeing oneself on a TV screen: it is hard to know how one is coming across without feedback about one's behavior (e.g., hostile patients may not be aware that they appear hostile, until it is pointed out to them).

e. Patients who have had considerable experience conning doctors and others may not start working on their problems until they find someone who cannot be conned.

Disadvantages

a. A confrontation may easily be seen as a criticism or a rejection, and a patient may become defensive, more hostile, or feel rejected.

b. If a person is "really hurting" and concealing it by hostility, a confrontation which identifies the hostile behavior, rather than the underlying hurt, may make the patient feel more alone and misunderstood (and lead to disaster in patient–physician interactions).

Application

a. Especially indicated with those patients whose motivation or commitment to treatment is dubious.

b. Often useful where a patient is making no progress in treatment, despite his alleged involvement in the treatment process.

c. May be absolutely necessary with those patients who have severe personality disorders that cause them to say what they believe the doctor wants to hear, rather than what they really believe.

d. Useful with patients with addiction problems who often agree to a program, but then spend a lot of time sabotaging it.

e. Useful with certain kinds of very reserved or "repressed" individuals who were raised to believe that everybody else's opinion counts except their own, but at the same time feel angry when other people give them advice or act parental.

THE ADVICE-GIVING STYLE

In their "medical role," most doctors are called upon to give advice: the proper medication, the correct surgical procedure, the number of sitz baths a patient should take, etc. In the psychological realm, patients rarely respond positively to advice that their physician gives them. The main reason for this is that for advice on psychological matters to be effective, it must in some way convey an empathic understanding of what the patient is experiencing and be seen as an unprejudiced offering of help to the patient in his dilemma, and not just an edict on what to do. Advice is often seen as a putdown, a desire by the physician for a quick solution when such a solution may not be possible, or a desire to get rid of the patient because "he takes up too much time." Some patients, of course, value specific alternatives and solutions if presented logically, and will welcome any input that contributes to a new perspective. Such input may certainly take the form of advice. In other words, for advice to be useful, it must fit the framework and context in which the patient himself defines the problem. Advice may also be more acceptable if it is given as an attempt to clarify alternatives, rather than as a strategy by the physician to promote his own particular alternative.

Guidelines

a. Listen thoughtfully to the problem presented.

b. Recall and describe a similar experience that you or someone you knew had to deal with. Explain what was done to solve it. If the help-seeker does not accept this solution and you still see it as valid, try to explain further (e.g., "Some people in your situation have considered vocational counseling....").

c. Recommend, in order, the steps you would take if you were in this situation. If the person does not accept some of these, make other proposals until you hit on something that is seen as helpful by both.

c. Outline, as you see them, the specific alternatives the person has, as well as the consequences of following these alternatives.

> "If you buy your wife a piano, it will cost more than you can afford. But, if you don't buy it, it sounds like she might divorce you."

Advantages

a. Brevity.
b. Ability to focus on a situation.
c. A chance for the patient to get another opinion in a hurry.

Disadvantages

a. In such a relationship the patient becomes dependent on your solutions, and this dependency and "need for supervision" may continue.
b. Advice-giving may easily stir up anger and resentment in the patient. If this occurs, the help and advice will doubtless be discarded.
c. Giving advice creates a hierarchy-authority position and establishes a greater emotional distance between you and the person seeking help, and the feeling

that the "doctor doesn't understand" may occur very easily. (Think of the many hours of advice about the dangers of alcohol which are given to alcoholics every year by physicians, and the relatively few instances when the advice is adopted, unless the person with the drinking problem participates actively in the planning.)

Application

Especially useful with those patients who require structure and a clear plan. Such patients may be those persons experiencing a "crisis," severely depressed or suicidal patients, patients recovering from psychotic illness, or patients with severe impairment of judgment or intellectual function resulting from organic brain damage or mental retardation.

"Body Language"

A primary physician, in his dealings with his patient, may talk with him from a variety of physical positions and postures: face to face, while examining the patient (standing over him, in back of him, below him, above him), while writing his prescriptions at the desk. In talking with the patient while he is supine in his bed, the posture is almost invariably one of gazing down.

Experts estimate that 80% of communication is nonverbal. Any posture not face to face, with eye contact on the same approximate level, is likely to be experienced as distant, parental, or unconcerned. Many patients are virtually unable to talk with a physician standing behind or above them—the posture is excessively reminiscent of parental hovering. Furthermore, an authority hovering over a patient or with his back to the patient may be perceived as critical and negative, feelings the physician may be unaware he is communicating.

To communicate effectively, the physician should be at eye level, lean forward, be at a "socially comfortable" distance (in the USA, approximately 2–3 feet, in Latin cultures, often less), and eye contact should be sustained during the interview. If at the patient's bedside, sitting in a chair next to the bed will facilitate the sense that the physician is personally concerned, and not the hovering authority, about to pounce or depart. Especially in dealing with children, communication with them at eye level promotes trust and disclosure. Looking up at a cluster of giant noses worn by parent, doctor, or nurse does little to promote a sense of security or a desire to confide.

ESTABLISHING AN OPEN RELATIONSHIP

Complementing the various techniques listed above is the ability of the physician to establish an open relationship with patients (or with other people in his life, such as his family). The *advantages* of an open relationship are that it usually allows both participants to feel close to each other, and is also usually a more personally rewarding way to communicate feelings of mutual understanding and sharing. The *disadvantages* include the substantial effort often necessary to maintain such openness, the possibility that the person with whom one is being open will not reciprocate, and the risk that attempts to be open may be misunderstood as some other kind of overture (such as sexual). Clinically, being able to develop an open relationship is particularly helpful if the physician intends to develop a colleageal relationship with the patient, e.g., have the patient be aware of the medical alternatives, share in the decision making, and be truly a part of the "informed consent."

At other times, even though the doctor's relationship with his patient may usually be more formal, the physician may decide to shift to a more personal, open relationship style as a way of reaching out to the patient who is in particular pain, sorrow, or grief. In primary care, the physician often has a long-term relationship with the patient's family, social situation, and support system in a way unavailable in other settings.

Table 4–1 outlines the dimensions of an open and closed relationship, i.e., specific time, specific information, personal perceptions, and the use of feelings.

Time Factor

In a closed relationship, people use generalizations and other kinds of data which are not time or person related. As one moves from the closed relationship toward an open one, the time focus narrows to the "here and now" and the topic narrows to the specific person.

Specific Information

Closed relationships use generalizations, jokes, and weather talk as a medium of exchange. The message is: "Let's agree to have this meaningless conversation since it will help pass the time," but the relationship is not important. Much of the social chitchat that occurs in most offices (including doctors' offices) consists of generalizations and maneuvers which serve to maintain distance between patient and physician. Such devices may be useful with brief, routine transactions, and

TABLE 1. *Dimensions of an open and closed relationship*

	CLOSED			OPEN	
Who is concerned about the **topic**?	A topic of concern to neither, e.g., weather talk.	A topic of concern to one of us.	A topic of concern to both of us.	The topic is our relationship, you and me.
What is the **time** frame?	No time perspective, e.g., jokes, generalizations.	Distant past or future.	Recent past or future.	Now...presently being experienced.
How do we use **feelings**?	Feelings are excluded as irrelevant or inappropriate.		Describing our feelings is viewed as providing helpful information.	
How **personal** will we be?	Generalizations...abstract ideas, intellectualizations.		Inner, private information, perceptions, feelings, thoughts.	
	CLOSED			OPEN	

Courtesy of Dr. William Barber, Eastern Washington State University, Cheney, Washington.

may even be crucial when it is necessary to terminate an interview or when the closeness seems excessive or sticky (as when a patient appears to be making a sexual advance, or is inappropriately seeking personal information from the physician which seems an invasion of privacy). As the relationship becomes more open, the information which is shared is specific, of immediate concern and intent to at least one of the persons in the transaction, preferably both.

Including Personal Perceptions

On the closed end of the spectrum of relationships, discussions focus on "objective" data and information. Personal perceptions and points of view are excluded as irrelevant and unnecessary. As one moves toward the open end of the relationship spectrum, an increasing amount of personal information and perceptions is shared by each.

Example:

The physician who has a pleasant but superficial relationship with an elderly woman to whom he prescribes antihypertensive medication on a regular basis may significantly change his style of relating to her during a bereavement period after her husband's death. Thus, rather than just commenting on medication dosages and schedules, the physician may express his personal concern for her personal health and his sympathy for her grief. He *may* even share some of the thoughts he had when he lost someone near to him and how the experience of grief must be painful to her, as it was to him.

The Use of Feelings

On the closed end of the spectrum, feelings are excluded as being irrelevant. On the open end of the spectrum, the sharing of feelings is seen as useful and appropriate. "Feelings" are different from perceptions, which are largely cognitive or intellectual. Feelings have emotional impact and affect attached to them. Thus, the more open the physician wishes to make the relationship with the patient, the more the physician will share his own emotional, "gut level" reactions to the situations being discussed. Being able to share feelings is particularly important when dealing with vulnerable individuals, such as those who are depressed, dying, the elderly in general, and little children.

COUNSELING IN PRIMARY CARE

Is counseling in primary care different from interviewing? Sometimes. Interviewing and the skills included in it can be applied to history-taking, data collection, system reviews, and diagnostic sessions. Counseling usually implies that a contract, explicit or implicit, exists between the patient and his physician, where both agree they will collaborate, usually over a specified period of time, on particular problems or issues. If counseling is to work in the primary care setting, certain aspects of the therapeutic contract must be clear: (1) What is the problem? Generally, the more specific, defined, and limited, the better it is to work on; (2) how long is each session between patient and physician?(15 or 50 min?); (3) over how long a period of time will sessions continue, and at what frequency? (once a month for 6 months?); and (4) how much is each session costing? (Physicians in primary care are often peculiarly reluctant to charge for their counseling time, labeling it "doing nothing," even though the patient finds it valuable.)

In making a counseling contract, it is crucial to keep in mind what kind of help is helpful. Often over time, with a particular patient, the help offered needs to change.

Example:

> For a person in an acute crisis (his child was badly burned and needs intensive care), information and direction may initially be far more helpful than empathy alone. For the same person suffering bereavement, advice may be out of place and offensive.

Specific kinds of counseling may have a different focus, and offer different kinds of help. The following are some examples.

A. Crisis Counseling (e.g., a patient is acutely overwhelmed or out of control).
  1. Establishment of a positive relationship.
  2. Review and understanding of the steps leading to the crisis.
  3. Ignore maladaptive behavior and emphasize positive behavior.
  4. Help patient recognize and defuse powerful feelings which are interfering with planning.
  5. Help patient evaluate actual crisis situation, prioritize action steps, mobilize coping skills, and mobilize support system.
  6. Establish a time limit within which you hope to help patient stabilize to his previous level of functioning.
  7. Consider additional sessions or referral as indicated.
B. Support Counseling (e.g., the patient is coping with the "empty nest," mobilizing to return to work, and increasing social life outside the home).
  1. Positive, empathic approach (respect, understanding patient's frame of reference, nonjudgmental).
  2. Communication and understanding in a language and vernacular in which the patient feels comfortable.

3. Genuineness.
4. Warmth.
5. Reinforce constructive client action, including talking about the situation.
6. Listening.
7. Consistency.
8. Non-defensiveness.
9. The therapist shares his own reactions.

C. Education as Counseling (e.g., the patient needs information about child rearing).
1. Assess the level of current understanding and information by the patient.
2. Assess what the patient expects as a result of increased knowledge and skills in a particular area. (Is it personally relevant?)
3. What is the specific clinical problem or anticipated problem toward which the education is directed? Can you and the patient both evaluate the effectiveness of the education in addressing the clinical problem?
4. Set up a process whereby the patient learns the new information, skills, or classifies his attitudes and values around a particular issue. (Can this be facilitated even more by assigning articles, books, or audiovisual materials?)
5. What are the factors facilitating or interfering with using the new information or skills?
6. Be aware of the patient's feelings of inadequacy or potential resistance to "expert advice."

D. Counseling for the Improvement of Emotional Conflict (e.g., the patient is torn between family and career obligations).
1. Time limited and focused.
2. Actively support the patient developing his own hypotheses, intuitions, and fantasies about his difficulties.
3. Clarification of patient's values (especially in relation to value differences between him and his family or employer).
4. Support the patient developing realistic alternatives for testing out possible hypotheses and courses of action.
5. Clarify alternative ways to see situation.
6. Concrete actions; develop in detail how the patient might try different alternatives.
7. Develop a force field analysis (which forces facilitate and impede implementing a new plan, life change, etc.).
8. Develop an accurate appraisal regarding job, educational, emotional options.
9. Appraisal of the support system.

To do justice to his role as counselor, the primary physician needs a number of approaches and strategies for interviewing his patients, developing a more open relationship if he chooses, and counseling the patient in a way that provides help for the kinds of problems experienced by the patient. Of course, no set techniques or rules are a substitute for the spontaneous, impromptu intervention, which may seem just right to both doctor and patient, and which may arise out of the long relationship between them. Ultimately, however, a range of interviewing and counseling options saves the time and energy spent retracing and retrying interviewing and counseling approaches which misfired the first time around.

5

Social Factors and Symptoms

Studies by Hollingshead and Redlich (1), Berlin (2), and others suggest that the way in which psychological symptoms are manifest may be related to socioeconomic, societal, and family style factors as much as dynamic factors. The lower the person is on the socioeconomic scale, the less educated and sophisticated he is, and the less sophisticated his background, the more likely it is that he will present psychological distress in somatic terms. Thus a rural working man may complain to his physician of fatigue, headaches, or back trouble; a person with more experience in examining his emotions and expressing his feelings may complain of anxiety or depression, feeling "blue," etc. It is certainly true that in symptom complexes such as anxiety and depression "vegetative symptoms" are often part of the syndrome or disorder, and, in the case of depression, these may include insomnia, weight loss or gain, constipation, early morning awakening, and so on. Nonetheless, a physician should consider that a somatic complaint may reflect a specific psychological state in his patient.

Example
"Doc, I'm really feeling tired. I've got this backache and headache that have been bothering me for about a month." The physician, after getting more history about the complaint, might inquire: "I wonder if you could tell me how things have been going in general. I mean, is there anything in your life that might be depressing you or upsetting you, or making you feel 'down'?"

If the doctor is lucky, the patient may respond, "Come to think of it, things have been really lousy between the wife and me recently. She's even been talking about taking the kids and leaving."

If the doctor is less lucky, the patient may reply, "Everything's fine. It's just my back that's killing me!" Many tests and pills later, the patient may be ready to start discussing his feelings.

Obviously, the examples above are unusually graphic, but the deeper meaning of psychological symptoms and the particular symptoms the patient believes are "okay" to present to his doctor must be kept in mind. Balint (3) described the way in which specific physical or emotional symptoms are "agreed upon" by both doctor and patient as the basis for their work together. The patient "offers" a particular symptom, which the doctor may accept or for which he may offer a substitute.

Conversion ("hysterical") phenomena occur when a psychological symptom or conflict is expressed through dysfunction, paralysis, disorder of voluntary musculature, or disorder of the senses (sight, hearing, etc.), without the presence of any demonstrable neurological basis for the malfunction. The degree of psychological sophistication of the patients varies; several factors determine whether the symptoms include hysterical or conversion elements. Thus children and naive, intellectually limited, or socially isolated adults may present with hysterical inability to move a limb, hysterical blindness, or sudden nonphysiological paresthesia, all without a neurophysiological basis. Such symptoms often respond promptly to strong suggestion, brief supportive contact with a physician, or sufficient exploration of the patient's life situation to make it apparent to both patient and doctor that the symptom may have some kind of special symbolic meaning.

In traditional sex roles (although these are gradually changing), boys do not cry, whereas girls are permitted to have and express painful emotions much more openly. Translated into adult patterns, women use medical and psychological services at a considerably higher rate than men do and complain more openly of anxiety, depression, or other dysphoric feelings, whereas men often feel it would be "weak" or a betrayal of masculinity if they complained of such emotions. Even strong men, however, are "allowed" to have backaches, and sometimes do, when experiencing sufficient emotional distress.

Symptoms presented to a doctor not only can reflect social expectations but may have a cultural or familial basis as well. In some American subcultures (e.g., Mexican-American or native American) feelings, moods, and emotions are simply not mentioned to a physician. The doctor deals in pills, fevers, injections, and surgery. Psychological disturbances—weird thoughts and feelings, discontentment—would be discussed with a respected elder or a close relative of the same sex, if at all. A similar, narrow perception of the physician's role occurs to a large extent among isolated, less-educated, or naive population groups. In some cultures (e.g., the Chinese), having a "depression" is seen as a familial blight, bringing disgrace on the family and making the individual less marriageable. Thus a patient may present with fatigue, tears, and vegetative symptoms of a depressive disorder but deny any difficulty with mood (4).

When approaching the treatment of somatic complaints for which there is no physical basis, the physician needs tact and an awareness of the orientation of the patient toward his symptoms. (For example, can such a patient talk about feelings?) It becomes crucial to assess the patient's understanding of his symptoms and his expectations of treatment before the physician outlines his assessment and treatment plans. Patient compliance is largely determined by whether the diagnosis and treatment plan correspond to the patient's expectations. If the patient stalwartly resists any hints that psychological factors may play a role in his condition, then strategies other than explicit counseling must be considered. These might include (1) a tranquilizer or even a placebo for the person who clings tenaciously to his "nerve trouble" or his tension headache; (2) brief supportive visits with the physician that focus on improved functioning or on life planning; (3) working in collaboration with a therapist who shares the patient's cultural values (or can at least work around these) and can act as an intermediary to facilitate patient compliance; (4) a behavioral program (often in collaboration with the patient's family) to reinforce other, healthier aspects of the patient's life and defenses against anxiety, ridding him of somatizing and hypochondriasis; and (5) referral to a therapy group where other patients may support and educate him about how emotions and physical symptoms are often closely linked. Many (if not most) patients come to a doctor for immediate symptomatic relief. Only those patients with some understanding of their emotional life can tolerate the notion that pain may come from emotional causes and not from "bad nerves," and that symptoms may be relieved through talking rather than through medications.

REFERENCES

1. Hollingshead, A. B., and Redlich, F. (1958): *Social Class and Mental Illness*. Wiley, New York.
2. Berlin, I.: Professor and Head of Division of Child Psychiatry, University of New Mexico, Albuquerque, NM (*personal communication.*)
3. Balint, M. (1957): *The Doctor, The Patient, and His Illness*. International Universities Press, New York.
4. Kleinman, A. (1980): Ethnicity and clinical care of the Chinese patient. *Physician Assistant Health Practitioner*, 4:60–68.

6

The Difficult/Problem Patient

Some patients are considered, because of their personal and interpersonal behavior with the physician, to be "problem" or "difficult" patients.

Such patients often make up a large portion of the primary care population, and yet many doctors blanch at the thought of dealing with them. Although these patients pose special difficulties because of their particular style of presenting themselves, the problem is often as much with the physician as with the patient himself. Being in close quarters with a difficult patient elicits feelings of "being in a foxhole." There is the pressure of a forced choice, a sense that one must do something right now, and do it despite one's feelings of shock, dismay, revulsion, or anger. A major reason that the problem patient often becomes the doctor's problem is because several of the basic value assumptions of the physician and his life are seriously challenged by the patient's behavior.

The first is "I am a rational, efficient scientist." When the patient's behavior is so distracting, hostile, or provocative, the assumption that the patient recognizes this "scientist" aspect of the physician is entirely thrown out.

A second assumption, "I am a 'kind' caregiver," is also seriously challenged, when the patient appears to disdain the physician's offerings and help.

The third, "A good physician should be in control of the doctor–patient interaction," is open to question, if it becomes clear that the patient, by various maneuvers, is controlling what is happening in the interaction, and the physician is powerless, or at least relatively so.

The fourth assumption, that the patient–doctor interaction is a human transaction, in which the skilled physician is using all of his empathy and intuition about human needs to respond to the patient, is shattered when the patient acts in a way in which the physician feels dehumanized.

What should be the stance of the physician dealing with the problem patient? Several tenets seem important to consider with any problem patient.

1. The physician should view the patient's behavior as a way of coping, rather than as behavior motivated by personal hostility or vindictiveness.
2. The physician should be aware of, and compensate for, his own feelings of hurt, anger, and being manipulated, and consciously decide not to do anything about such feelings except know that they are there. Retaliation is almost always untherapeutic.
3. The physician should acknowledge the patient's feelings of discomfort which often underlie the patient's need to be difficult.
4. The physician should begin to search for alternative choices and strategies with the problem patient.
5. The physician should, if necessary, explicitly define and clarify his role with the patient.
6. The physician should ask himself, "Despite how the patient is acting, what does he really want: Is there nonverbal and covert behavior indicating that he wants help, even if he is saying that he doesn't? (Often the physician's intuitive sense is the guide to determining this answer.)
7. What do you, as a physician, feel that the patient needs?
8. What is the patient's milieu—his "system"—of which this is a part. (Why would the patient need to act this way with you? What else is going on in his life?)

THE HOSTILE PATIENT

A myriad of reasons may occur to the experienced physician to explain why a patient might openly express hostility toward a physician either in the office or at the hospital. There may be a "realistic" cause, such as having to wait two hours in the waiting room or being treated brusquely by a nurse or receptionist. Or this may be a characteristic way in which this patient deals with the world, trying to dominate or challenge a threatening person or situation. On the other hand, the hostility may be an expression of the fear, depression, or grief which the patient experiences because of his real or fantasied illness. He may also fear and resent having to accept help from and depend on another person for his comfort. With either this fear of accepting help or this need to dominate in threatening situations, the patient may be transferring to the current situation old feelings which originally were present in his childhood; such behavior is not dictated by "personal" feelings toward the doctor.

Still another cause for anger is a fantasied loss which an illness may imply: a loss of independence, self-respect (if there are any physical limitations), and, with surgery, a loss of a part of oneself which may be seen as precious by the patient, even if seen as "diseased and defective" by the physician. All of these emotions—fear of illness, fear of dependency, depression, grief, anger about losses—may crystallize in a hostile reaction of a patient toward the physician. It is the doctor who is the "bearer of bad news," and the "man in charge," and the person who can be active and "help," while the patient feels helpless. It is a rare patient who, in moments of anger, can analyze his behavior and seek out the feelings behind his own anger (and an equally rare physician who will accept the patient's anger with compassion).

Strategies and Approaches

Most of us have learned that when somebody gets mad at us we are entitled to get mad in return. Especially with the American male, there is a macho tradition of "not taking anything off of anyone," and "standing up for yourself." Such attitudes are both useless and destructive when a doctor sees a hostile patient and feels compelled to act out such beliefs. The only practical way to deal with the patient's hostility is to avoid becoming hostile in return. When two people are fighting mad, it is almost impossible to do any constructive problem-solving: one of them should remain calm enough to figure out what to do.

In an encounter between an angry patient and a physician, the physician must remain calm, even if he feels like punching the patient in the mouth, or telling him to go away (and maybe not come back). A tactful confrontation technique in which the doctor calls attention to the patient's anger and inquires about it is a useful way to begin. The doctor may want to offer the patient the option of continuing to see him or seeking another physician. Or the physician may soothingly empathize with the pain and discomfort which must be producing the patient's anger, and stress the support he is willing to give during the patient's ordeal. Thus, to the patient's comment, "The medicine you give me for my cough isn't doing a thing for me! What kind of a doctor are you, anyway?", the doctor might reply, "Gee, you certainly seem angry with me. I wonder why you're so mad." Or, "It must be hard for you to continue to have all these troubles without feeling that anything I do is helping you." Or, "Are you saying that you've lost confidence in me? Would you like to see somebody else?" The difficulty with the last kind of statement is that when a patient feels angry about what is happening to his body and is doubting whether it will ever work smoothly again, his judgment may be unreliable and his actions self-destructive. If such a patient "fires" his doctor, the immediate consequences may be harmful and injurious to the patient. For example, he may decide he can manage his own illness and delay treatment until it is too late. As a long-term consequence, he may rationalize the encounter by perceiving it as a rejection by the doctor. At the same time, one should remember that patients *do* have ultimate authority over their own lives, and that it is their legal and personal prerogative to reject the doctor and his advice.

The strategies for dealing with hostility involve patience, forbearance, acknowledging and defusing the anger, clarifying the issues, focusing on those aspects in the patient's life that are giving him/her real pain, clarifying your role as physician, and embarking on mutual-problem-solving to help the patient feel better. Sometimes just having the patient talk for a while with an attentive audience is enough to defuse the hostility ("Don't just do something, stand there!"). Sometimes nudging the conversation toward a less irritating topic than the presenting complaint may also dissipate the anger, and permit the attack to evolve into a more human interchange. A verbal sparring match is useful neither to the patient nor his doctor, even if both momentarily feel that's what they'd like to do. This is not to say that if there is a firm therapeutic relationship, that angry feelings or disappointment may not legitimately be expressed: they can and should (and may also be valid!). The caveat is not to turn a hostile beginning into an escalating exchange of irrevocable insults. The doctor who says, "I don't have to take this from you. Go find yourself another doctor," is likely to be countered with, "I think you're incompetent and irresponsible: I plan to report you to the Medical Association. A doctor who insults his patients ought not to be practicing." From a selfish point of view, not fighting with a hostile patient may be a practical preventative measure against a future lawsuit. (Lawsuits are provoked as much by the patients' feelings that their doctor did not understand and care about them, or rejected them, as they are by "legitimate" issues of incompetence and neglect.)

But, hostility may be legitimate. Like the amateur lepidopterist looking for a rare specimen, the wise physician will continue to search for the justifiably hostile patient; the one who waits interminably in his waiting room (with butterflies in his stomach), who is somehow passed over in line, who is the recipient of tactless or rude remarks by the staff, who is forgotten as he or she shivers in his/her short gown in the dim examination room, reading the Snellen chart for the 200th time. The same wise physician will periodically look to see how much his office revolves around patient comfort, and how much around staff convenience. Long hours in the waiting room may be avoided by hiring a physician's assistant or nurse practitioner or associate to do much of the screening or routine history-taking and system review. The waiting room atmosphere (see Chapter 2) can help the patient feel he is being treated to a period of rest and relaxation rather than being held prisoner. Patients (unless certified masochists) universally dislike long waits in flimsy gowns in examining rooms. Adequate scheduling (and a competent scheduler) should prevent excessive waiting. If a long wait is somehow inevitable, a nurse popping in with an apology and a magazine can turn off the mounting hostility.

Patients have been known to change physicians because they dislike a nurse or receptionist. A cold, brusque, unhelpful nurse will, at the very least, guarantee that a high proportion of angry, hostile, resentful patients finally face the doctor in the examining room (requiring more time, of course, to soothe).

Office personnel answering the telephone should make it clear to patients the time when the doctor will most likely be able to return their calls. A 9:00 a.m. inquiry not answered until 5:30 p.m. produces an angry patient who would have been much less angry had he been told that the doctor could not return the call until late in the day, and *not to wait around*. Most important, calls *should be returned*! The doctor may decide that the patient's complaint is trivial and can be dealt with at the appointment next week, but the patient will conclude that the doctor cares nothing for his health and peace of mind. An unanswered inquiry may result from a nurse not passing on the message, but the patient will naturally place the blame on the doctor. Everyone loses when the patient becomes and remains hostile. But, it is the physician who, if not able to salvage the situation, can at least train himself and his staff to prevent it from occurring.

THE DEPENDENT PATIENT

Dependent patients are in many ways "good" patients, but can drive a physician to distraction. Dependent patients take their medicine, listen eagerly to the doctor's advice, and show up faithfully—sometimes too faithfully—for appointments, and improve by miniscule amounts. What irritates physicians about such patients is their clinging quality and the peculiar role into which they force a doctor: being omnipotent, omniscient, infallible, and (hopefully) perpetually available. This combination of clinging obedience and childish adulation churns up a mixture of emotions in most doctors. The compliance is welcomed, but the doctor can't help but complain to his colleagues that he wishes his patient would "grow up."

Strategies and Approaches

A first and necessary step in evolving an effective strategy to deal with a dependent patient is to figure out why the patient is dependent. Is it a life-long pattern involving every authority figure? Is it a way of seeking affection and attention from the physician? After assessing which is the most likely alternative, the physician can take the following steps:

1. If the patient has had a long history of dependency on a series of authority figures, the physician must determine just how much contact with the patient is optimal, and then set limits accordingly. Doctor–patient contact might be weekly visits of five minutes or semimonthly visits of half an hour, but imposition of a "structure" will help both patient and physician build a relationship in which dependency is minimized.

2. If the dependency springs from the difficulties attendant upon a major or chronic illness (such as diabetes, a malignancy, or chronic lung disease), the physician can establish a frequency of visits to best meet the psychological and physical needs of the patient. For example, a patient with chronic emphysema may need to be seen once a month for medical reasons alone, but for psychological reasons (support, reassurance, coming to terms with the disability) needs telephone contact once a week. Specifying this arrangement in advance avoids the pitfall of return visits on a p.r.n. basis, which the dependent patient will use as a reason to turn up every week, even if he does not have a medical problem. If addressing the patient's psychological needs requires more time than the primary physician has available, he can either make a referral to an appropriate mental health agency, train one or more of his staff to provide the necessary emotional support, or act as triage to the community support persons and groups who could assist the patient.

[NOTE: Although both (1) and (2) above suggest establishment of specific limitations on doctor–patient contacts, the purpose of these limitations differs. In (1), the patient needs to be prevented from forming a dependent relationship with the doctor, since it serves no useful medical or psychological purpose. In the case of the second (2) patient, however, some degree of dependency is natural, inevitable, and desirable. The concern is to prevent it from becoming crippling for either doctor or patient.]

3. If the patient uses clinging and compliant behavior as a way of seeking attention and affection from the physician, it is often because no one else will meet those needs. A healthier thrust with this kind of dependency and dependent patient is helping him gradually establish for himself more viable support mechanisms. The doctor can investigate other community resources which might meet the patient's needs, recommend life planning, or serve as a bridge between the patient and appropriate support groups. This means, of course, that the physician must assemble his own resource lists, including agencies, and specific people who might themselves provide or know people who could provide what the patient needs. Thus, in the case of a geriatric patient who insists that the doctor stop by for a blood pressure check, even when the blood pressure is fine, the doctor has the option of (a) continuing to stop by and giving the patient emotional support under the guise of a medical service; (b) arranging for a community health nurse or a clergyman to stop by from time to time to see how the patient is; (c) contacting an agency in the community which does volunteer work with the elderly to see if someone would be available to visit on a regular basis, perhaps to take the patient shopping or for rides if poor vision or partial disability is a factor in the social isolation; or (d) sending one of his own nurses to talk with the patient with instructions to encourage gradual resumption of contact with the existing friends and family. This contact can also be facilitated by the physician or his nurse, with the patient's permission, phoning the family to talk about increasing or changing their contact with the patient.

The doctor or his nurse can also keep in contact with a patient by telephone. If community outreach agencies are few, and if the physician has many bedridden, geriatric, or infirm patients, he might find it useful to organize his own corps of volunteers to phone and visit these patients. Alternatively, such a project might be set up through a church service group, the leader of which could report to and receive instructions from the doctor periodically. All of these strategies may be temporary; the goal is to provide short-term support for a dependent individual while encouraging him to make contacts in the community to provide a wider support network and lessen the need to depend on one individual, alone. In some withdrawn, fearful, or reticent individuals, the link to the world—their bridge to life—may still be through the physician and his staff.

If the patient is infirm and needs more medical or supportive care than the doctor or any outpatient program can provide, the physician will need to work with both the patient and his family on placement either in a nursing home or in an appropriate part-time facility. Alternatives could include a nursing home day-care program, where the patient comes to the nursing home during all or part of the day for socialization and medical care and returns to his own home at night; periodic admissions to a nursing home facility in order for drugs to be regulated and to allow the family, if they are taking care of the patient, to have a respite. In some nursing homes, arrangements can be made for the family to receive on-the-spot training in physical rehabilitation programs which they can use with the patient at home. Some nursing homes also provide a continuum of services (with medical backup) ranging from total intensive nursing care for physical and emotional needs, to partial nursing home care, day-care programs, and retirement homes attached to or affiliated with nursing homes which have such services. This range of services is often extremely useful for the physician who may wish to combine occupational therapy, social work services, nutritional management, and medical-nursing care for his elderly patient. For such a program to work well, the physician should make specific recommendations and prescriptions for the physical, rehabilitative, and emotional problems or concerns of his patient rather than leaving the program definition entirely to the discretion of other health personnel.

To sum up, it is helpful to view a patient's dependency as not only a "problem" but also as an idiosyncratic adaptation or maladaptation. This attitude permits the physician to do some constructive problem solving about the diagnosis of the patient's present and previous level of functioning and the extent of his social and support system. Ultimately, the goal is for the patient's medical and psychological needs to be met in an adequate way, and yet hold in reasonable balance the patient's desire to be dependent.

The Rigid, Competitive, and Perfectionistic Patient

What characterizes all three of these kinds of patients is an insistence on "being in control." For many patients, the idea of having someone tell them what to do, even if it is someone who has been "hired" for that purpose, can produce a great deal of discomfort and anxiety. The patient may react to such a situation as if it were a repetition of some early experience when he had to struggle with some other authority, perhaps a parent or teacher, to maintain his own self-esteem and independence. If the patient is transferring these feelings inappropriately to the present situation, such behavior does not have the same implications for the doctor as if the behavior were intended as an attack on the physician's personal or professional integrity. When a rigid and perfectionistic patient complains to the doctor that orders were not spelled out precisely enough or that the doctor did not warn him about all the possible side effects of the medications, this may be another way of saying, "Doctor, I have to depend on you medically, but I want you to know that I don't entirely acknowledge your control over me. I'm still free to evaluate your efforts and I'm still in control of my life." Even when the physician achieves an intellectual understanding of the motives underlying the patient's actions, such patients are still difficult. They frequently appear hostile, argumentative, and continually dissatisfied, even if their medical care is excellent. Strategies which may decrease the personal struggle between patient and physician include the following.

Strategies and Approaches

Details of the Treatment Plan in Writing

For a perfectionistic patient, a fuller explanation than usual of the treatment regime is necessary. If the explanation is in writing (such as a list of the procedures to be used, the specific outcomes expected from each, etc.), this at least provides a common area of agreement and a reference document. Many patients who are anxious about their physical condition do not hear or fully comprehend the doctor's explanations. Putting the explanation in writing and setting up further visits to clarify questions and information is often helpful.

Involvement of the Patient in Setting Up His Own Treatment Program

If the treatment regime involves some inconvenience or discomfort to the patient, another useful strategy is to negotiate with the patient about some of the options which may not be essential for the medical management of the illness, but which definitely affect the patient's comfort level. For example, a perfectionistic patient who must follow an ulcer diet, or take medications and avoid specific foods because of his spastic colitis, may feel more secure and complain less if the treatment plan (including the optional medications and foods) is first negotiated with him. The final treatment plan can then be drawn up as a formal contract. In this way, the perfectionistic patient has helped define both the physical and psychological dimensions of his treatment regime.

Counting the Symptoms

Perfectionistic patients often do better when they have a "specific task" that relates to their treatment plan. Counting particular symptoms, especially those related to improvement, is such a specific task. For instance, patients on p.r.n. medication might record when they take each pill, noting what effect the medication had, what feelings they were having at the time to justify the need for the medication, and what alternatives (such as relaxation exercises, or a hot bath) had occurred to them. In the same way, patients who are experiencing the kind of chronic pain that strongly suggests psychological causation can be requested to make charts, recording every fifteen minutes when they are not in pain. Such charting meets a perfectionistic person's need for knowing what is going on, gives him something specific to do which is helpful to the treatment, and allows his compulsive need to worry and "object" to be deflected from the physician. Keeping such a diary and charting behavior is also helpful in carrying out a behavior modification program. (See Chapter 20.)

A patient who is competitive with a physician must be approached in the same way as a hostile patient. The doctor refuses the provocation and instead includes the patient as much as possible in the design of the treatment plan. To a large extent, such management puts the patient "in charge." A patient's competitiveness may be his way to assert control over a situation that is frightening and beyond his depth. If it transpires that the patient's competitiveness is sabotaging treatment, this must be pointed out tactfully. The patient can then be given the choice of accepting the physician's recommendations, obtaining a consultation, or being referred to another doctor (where the same unfortunate cycle of challenging and disputing the doctor's orders, and "being difficult" is likely to occur once again). If the physician can view the patient's competitiveness as a problem to be solved, rather than a personal affront, the physician may be in a better position to tolerate the patient and his irritating behavior. The most notoriously competitive patients are, of course, physicians themselves, all of whom need medical care at one time or another, but who frequently fight and challenge it all the way.

THE SEDUCTIVE PATIENT

Individuals of both sexes and all shapes and ages can be seductive patients. The male patient might say,

>"Doctor Hancock, I find talking with you fascinating, and I find myself very attracted to you. I wonder if you might join me for a drink after you finish, today?...."

The female patient in the doctor's office might say,

>"....Doctor, you're so understanding. The person I live with doesn't seem to have time for me the way you do.... Sometimes I feel so lonely.... Don't you ever feel lonely?..."

In either of these situations, if the patient is of the opposite sex, the doctor may find himself, or herself, squirming. If the patient is of the same sex, the doctor may be squirming even more. In either case, the doctor usually wants to stop the seductive behavior of the patient so that the business of "doctoring" can continue. On the other hand, all of this is pretty exciting and flattering. And what to do about it?

The meaning of the seductive behavior of a particular patient is variable and idiosyncratic. One patient may wish to be "special" to a physician, rather than "just a number"; the seductive behavior may be an overt way of seeking this recognition. Another patient may feel insecure, lonely, or depressed; being seductive is a way of actively concealing and controlling such feelings in a social context. Still another elderly patient, by bringing cookies or physically or emotionally flattering the doctor, may be wishing to insure that the physician will not abandon the patient, as old age advances. Other motivations may include hostility, a desire to control the physician or the medical transaction, to "make a sexual conquest" of a "powerful" person, or as a way of "putting on" the doctor. Depending on the perceived motivation, the physician should try to explore and clarify the motivation behind a patient's behavior. If the patient has a desire for sexual conquest, "teasing" the physician, or acquiring power through a sexual transaction, the patient is doubtless responding and "transferring" to the doctor–patient relationship something from his/her own past, and previous experience with powerful people (perhaps parents or other authorities from childhood). Such a patient may be playing out a fantasy for recognition, affection, or revenge with the doctor never able to be played out with the original authority. The behavior may not really be intended for the doctor himself, but instead the patient may be "using" the doctor as one of the characters in a childhood play being reenacted. Clues to this kind of behavior should be apparent to the doctor if he considers whether the patient really knows the doctor well enough personally to behave the way he/she is doing, or whether the behavior in some way seems "phony" or contrived to him. To clarify the situation, the doctor may want to try some of the strategies listed below.

Strategies and Approaches

Confrontation

The doctor may confront the patient. This may be done by a clarifying question such as,

> "Are you suggesting that our relationship should no longer be a professional one?"

or, in a more subtle way, by the doctor clarifying his own role,

> "I do feel lonely sometimes, but what you are saying is making me rather uncomfortable. As you know, I'm your doctor, and I think that to continue to act as your doctor, we'll have to keep relationships on a professional basis...."

or,

> "I appreciate your invitation, but I find it difficult to take care of patients when I'm involved with them socially."

The *advantage* to this approach is that it does clarify the issue and reduces the pressure long enough to allow completion of the medical transaction. The *disadvantage* is that the patient may be unaware of how seductive the behavior appears, and may feel affronted or rejected.

Acquiescence and Deflection

The doctor may acknowledge the seductive maneuver, respond perfunctorily to it, and yet continue the professional role. For instance, he might smile and say,

> "You're an attractive person, Mrs. X, and I'm sorry that you're feeling lonely. Perhaps you could tell me more about it."

In this way the doctor preserves his dignity and that of the patient. At the same time he provides the patient with some of the flattery and sexual recognition apparently being sought.

Advantages

The patient's needs for both personal and professional recognition can be met.

Disadvantages

The maneuver may be so subtle that the patient may interpret it as one more step in the seduction process and may miss the doctor's attempt to maintain his professional stance.

Problem Clarification

The doctor can take the nonsexual aspects of the patient's communication, such as her feeling lonely, and respond appropriately and empathically to these. For example, he might say, "It must be hard for you to feel so lonely," and then go on to explore not only her feelings, but also how she spends her day, what her relationships are with other people, including her husband, and whether she used to enjoy things more. Implicit in this approach is the notion that seductive maneuvers, in and of themselves, may not mean a great deal, and should be used as the invitation to explore other concerns, such as the painful and humiliating problem of being ignored and neglected by a spouse.

Advantages

Clarifying the problem and the posture that the doctor is going to take toward it, may be helpful to the patient. Once the physician has established a role and position in this particular transaction, the patient may be able to look at his/her own behavior, and reassess whether this is the way the patient wants to appear to the outside world—always "on the make"—or whether a different stance is indicated.

Disadvantages

By ignoring the sexual implications of the patient's maneuvers, the doctor may be inviting more of the same.

The Doctor's Own Behavior

Patients are not always seductive in a vacuum. The doctor's discovery that he is very attractive to someone (while probably not feeling as passionately appreciated at home) may subtly lead the doctor into reciprocal seductive maneuvers toward the patient. If this mutual seductiveness culminates in an overt sexual encounter, the doctor has put himself in a very precarious position, with some of the following implications:

a. He has violated professional ethics, and has taken advantage of his professional role to gratify his own personal needs.

b. The doctor may be doing personal and psychological injury to the patient, even if at the moment the patient is the aggressor.

c. The chance of getting embroiled in a sticky relationship in which he is the "other party" who has alienated a mate's affection is real, as is the chance that the doctor's spouse may learn of the entanglement.

d. The physician runs the risk of being kicked out or censured by his medical society for unethical practices. (With the new statutes throughout the county on mandatory reporting of unethical conduct, the state licensing agency may also become involved.)

e. If his patient develops regrets about the doctor responding rather than merely flirting, the doctor may be accused of rape or indecent liberties by a guilt-ridden patient.

f. The doctor himself may regret such an impulsive act when he/she has had a chance to think about whether this particular relationship was really one he/she wished to change from doctor–patient to doctor–lover.

Caveat. If the physician finds himself besieged by an unusually large number of seductive patients, the next step might involve looking at his/her own behavior, which itself may be seductive. There are doubtless times in the life of every physician where "a little kindness" is appreciated, and where the physician may respond to flattery and flirtation with mirroring behavior. Misperceiving his professional role, the patient's intent, and the patient's real needs, however, and meeting seduction with seduction, is likely to lead to disaster.

THE PATIENT WITH SOMATIZATION, HYPOCHONDRIASIS, OR CHRONIC PAIN COMPLAINTS

Perhaps the most difficult of the "difficult" patients to treat are those patients with psychogenic pain or physical complaints, or those who misinterpret or are preoccupied with physical signs and sensations, fearing and believing that they represent disease. Such patients consume an inordinate amount of physician time in "ruling out" organic disease, and often lead physicians "down the garden path" of tests, repeated tests, multiple laparotomies, and the sinking feeling that when one complaint seems to abate, another arises full-blown from the head or belly of the ever-complaining patient. Causation is often multidetermined, depending on social reinforcement, learned behavior, lack of social support, identification with important figures who have also had such complaints, and because of social or familial expectations that psychological conflict be expressed in this way rather than in a more direct or overt fashion. All three kinds of patients share the unfortunate and immensely frustrating characteristic of tending to retain and maintain their complaints and ways of relating to the world through physical symptoms, regardless of the competence of their physicians, the intervention of mental health consultation or psychotherapy, and the use of medications. Technically, the classification of the disorders, and their predominant symptoms [according to the Diagnostic and Statistical Manual (DSM III) (1) of the American Psychiatric Association] are as follows.

Somatization Disorder: Occurs almost exclusively in females, begins before the age of 30 (often with menstrual symptoms), with complaints presented in a dramatic, vague, or exaggerated way, or as part of a complicated medical history in which many physical diagnoses have been considered. Complaints include the neurological, G.I., female reproductive, psychosexual, pain, cardiopulmonary systems, and patients are often receiving simultaneous treatment from a number of doctors. Often, depression and anxiety are present. Because of constant seeking out of doctors, numerous evaluations and unnecessary surgery are undertaken.

Psychogenic Pain Disorder: The complaint of pain, in the absence of adequate physical findings (either not consistent with an anatomic distribution of the nervous system, or, if mimicking disease, cannot be accounted for by adequate pathology, after extensive evaluation). Psychological factors related to the etiology of the pain are inferred by the temporal connection between an environmental situation reflecting a psychological conflict or need and the occurrence or worsening of the pain, or the pain permitting a person to avoid or leave a situation that is feared or unpleasant, or the pain eliciting support from the environment, where the support would otherwise not be forthcoming. There are frequent doctor visits for pain relief, excessive use of analgesics without relief, requests for surgery, rejection of any role of psychological factors in the pain, and assumption of the invalid role. Usually arising in adolescence or early adulthood, the disorder is diagnosed more frequently in women than men. Severe psychosocial stress is a precipitating factor.

Hypochondriasis: In this condition, there is an unrealistic interpretation of physical signs or sensations as abnormal, leading to the preoccupation with having a serious disease. Physical examinations do not account for the physical signs or sensations or the individual's interpretation of them. Fears or belief of having a disease persists despite reassurance, with social or occupational impairment. Preoccupation is with bodily functioning or a minor physical abnormality. Medical history indicates a great deal of doctor-shopping, dissatisfaction with previous medical treatment, and refusal to consider emotional factors. Social relationships are often strained (with family, doctors, and employers). The disorder is equally common in men and women.

Strategies and Approaches

What is the primary physician to do, once he has an inkling that the complaints are not organically based? A strategy might include the following (with the assumption that "cure" may not be a realistic expectation, in any case, but that "decrease and management" of symptoms may be more realistic).

1. Take a thorough personal and family history. Such symptoms tend to run in families, begin early, and persist, to a greater or lesser extent, throughout the life cycle, often aggravated by stress. Tally the number of diagnoses, doctors, hospitalizations, medications, and surgical procedures, plus the number of different complaints (and number of organ systems), and the diagnosis may suggest itself with greater certainty.

2. Do a comprehensive assessment of the patient's "life space," to determine the adaptive role such symptoms play. If the patient is isolated, lives alone, and is frightened to initiate social contact in the community, having medical complaints to present may be the most legitimate way the patient can relate to the world. Asking the patient to "give up" his symptoms may be asking him to give up his one source of support.

3. Set realistic goals. While functioning as the patient's doctor, avoid confrontation about the symptoms themselves. Instead, try to get the patient to increase his activity level, social contacts, level of psychological functioning, and to increase the length of time that is symptom-free (or, at least, has fewer symptoms). This may have to be done by specific contract: to walk around the block each day; to accept visits by the community health nurse; to volunteer for outside activities; to increase social contacts. The family must be enlisted to support the positive, non-symptomatic behaviors of the patient, rather than fighting or supporting the patient solely around his complaints.

4. The physician utilizes the supportive, "holding" atmosphere of the office setting, instructing his personnel to accept and tolerate the patient's complaints for a limited prearranged time (e.g., five minutes each visit), inquire about specific contractual arrangements (e.g., diet, medications, exercise), and try to increase the repertoire of the patient's activities (e.g., bringing in home-grown flowers and home-baked cookies).

5. Consider asking a psychiatrist or mental health colleague for some ideas. Although such patients are notoriously poor at following through on a psychiatric referral, viewing their symptoms as entirely somatic, they may be willing to form an alliance with someone whom they see as "medical" in orientation—an orientation shared by the patient, his family, and his friends. Nowadays, even such patients are somewhat amenable to the notion of illnesses caused or aggravated by "stress." So a primary physician may be able to form an alliance with and maintain such a patient with vitamins, placebo medications, and supportive psychotherapy in his office. Though not the kind of "cure" for which one might hope, it is a far more desirable outcome than one or two more decades of doctor-shopping, a barrage of CT scans, and a laparotomy or two.

REFERENCE

1. *Diagnostic and Statistical Manual* (1980): third edition, pp. 241–252. American Psychiatric Association, Washington, D.C.

7

Children's and Adolescents' Issues

A variety of psychiatric issues related to primary care arise in relation to children. Specific expertise, diagnostic approaches, and strategies must be available for every primary care physician to interview and assess children. This chapter will address a number of diagnostic treatment issues on children, but is by no means comprehensive. When in doubt, it is always wise to get a consultation from an expert in children. That expert may, at times, be a teacher, a developmental specialist, a child psychiatrist or psychologist, or a social worker with specific training in working with children.

DIAGNOSTIC ISSUES AND TREATMENT IMPLICATIONS

Why interview and assess children, anyway? Why not take the observations and concerns voiced by parents, teachers, and other adults, and assume they are correct? Well, for one thing, observations by adults with an axe to grind rarely reveal accurate data. Parents usually want to control rather than necessarily understand their children. Furthermore, unless an assessment and a tentative diagnosis can be made by an informed, but unbiased observer, interventions are often haphazard and nonspecific. A large number of problems presenting in primary care settings are healthy responses (the parents are uninformed that many two-year-olds are negativistic) or responses to a developmental or situational crisis (a move, an illness in the family, a change of schools, the birth of a sibling, an entry into junior high school). A therapeutic response to these situations might be counseling and education for the parents and reassurance and environmental manipulation for the child (e.g., the six-year-old supplanted by the new baby in the family needs some special privileges and perogatives for "being more grown up"). Another large category of referrals to primary physicians is children who have a specific external conflict, usually to a specific person. The antagonist may be a sibling, a punitive parent, or a harsh teacher. Again, environmental manipulation, negotiation, specific suggestions, and supportive counseling may be indicated. A third category of common problems, especially with young children, is developmental delays or deviations, where it is unclear whether there will be a continuing problem or one that the child will outgrow. Being able to assess and follow early speech and language development, record baseline data, identify whether the child is receiving sufficient stimulation and encouragement to speak, and knowing which experts can assess which developmental lags is also important.

In addition to these problems, many of which will clear up by themselves or with minimal intervention, there are other more severe disorders of childhood. Using DSM-III (The Diagnostic and Statistical Manual of the American Psychiatric Association), the most common of these disorders presenting in childhood include the following:

a. *Mental Retardation:* Significant subaverage general intellectual functioning: IQ of 70 or below together with a concurrent impairment in adaptive behavior. Onset before age 21.

b. *Attention Deficit Disorder:* Developmentally and age-inappropriate lack of attention, impulsivity, with or without hyperactivity. (For more detailed diagnostic and treatment considerations, see below.)

c. *Conduct Disorder:* A repetitive and persistent pattern of aggressive or non-aggressive conduct in which the basic rights of others are violated or age-appropriate societal norms or rules are violated. (Such patterns are extremely difficult to change, especially after they have occurred for a considerable period of time: a significant number of children who have this disorder develop an antisocial personality disorder as adults.)

d. *Anxiety Disorders of Childhood or Adolescence:* Excessive anxiety concerning separation or age-appropriate social relationships or the presence of generalized and persistent anxiety. Specifically, such anxiety may occur on separation (e.g., when a child has to go to school or the child is left with the baby sitter); may occur in relation to strangers or new situations, or may occur as a generalized pattern of worry and anxiety in many familiar and unfamiliar situations. Separation anxiety disorder, itself, appears to respond to imipramine; generalized anxiety disorders, even in childhood, may require a number of strategies mentioned in the chapter on anxiety, including medications (see Chapter 12).

e. *Oppositional Disorder:* The onset of this disorder is after 3 and before the age of 18, and includes a pattern of disobedient, negativistic, and provocative opposition to authority figures for at least six months. (Although irritating, such children do not violate the basic rights of others or age-appropriate societal norms, except for their oppositional patterns.) A certain number of these children with this disorder develop passive–aggressive personality disorders as adults.

f. *Pervasive Developmental Disorders:* including infantile autism and childhood onset pervasive developmental disorder. Both subgroups involve gross and sustained impairment in social relationships, language; inappropriate affective responses, clinging, resistance to social changes, oddities of motor movement, or self-mutilation. Infantile autism begins before 30 months; childhood onset pervasive developmental disorder after 30 months and before 12 years. Both conditions are extremely difficult to treat, and favorable prognosis correlates with language development and level of intelligence.

g. *Eating Disorders:* Including anorexia nervosa, bulimia (binge eating), pica (eating of non-nutritive substances).

h. *Stereotyped Movement Disorders:* Including transient tic disorder [recurrent, repetitive, rapid, purposeless motor movements (tics) for more than 1 month but less than 1 year]; chronic motor tic disorder (tics for more than 1 year); and Tourette's syndrome (tics plus vocal tics, often including the use of foul language). The latter condition responds specifically to haloperidol.

i. *Other Disorders with Physical Manifestations:* Stuttering; functional eneuresis (involuntary voiding of urine day or night, $2\times$/month if ages 5–6, or $1\times$/month over 6); functional encopresis (involuntary fecal passage in inappropriate places, $1\times$/month after age 4).

As one can see, the range of diagnostic possibilities is vast. The ability to talk with a child as well as the parents is crucial to settle on a specific diagnosis. Distinguishing which disorders are likely to disappear by themselves ("the child will outgrow it") and which ones require referral or other interventions is often the primary physician's role.

INTERVIEWING CHILDREN

Interviewing children should be easy, one would think, but many primary care physicians find it excruciating for themselves and for their patients. The physician is often nervous, and has the feeling, often justified, that he is making the child as nervous as he is. For this reason, many physicians resort to interviewing parents and assume that the parental view of the child's difficulties is accurate. When the physician acts primarily as the parent's "agent," however, a significant bias is introduced into the transaction. The child, even if he finds it difficult to articulate his point of view, becomes resentful that he is not being heard. The following are some general guidelines for interviewing children that may help the interviewer. (The assumption is that one may have a fair amount of time in which to conduct the interview; if the interview must be much more brief, the guidelines must, of course, be shortened.

1. Before seeing the child, decide on a strategy that might be useful for the specific situation. For example, with a preschool child, seeing the child with the parents for part of the time (or possibly all of the time) permits you to see how they interact, and allows the child to become comfortable in the setting before trying to engage the child. A premature move by an authority (especially a doctor) toward a young child often frightens the child (who often expects a "shot"). An adolescent or a latency child on the other hand, especially if the child is in some conflict with the parents, may need to be seen first, simply to establish that you

are not "taking sides." In other situations, such as with a latency child who is *not* angry, seeing the parents first permits you to get some history and learn why they are there and what their concerns are. The source of referral—who wants you to see the child—often determines the psychological stance of the child and his family. A child referred by his school because of "bad behavior" and as a condition for reentry into the school program often enters with a hostile set of assumptions about what is to occur with you. In contrast, a depressed child who refers himself, is aware of being unhappy, and wants to "talk to someone," may present himself more willingly. Anticipating hostility and acknowledging it, while clarifying your role at the outset ("I'm here to understand and try to make things better"), may allow the tension and hostility to dissipate a bit.

2. As you greet the child in your waiting room and walk back with the child to your office, it is often the first order of business to decrease anxiety with small talk, asking the child's name, his age, the school he attends, his grade, etc. It is frequently possible to put the child at ease by the time you reach your office.

3. Who you are, the purpose of the interview, and what you do should be explained. As mentioned in No. 1, children often have odd misconceptions about what is to happen when they go to any doctor—and in a primary care setting, the first expectation may be a physical procedure, a shot, or something equally unpleasant. Explaining to the young child that you understand his parents are concerned about him, and that you will be talking and playing with him to try to understand how to help him, may set him at ease. Some physicians ask children why they believe they are coming; others explain in a general way some of the concerns that their parents have revealed, for example, "I talked with your mother, and she seemed worried about you. She thought perhaps you were unhappy or angry about something, and that's why your grades have gone down this year."

4. Initially, an *unstructured* time should be provided for a younger child to choose toys to play with, activities to engage in, or to talk. Younger children often are interested in clay, paints, magic markers, puppet play, dolls and a doll house, trucks, soldiers, and Legos™. Older children like Legos™, board games (such as checkers), darts, tossing Nerf balls™, or making models. The purpose of the unstructured time is to develop a relationship with the child, as well as to assess specific areas: the child's appearance (sloppy, inappropriately dressed); mood (sad, carefree); coordination (peculiar gait, problems with position in space); activity level; impulsivity; attention span; and anxiety around a stranger (some anxiety is normal). One also observes the level of selfishness and social maturity (does the child play cooperatively or "want everything for himself" and does the child "have to win"). Other observations include unusual symptoms (tics, stuttering, seductiveness) and whether the child gradually warms up or whether the child is very suspicious and guarded with you, even after a considerable period of time.

Following unstructured play, an evaluation should have a period of structured play and activities to try to acquire additional information about whether the child is cooperative or oppositional, whether the child behaves differently when you are in charge, rather than he. Structured questions also serve to uncover the nature of the child's fantasies and concerns about himself, his relationships to his family, and his relationship to peers. To elicit fantasies (which otherwise might not emerge), the following questions are often useful:

1. "Magical Wishes." If you had magical powers and could have 3 magical wishes, what would you wish for? (Surprisingly, even adults find this question intriguing.)
2. "Changes." If you could change one thing about your family to make it happier for you, what would it be? If you could change one thing about your (father, mother, self), what would it be?
3. "Animals." If you could be any animal, what animal would you be?
4. What kind of animal would you hate to be?
5. "Desert Island." If you could take one person to live with you on a desert island, who would it be? (2 persons, 3 persons, etc.)
6. "Money." If you won one million dollars on a TV quiz show, what would you do with it?
7. "Best Thing." What is the best thing that ever happened to you?
8. "Worst Thing." What is the worst thing that ever happened to you?
9. "Another Person." If you could be any other person in the world, who would you be?
10. "Age." If you could be any age, what age would you be (and why?). (This question can sometimes lead to a discussion of being 21 and "totally on my own" or being one year old and "still be carried around by Mom.")

If there is sufficient time, another quasistructured way to elicit and assess a child's fantasies is to use the Mutual Story Telling Technique, developed by Dr. Richard Gardner as a psychotherapy technique (1). Using a tape recorder, you introduce the child, as if introducing a radio or TV announcer, coaching the child to tell an original story which has a "beginning, middle, end, and a moral." The interviewer can then take similar themes and elaborate them into a story with a different ending or moral, thereby teasing out the child's point of view around important family and personal issues. Another structured activity to elicit a child's fantasies is to use Dr. Gardner's "Talking, Thinking, and Feeling" game, which is a structured board game that, in a nonthreatening way, has children draw cards which instruct them to do certain things ("Say what you like best about your mother"), and thereby permits the rapid uncovering of a great deal of feeling and personal perception (2).

Another structured activity is to have the child draw. Having a latency age child draw a car, for example, gives you an interesting view of the child's world: enthusiastic, outgoing children often draw dramatic or flashy racing cars; depressed children tend to draw monochroic, unsubstantial-looking, tiny cars. Having a child draw a picture of everybody in his or her family doing something is a projective technique described by Burns and Kaufman as Kinetic Family Drawing (3). Having a child draw a picture of him/herself "all grown up" also at times reveals current sexual or other preoccupations. An old standby, having a child draw a house, tree, and person, and make up a story about them, may also reveal additional fantasies. This latter test has been described in some detail (4). All of the drawings, of course, have no "absolute" meaning, and only suggest important themes and hypotheses to be elaborated or confirmed in the clinical interview itself.

Board games, such as checkers or Candyland (for younger children), are a good way to get a rough impression of the child's cognitive capacities, ability to understand rules, the child's attitudes about competition, and the need to cheat. The degree of vulnerability of the child's self-esteem may only become apparent during such competitive play (who wins, who goes first, can one stand to lose, etc.) (Incidentally, if the child cheats, moralizing or reprimanding the child will only destroy your rapport and probably not stop the cheating.)

Tossing a Nerf™ baseball or basketball around is often a way to "warm up" a child, as well as to test age-appropriate gross motor coordination. Many children feel much more comfortable during or after they are having a playful athletic interchange with the physician; a Nerf-ball game of catch accomplishes this and can be done safely in your office.

Play materials nonverbally communicate that "the medium is the message." Messy materials (clay, finger paints, water colors) invite messy or regressive play. More structured materials (Legos™, blocks, magic markers, crayons) elicit more structured play. If you believe that a child has some sort of conflict about neatness or messyness, you may deliberately want to provide such materials to see what the child does with them. On the other hand, if you want to assess the fine-motor abilities of the child, materials which can be controlled and require dexterity (small Legos™, colored pencils, fine point magic markers) may be more in order.

Confidentiality, particularly with older children, is an important issue. Unlike working with adults, however, an assurance of confidentiality in the assessment period may be both unwise and unwarranted, if you have to have the parents accept a referral to someone else, or must dictate a report to the juvenile court or another referral agency. If you take the child into counseling yourself, however, a contract of confidentiality may be very important.

As will be mentioned elsewhere in the book (see Chapter 22), assessment of the family is often crucial to an understanding of the problems of a child, or another family member, and may determine your therapeutic recommendation. Observing how a mother and child relate to each other in your presence, or how the father insensitively criticizes his child in the child's presence, gives a totally different kind of information from what you might conclude from individual observation. A family session, if only for ten minutes, is usually a necessary part of a comprehensive assessment of each child.

ASSESSMENT OF ATTENTION DEFICIT DISORDER IN CHILDREN

It has been estimated that approximately 10% of children have what has been called Attention Deficit Disorder. The disorder occurs ten times more often in boys than girls, and is characterized by: (1) inattention (distracted easily, fails to finish things, difficulty concentrating, often seems not to listen); and (2) impulsivity (acts before thinking, shifts excessively from one activity to another, needs a lot of supervision, calls out frequently in class, has trouble waiting for his turn, difficulty organizing work). In addition, approximately half of these children have hyperactivity (difficulty sitting still, fidgeting excessively, running about or climbing on things excessively, moving excessively during sleep, trouble staying seated, always "on the go") (5). Schools are often the major referral source, since many of these children become more symptomatic in situations requiring concentration and sitting still. Also when starting school children first come to the attention of adults other than their families, who may have labeled the child's behavior as "all boy." Hyperactivity, inattention, and impulsivity are not specific symptoms, and the differential diagnosis of the syndrome includes acute stress, mental retardation, a psychotic child, and family chaos. An assessment for this condition should include the following.

1. A careful and complete history. Prematurity, pre- and postnatal complications, a family history of school-related problems or hyperactivity, and the chronology of the parental observations about the child from an early age (e.g., he "got up and ran at 11 months, and never stopped..."; he "hits other kids and doesn't understand why they get mad..."; he "can't ever remember what he's supposed to do, even though we've gone over and over it..."). A history of irritability, aversion to being held or touched, and unpredictable sleep patterns is also sometimes found.

2. A clinical observation. In its most graphic form, children impulsively may dart around the office, opening desk drawers, spilling objects everywhere, and becoming increasingly out of control. (Normal children of three may also do this, sometimes.) In a more subtle form, a child may have much more trouble remembering what you ask him to do or remember, may be slightly distracted during conversation, may impulsively approach paper and pencil tasks you ask him to do (e.g., a house is impulsively drawn on paper, with no planning at all); and may reverse letters and write them in a random fashion about the page. Neurological examination may reveal a number of "soft" neurological signs (disdiadochokinesia, nystagmus, problems with finger-thumb apposition, tremor with finger to nose testing, abnormal gait, abnormal reflexes, dysarthria, abnormal tandem gait), the presence of any of which can be associated with the syndrome.

3. Observation or using data about the child's behavior in a "normally distracting" situation, such as a schoolroom. Teachers are expert at observing children, and a teacher rating scale developed by Dr. Keith Connors (6) and available through Abbott Laboratories (7) is often useful to distinguish those children who are constitutionally boisterous from those children whose attentional problems are likely to lead to academic or social difficulties.

Treatment of Attention Deficit Disorder

1. A structured home. Children with this disorder do better if their lives are reasonably predictable, and sufficient structure exists that they don't need to make

dramatic adjustments from day to day. Posting a schedule, and rewarding a child for following it through a behavior modification program (see Chapter 20), often helps the child focus his attention more on his own behavior. Stressing parental consistency and follow-through on promises and rules helps the child control his own impulsivity better.

2. A structured school situation. As with the structure in the home, the school structure often helps a child organize his life. Because of distractions, a child may often have trouble listening to and remembering instructions given orally. Writing these instructions and rules down, and having the schedule and expectations posted will help many of these children stay more in touch with what is happening. Children with attention problems usually do much better in self-contained classrooms, rather than in open concept classroom situations. If a child, because of impulsivity, leaves his seat, starts whispering, or gets off task, a reminder of expectations should be made by the teacher, followed, if unsuccessful, by a "time out" interval. A "time out" strategy usually works better than excluding the child, or placing him in the hall for long periods, or sending him to the principal. Many of these latter interventions do not refocus the child, who often does not understand them, and views them simply as retaliation by a "mean teacher."

3. Medications. 80–85% of these children respond to one or another of the stimulant medications commonly used: methylphenidate (Ritalin®), dextroamphetamine, and pemiline (Cylert®). Both methylphenidate and dextroamphetamine are short acting (3–4 hr), should be given on an empty stomach, and in high doses may interfere with appetite, weight gain, and growth (compensated for, however, by growth spurts during "vacation periods" off the medications). Though addictive in adults, they do not appear to be addictive in either children or adults who have this disorder, and may be prescribed safely for long periods of time, provided the medication is monitored by height and weight checks every several months. For school-related attentional problems, the medications are usually given in a morning and noon dose, with the noon dose often somewhat smaller than the morning dose (e.g., a ten-year-old boy might get 10 mg of methylphenidate before breakfast, and 5 mg of methylphenidate before lunch on school days). Pemiline is usually given once a day in the morning. For dosage regulation, the dosage is usually started at 16.75 mg/day for the first week, 37.5 mg/day the second week, and increased in this manner, until a therapeutic response is noted. (Check the insert literature and P.D.R. for dosage recommendations.) Clinical response to both medications is usually monitored with Connors rating scales, which are excellent at picking up subtle changes.

Parent Education About the Effects of Medicine

Using a hand-out about the effects of the medications you are using with a child often serves to reduce the time explaining the therapeutic and side effects of the medications, as well as offering the basis for "informed consent" to prescribing the medication. One such sample is the following (for dextroamphetamine).

Dexedrine

The medication that I am prescribing for your child is Dexedrine, or dextroamphetamine as it is called chemically. This medication, which acts as a stimulant in adults, acts in quite a somewhat different way with children who have an attention deficit disorder (usually characterized by short attention span, distractibility, impulsive activity, poor social relationships and awareness, and sometimes hyperactivity). The specific behavior we hope to elicit, using this medication, would be to lengthen the attention span, decrease the impulsivity and decrease the hyperactivity. Sometimes children who have memory problems also have been aided by this medication, and some children become socially much more aware and compliant. This medication in children is not addictive and other side effects sometimes seen in adults, such as increased blood pressure, are not usually seen in children. Because, with both children and adults, this medication may decrease appetite and hence may affect both height and weight, children must be weighed and have their height measured on a regular basis. Usually during school and summer vacations, medication is discontinued, at least on a temporary basis, to see whether the child still requires the medication and also to allow for a growth spurt. An occasional side effect of the medication is excessive sedation. If this occurs, the chances are likely that the child is receiving too much medication and the medication should be reduced. The duration of a single dose of Dexedrine is usually approximately 4 hr, and works best if taken on an empty stomach (½ hr before meals, or ½ hr after meals). On a totally empty stomach, some children develop a stomach ache if given the medication. If this should occur, giving medication with a piece of toast or a glass of milk may be useful. If you have any questions about the effects of the medication, please stop it immediately and contact me.

4. Psychotherapy. Although not particularly useful for the attentional difficulty, itself, individual or group therapy is sometimes useful for the secondary depression or low self-esteem which many of these children have. Explaining the condition to the child, so that he does not feel so much "like a freak," can often be helpful in gaining greater cooperation of the child with such a program (since many children cannot notice the things about their behavior which other people notice).

5. Social skills training. As developed by Trupin (8), social skills training for children with attentional problems may be very helpful, since it significantly increases the child's focus on his own impulsivity and the options available in new or difficult social situations. Trupin believes that many of these children lack the ability to plan ahead, and have a very limited repertoire of options, especially when they are angry or put under pressure. A SIGEP program teaches such skills. SIGEP is an achronym meaning *S*top, *I*dentify [the problem(s)], *G*enerate (new solutions and options), *E*valuate (which is the best option or choice), and *P*lan (how are you going to implement this option). Used with preschoolers, latency children, and adolescents, the SIGEP program has been effective in significantly changing the problematic behavior of such children. Detailed information about teaching children to practice and critique their behavior and strategies through using SIGEP may be obtained from Trupin (9).

> An impulsive boy of ten who is continually getting into fights is asked to role play a typical situation which would result in a fight. An example might be when another boy comes up and pushes him inadvertently. The patient would be asked

to *Stop, Identify* the problem (I want to let the boy know I'm angry; I want to hit him; I don't want to get pushed around). *Generation* of new solutions might take the form of brainstorming different things to say to the boy who pushed him ("Hey, stop, you fucker; Don't do that; Please stop pushing me!"). *Evaluate* these possibilities (the boy chooses, "Stop pushing me"). Then the boy plans through role play just how he can use his idea the next time he needs it.

REACTIONS OF CHILDREN TO ILLNESS AND HOSPITALIZATION

Although many hospitals are becoming more aware of the special psychological needs of their pediatric patients, a few points about the reactions of children to serious illness and hospitalization should be remembered. An informed and sensitive physician may often be consulted about emotional problems a child is displaying while in the hospital. Some of these points may be useful to the primary physician, both in the role of consultant, and as the personal physician of a child:

a. Enforced passivity and isolation, whether because of intensive burn treatment, being in a body cast, or being isolated because of medical concern about bacterial contamination, may produce regressive behavior, at times of psychotic proportions (e.g., with mutism or incontinence). Young children, especially, regress without extensive sensory and interpersonal stimulation.

b. Fears of mutilation and concerns about body intactness are particularly prominent when a child is 4–6 years old. Urological surgery for boys, hernia repairs, or any kind of disfiguring surgery which has a visible effect on appearance at this age may be extremely upsetting for the child.

c. Children adjust their level of activity and physically define themselves by what their environment and their own physical stamina and constitution will permit. When this changes, such as when a child with cyanotic heart disease has successful corrective surgery, the massive increase in energy available to the child is often perceived as frightening, unmanageable, and almost like a psychotic, altered state. It is useful to prepare both the child and parents for what they may expect, as well as helping the parents impose appropriate external limits.

d. Both stranger anxiety and separation anxiety are at their peaks between 18 and 30 months. If surgery or hospitalization is necessary during this time, maximal attention should be paid to having the mother available as much as possible for the child.

e. Hospital routine, in order to be therapeutic for the child, must be somewhat tailored to the child's emotional needs and developmental level. Being "quiet and clean," for example, is usually a goal of the staff far more than for the young child. The child often needs to play and interact with other children, with some boisterousness and messyness to feel that the hospital is a reasonably normal and safe place. The child also needs to play out his fears and concerns about being hospitalized (and this play may not always be quiet and neat). If at all possible, children should be encouraged to talk about and play "doctor" with dolls and drawings, and to release or reenact their fears about surgical and medical procedures. For the child to protest being in the hospital, especially with staff and through play, is natural and healthy.

f. Questions that concern a preschool child being hospitalized or undergoing surgery include, "Will it hurt? Will someone I trust be near me? Will I be safe?" It is important that someone whom the child knows and trusts be available to the child, to comfort him, explain what is going on, and what is to occur.

g. Children often blame and are angry with their parents, both for being abandoned in a hospital as well as for the pain or discomfort of any of the medical or surgical procedures. Parents must be prepared for this, view it as normal and adaptive, and not retaliate.

h. Parents often feel guilty about the pain that illness or hospitalization imposes on a child, and deal with this guilt by withdrawing, making unrealistic promises to the child, or treating the child in an infantalizing or unrealistic way to compensate for their guilt. This guilt may also take the form of challenging or being uncooperative with the medical staff. The primary physician can recognize and help parents deal with such feelings, rather than retaliate toward them.

i. With a dying child, staff and parents are both uncomfortable and guilty. Children who are dying experience and express to a greater or lesser extent the FAGS syndrome (*F*ear, *A*nger, *G*rief, *S*adness) (M. Rothenberg, *private communication*). Younger children are usually much more concerned about pain and being abandoned than are older children who may deal with their feelings more directly. The primary physician can help the child with whatever emotion he is experiencing at the time, as well as give support to the staff and parents who are frequently experiencing equally painful feelings. As outlined in Chapter 10, an important role is to establish regular contact with the parents of a dying child to help them deal with their own feelings, especially the guilt which they may feel, and which may be transmitted to the child (who already may view his illness as a punishment or divine retribution). The siblings also may be experiencing significant reactions to the impending or actual death (10). With a preschool sibling, there is a sense of loss of love and withdrawal; for a sibling age 5–10, a concern and fear for themselves, and later they experience a survivor guilt. The primary physician may be very helpful in explaining the medical situation to siblings. For example, using Lewis' model, describing that "the child is very ill, everyone is trying to make him as comfortable as possible, the illness could not have been prevented and was no one's fault, and everyone together has to figure out how to help" (11). The primary physician may also be of great use to the staff, whose reactions may be fully as intense as those of the parents.

SEXUAL ABUSE IN CHILDREN

Although child abuse is now a commonly discussed area, with considerable literature now available geared for primary care physicians (12), less is available for the role of the primary care physician in interviewing child victims of sexual molestation. Estimates suggest that one-quarter of all girls and one-tenth of all boys are molested before the age of 18, and that the vast majority of these are molested by someone they know. Fathers (about one-half biological fathers and one-half stepfathers) (13) represent the most common offenders. In the majority of cases, the offender does not commit a sexual act which injures the child, but because of the natural authority of adults over children, force is rarely necessary to enlist cooperation of the child. Two-thirds of the children victimized are pre-teen when the abuse is discovered, and about one-quarter are younger than 6 years. Children are afraid to report the abuse, fearing they will be blamed or disbelieved. The repercussions for sexual and psychological problems in later years are very great, particularly if the sexual abuse is chronic. Regarding the offenders: one-third of them were molested as children themselves or observed this; a large majority were physically abused during childhood and adolescence. Except for the abuse, most of the men commiting such offenses are not criminal or antisocial in the rest of their lives. Many have good jobs and are actively involved in their communities, although having few friends. Most are socially inadequate and form few close relationships. Many feel ashamed or bad about themselves, which they cover up by an excessively domineering or macho exterior. (The similarities to the child abuser are striking: lonely, low feelings of self-esteem, socially isolated, impulsive, and an unrealistic expectation of the child to gratify their needs.)

In interviewing a child who has been sexually molested, the following guidelines, developed for criminal justice personnel (14), apply equally well to a physician or someone on his staff who may want to take a history from the child: *Interviewing Child Victims—Guidelines for Criminal Justice System Personnel.*

Background Information

The following issues affect the child's ability to give a history of sexual assault and influence the cooperativeness of victim and family.

1. Child's Developmental Level: A child's cognitive, emotional, and social growth occurs in sequential phases of increasingly complex levels of development. Progression occurs with mastery of one stage leading to concentration on the next.
    a. *Cognitive*—preconceptual, concrete, intuitive thinking in the young child gradually develops toward comprehension of abstract concepts. Time and space begin as personalized notions and gradually are identified as logical and ordered concepts.
    b. *Emotional*—the young child perceives her/himself egocentrically with little ability to identify her/himself in a context. She/he is dependent on the family to meet all needs and invests adults with total authority. The child often reflects the emotional responses of the parents. She/he gradually shifts to greater reliance on peer relationships and emotional commitments to people outside the family.
    c. *Behavioral*—the young child is spontaneous, outgoing, and explosive with few internal controls and only a tentative awareness of external limits.

She/he has a short attention span. A child most often expresses feelings through behavior rather than verbally. As the child grows, she/he develops internal controls and establishes a sense of identity and independence. Peers and other adults have increasing influence on behavior.
2. Sexual Assault: Characteristics of the assault affect the child's emotional perception of the event and to a great extent determine the response. The closeness of the child's relationship to the offender, the duration of the offense, the amount of secrecy surrounding the assault, and the degree of violence are the factors which have the greatest impact on the child's reaction. The child may very well have ambivalent feelings toward the offender or be dependent on him for other needs.
3. Response to Child: The child is fearful of the consequences of reporting a sexual assault. The response of the family support system and official agencies will directly affect the resolution of the psychological trauma and her/his cooperativeness as a witness. The child fears she/he will be disbelieved or blamed for the assault and almost always is hesitant about reporting.

Interviewing Child Victims

1. Preparing for Interview: Prior to interviewing the child, obtain relevant information from parents/guardian, and if applicable, Child Protective Services caseworker, physician, and/or Sexual Assault Center/Rape Relief counselor.
    a. Explain your role and procedures to above personnel, and enlist their cooperation.
    b. Determine child's general developmental status: age; grade; siblings; family composition; capabilities; ability to write, read, count, ride a bike, tell time, remember events; any unusual problems: physical, intellectual, behavioral; knowledge of anatomy and sexual behavior; family terminology for genital areas.
    c. Review circumstances of assault (as reported by child to other person): what, where, when, by whom, and to whom reported; exact words of child; other persons told by child; how many have interviewed child; child's reaction to assault; how child feels about it and what, if any, behavioral signs of distress (nightmares, withdrawal, regression, acting out) have occurred.
    d. Determine what reactions and changes child has been exposed to following revelation of the assault(s): believing; supportive; blaming; angry, ambivalent; parents getting a divorce; move to a new home.
2. Beginning the Interview:
    a. Setting—the more comfortable for the child, the more information she/he is likely to share.
        i. Flexibility—a child likes to move around the room, explore and touch, sit on the floor or adult's lap.
        ii. Activity—playing or coloring occupies child's physical needs and allows her/him to talk with less guardedness.

iii. Privacy—interruptions distract an already short attention span, divert focus of interview, and make self-conscious or apprehensive child withdraw.
iv. Support—if the child wishes a parent or other person present, it should be allowed. A frightened or insecure child will not give a complete statement.

b. Establishing a relationship:
i. Introduction—name, brief and simple explanation of role, and purpose: "I am the lawyer (or legal person) on your side; my job is to talk to children about these things because we want them to stop happening."
ii. General exchange—ask about name (last name), age, grade, school and teacher's name, siblings, family composition, pets, friends, activities, favorite games/TV shows. (It often helps to share personal information when appropriate, e.g., children, pets.)
iii. Assess level of sophistication and ability to understand concepts—does child read, write, count, tell time; know colors or shapes, know the day or date; know birthdate; remember past events (breakfast, yesterday, last year); understand before and after; know about money; assume responsibilities (goes around neighborhood alone, stays at home alone, makes dinner, etc.).

3. Obtaining History of Sexual Assault:
a. Preliminaries:
i. Use language appropriate to child's level; be sure child understands words. (Watch for signs of confusion, blankness, or embarrassment; be careful with words like incident, occur, penetration, prior, ejaculation, etc.)
ii. Do not ask WHY questions ("Why did you go to the house?" "Why didn't you tell?"). They tend to sound accusatory.
iii. Never threaten or try to force a reluctant child to talk. Pressure causes a child to clam up and may further traumatize her/him.
iv. Be aware that the child who has been instructed or threatened not to tell by the offender (*especially* if a parent) will be very reluctant and full of anxiety (you will usually notice a change in the child's affect while talking about the assault). The fears often need to be allayed.
—"It's not bad to tell what happened."
—"You won't get in trouble."
—"You can help your dad by telling what happened."
—"It wasn't your fault."
—"You're not to blame."
v. Interviewer's affective response should be consonant with child's perception of assault (e.g., don't emphasize jail for the offender if the child has expressed positive feelings toward him).

vi. Ask direct, simple questions as open-ended as allowed by child's level of comprehension and ability to talk about the assault.
b. Statement:
 i. WHAT
 —"Can you tell me what happened?"
 —"I need to know what the man did."
 —"Did he ever touch you? Where?"
 —"Where did he put his finger?"
 —"Have you ever seen him with his clothes off?"
 —"Did you ever see his penis (thing, pee pee, wiener) get big?"
 —"Did anything ever come out of it?"
 Once basic information is elicited, ask specifically about other types of sexual contact.
 —"Did he ever put it into your mouth?"
 —"Did he ever make you touch him on his penis?"
 ii. WHO
 Child's response here will probably not be elaborate. Most children know the offender and can name him, although in some cases the child may not understand relationship to self or family. Ascertain from other sources what is the exact nature/extent of the relationship.
 iii. WHEN
 The response to this question will depend on child's ability, how recently assault happened, lapse between last incident and report, number of assaults (children will tend to confuse or mix separate incidents). If the child is under six, information regarding time is unlikely to be reliable. An older child can often narrow down dates and times using recognizable events or associating assault with other incidents.
 —"Was it before your birthday, the weekend, Valentine's Day?"
 —"Was it nighttime or daytime?"
 —"Did it happen after dinner, 'Happy Days,' your brother's bedtime?"
 iv. WHERE
 The assault usually occurs in the child's and/or offender's home. Information about which room, where other family members were, where child was before assault may be learned.
 v. COERCION
 What kind of force, threat, enticement, pressure was used to ensure cooperation and secrecy?
 —"Did he tell you not to tell?" "What did he say?"
 —"Did he say something bad would happen or you would get in trouble if you told?"
 —"Did the man say it was a secret?"

c. Assessing credibility and competency:
   i. Does child describe acts or experience to which she/he would not have normally been exposed? (Average child is not familiar with erection or ejaculation until adolescence at the earliest.)
   ii. Does child describe circumstances and characteristics typical of sexual assault situation? ("He told me that it was our secret"; "He said I couldn't go out if I didn't do it"; "He told me it was sex education.")
   iii. How and under what circumstances did child tell? What were exact words?
   iv. How many times has child given the history and how consistent is it regarding the basic facts of the assault (note times, dates, circumstances, sequence of events, etc.)?
   v. How much spontaneous information can child provide? How much prompting is required?
   vi. Can child define difference between truth and a lie? (This question is not actually very useful with young children because they learn this by role but may not understand the concepts.)
4. Closing the Interview:
   a. Praise/thank child for information/cooperation.
   b. Provide information:
      i. Child—do not extract promises from child regarding testifying. Most children cannot project themselves into an unknown situation and predict how they will behave. Questions about testifying in court or undue emphasis on trial will have little meaning and often frightens the child (causing nightmares and apprehension).
      ii. Parent—provide simple, straightforward information about what will happen next in the criminal justice system and approximately when the likelihood of trial, etc.
   c. Enlist cooperation: Let them know who to contact for status reports or in an emergency; express appreciation and understanding for the effort they are making by reporting and following through on process.
   d. Answer questions; solicit responses.

Although many adults, including physicians, are outraged when they hear of an incident of sexual abuse, the crucial issue is to conduct an interview with the child which can help the child recover from the experience and not be traumatized further. Many children (and their families) need support, and treatment, often in therapy, where the possibility of discussion of feelings can be done without feeling "like a freak." With younger children, playing out the fantasy (if it occupies a prominent part of the child's concerns), or leaving it alone if the child has "forgotten" about it may be indicated. As with the dying child, one should be responsive to "where the child is" and the child's concerns, and not be intent on dredging up details, come hell or high water.

ADOLESCENT PROBLEMS AND THEIR MANAGEMENT

In approaching the recognition and treatment of any adolescent problem, the physician should keep in mind that adolescence is characteristically a period of a great deal of change, in which children must separate from their parents, find their own sexual identities, make an appropriate adjustment to members of the opposite sex, choose vocational goals, and find persons other than their parents to love, be close to, and identify with. The adolescent is in the process of changing from a submissive person who accepts the authority of parents and elders in major matters to an independent individual who can make his own decisions and choices about life-styles, ethics, morals, sexual behavior, etc. The necessity for such changes produces some unrest in adolescence, although the old belief that adolescence is always a period of "turmoil" does not appear to be true: about one-third of adolescents do have turmoil and struggle, one-third have an occasionally difficult period of struggle and rebellion, and about one-third pass easily from childhood into adulthood without major tumult or difficulties (15).

Compounding these "normal" changes is an awareness on the part of practically everybody who watches television of the value shifts and changes—cultural, spiritual, sexual, and ethical—which affect the behavior and expectations of both adults and children in our society. Thus, one adolescent talking to a physician may speak of all his friends "dropping acid" and everybody "swinging." He may mention dropping out of school to "find a new life-style." Another adolescent may seem extraordinarily religious—far more than the physician may anticipate—and suggest that all women return to the home and hearth, that many well-known books should be banned, and that sex education be eliminated altogether from the public school curriculum. Between these two extremes of adolescent values the primary physician must tread a perilous path, deciding what is personal belief and what pathology, and maintaining a nonjudgmental acceptance of the person, in any case. An adolescent who assaults the physician with a set of ironclad beliefs (either radical or conservative) may be "putting on" the adult just to see what kind of reaction he gets, and also to see just how prejudiced and judgmental the adult (whether parent or doctor) is. Looking carefully at what is behind the value system espoused by the adolescent is crucial if the doctor is not to become inadvertently an agent of repression in the patient's eyes—a person who, like parents, police, and teachers, is suspected of being dictatorial, condemning, and hypocritical.

Parents are usually the culprits, the persons who decide that "Johnny has a problem," and bring the reluctant teenager to the doctor for a checkup or a lecture. Problems which frequently bestir parents to action are the following:

1. Deteriorating communication and escalating hostility between the adolescent and his parents, with both sides blaming each other: "I'm leaving home! You can't stop me, and besides, it's all your fault!"
2. Sudden displays of independence, including, at times, rebelliousness, which parents have difficulty reconciling their previous view of their child as pri-

marily submissive and obedient: "If I want to picket the supermarket or the Federal Building, I don't see that it's any of your business!"
3. Overt sexual activity, often perfectly normal and sometimes highly exhibitionistic and provocative. The norms for sexual behavior continue to change, but discovering that one's "little child" is now sexually active causes many parents to fear the worst. The parent often wants the physician to "talk to" (stop or scare) the child, who may innocently state, "Bill and I love each other, so of course we want to sleep together, too."
4. Drug usage, which may range from mild experimentation with marijuana and alcohol, to habitual and heavy usage of marijuana, amphetamines, barbiturates, psychedelics, and even (rarely) "heavy narcotics" such as heroin or morphine. Both infrequent and heavy usage may be detected by parents or come to the attention of physicians through school officials or law enforcement authorities.
5. Strange or deteriorating behavior, appearing either at home or at school, and having either an antisocial or psychotic flavor. Sometimes this behavior may take the form of bizarre activities such as dressing peculiarly, appearing incoherent, sudden or gradual deterioration in school performance, progressive withdrawal from friends, and a fixed conviction that "something terrible is wrong with me." The change may also be much more subtle, with a neat person becoming progressively more sloppy and disorganized. (Sloppiness, a hallmark of adolescence, is not necessarily pathological, however.)
6. An escalation of turmoil in the child, with enormous mood fluctuation, problems concentrating, severe unhappiness, and deterioration or avoidance of usual social, academic, and extracurricular pursuits or interests.
7. A clearly defined move on the part of the child to break away from the nuclear family, and establish his own life, while the family feels he is still "too young to leave home."
8. A severe depression (also see Chapter 11), or a severe anxiety disorder, including panic attacks, in response to the impending separation or following a separation from home and family, such as leaving for college, and taking a job in another city.
9. The appearance of strong hostile and affectionate emotions which the previously "good" and compliant child now shows toward his parents. The parents are upset by the mood swings, particularly the hostility, and bring the youth to the doctor to be "straightened out" (made compliant again).
10. The development of a new psychophysiological disorder or if an old physical disorder is getting worse because of psychological factors (e.g., the child begins to lose enormous amounts of weight, because of the belief that she is "too fat" and comes to you with possible anorexia; the child with diabetes under reasonable control goes off his/her diet and goes out of control because he/she wants to be "normal like other kids").

THE PHYSICIAN'S ROLE

A doctor who is armed with knowledge about the normal processes of adolescence and has seen many teenagers exhibiting "typical" adolescent behavior can serve as a mediator between parent and child. However, since physicians are often contemporaries of the parents, communication is at times difficult. The doctor finds himself drawn to the moral position taken by the parents, rather than remaining as a more objective and neutral outsider. The following principles may help maintain this neutrality and objectivity.

Rapport and Deescalation

The physician should try to establish rapport with both the parents and child so that the adolescent does not feel that the doctor is the "hatchet man" for his parents. This rapport can sometimes be achieved by seeing the child first, without his parents, if only for a few minutes. It is crucial during this initial contact to clarify that regardless of the reasons the parents have for wishing you to see their child, that you are there to help make things better for everyone. The doctor may want to ask the adolescent not only about why he personally may be interested in coming, but also inquire about what is worrying or puzzling the parents that they think the child should be seen. If there is hostility between a child and his parents, usually the child is eager to tell someone about it. Once rapport is established with the parents and child separately, a conjoint interview (seeing them all together) is often indicated. The interaction together lets you see the quality of the interactions (friendly, anxious, hostile) and answer some questions. Who talks to and for whom? Who blames whom? What alliances are there in the family (e.g., mother and son against father). Is there an underlying cohesion and affection among family members, or just hostility? (However, seeing a hostile family together may simply be an invitation for them to fight. The doctor should feel free to "break it up" and see the different factions and individuals separately.) If planning for or about an adolescent is to occur with the parents, this planning should be shared as much as possible with the child himself present, who should participate as actively as he can. If arguments emerge within the conjoint session between the child and parents and threaten to disrupt or destroy the problem-solving focus, one or more of the following strategies may be adopted.

1. Insist that the rest of the family be silent while each complaining family member in turn tells what he thinks are the difficulties in the family, what changes would make the family life better for him, and what would promote a happier family life in general.

> "I wish Dad wouldn't always yell at me when he wants me to do something. It makes me mad, and I feel like punching someone..."

2. If taking turns doesn't work and everybody verbally abuses everybody else, insist that each family member put in writing what he sees as the problem and what he thinks would help. The doctor can then read these anonymous statements aloud.

Values Clarification

Bringing out and trying to clarify value differences within the family may be useful. For instance, it may emerge that the 17-year-old son smokes marijuana periodically because he enjoys it and it makes him "feel good." A question to the parents may elicit the information that they periodically get high (on alcohol) at a party because it makes *them* "feel good." It is now clear that son and parents have quite different values about what is "legitimate" relaxation, and discussion of these different points of view may be quite helpful if the physician feels capable of dealing objectively with values which are not his own. Many physicians, of course, may feel strongly that marijuana is in no way comparable to alcohol, so such an intervention dealing with this issue would not be advisable.

In another instance, a teenage boy may be having sexual intercourse with his girlfriend, and his parents are uncomfortable about this. The doctor might ask the parents, in the son's presence, how they felt about premarital sex when they were growing up: what did they and their friends actually *do*? What often emerges is that today's conservative parents may have raised a little hell in their own youth, and might have raised more if pregnancy had been less of a danger. This open discussion of value similarities and differences between parents and children may be a point of departure for considering in a more realistic way the pros and cons of experimentation. For instance, in favor of sexual experimentation may be that it feels good, is exciting, and promotes closeness. Against it may be the danger of pregnancy or venereal disease, guilt, necessity for concealment from parents and family, and a too-rapid entry into adulthood before one feels emotionally ready (16,17).

Friendly and Objective Counseling

Many adolescents are willing to view a physician as an interested and reasonably objective scientist, who can provide information on emotional as well as physical problems. A teenager might very well decide to consult his doctor about the pros and cons of birth control pills, whether to drop out of school, what to do about under- or over-development, or what to do about low self-esteem related to "being ugly" or "having pimples." If the physician is careful to suggest appropriate options in a nonjudgmental, supportive, and interested way, his advice may often be listened to, although the same advice from a parent might be rejected. The danger is that the physician may give advice to a question he is not asked, such as in a discussion about dating, the doctor may say, "You're too young to think about getting married," when what the teenage girl was leading up to is, "How can I avoid getting pregnant, if I go to bed with my boyfriend?" Even one misunderstood question may sabotage the relationship between the doctor and his teenage patient, and the neutral scientist becomes "the enemy." Advice to teenagers must often be given by indirection—kids may respond to the folly of wrecking their car while intoxicated although they may dismiss the dangers of excessive drinking, per se.

Reaction of Adolescents to Physical Illness

Most older children, and particularly adolescents, become very conscious of how their peer group views them and worry about whether they, in some awful way, are "different" from their friends. Children are extremely self-conscious about their looks, about whether they have acne or are too fat or too thin, whether they have too much or too little body hair, whether the size of their genitalia (boys) or breasts (girls) is adequate. Because of this concern with the suitability of their bodies, an illness is particularly distressing to an adolescent, especially a chronic illness which requires some special diet, procedures, or physical rituals.

In American culture, the normal, healthy adolescent child is seen as full of energy, outgoing, capable of doing almost everything and fitting into almost every situation. Discovering that he has a severe physical limitation, even if it will be temporary, produces in the teenager emotional reactions like those seen in persons who are dying: a sequence or combination of denial, anger, depression, guilt, and often self-deception. For instance, children with diabetes, when they reach adolescence, may go out of diabetic control, because of resisting their diets, fighting medical advice, and skipping urine checks. Understanding what is behind their behavior rather than rejecting or criticizing the child (either verbally or nonverbally) can lead to productive discussion between the doctor and his adolescent patient about just what the realities of the illness are.

In their attempt to protect themselves from their fears about their illness, adolescents often simply do not assimilate basic information about their illness, despite having heard "lectures" time and time again. In exploring the feelings that an adolescent might have about his illness, a good approach is to ask him first to tell you what he knows about his illness. One can then focus on what a person with such an illness can as well as he cannot do. Being able to talk about the lives of some famous athletes who have had diabetes may be quite reassuring to the adolescent diabetic patient. Because many adolescents, well or ill, occasionally engage in activities which adults regard as life-threatening, dangerous, or defiant, the perception of many adolescents is that they are continually receiving lectures, admonitions, and anger from authorities in the adult world. It is especially important for them to find in their doctor an adult who can empathically understand and share their concerns about being different or "crippled," who realizes how annoying and inconvenient their illness must be, and who, at the same time, is willing to plan and discuss with the patient how he can lead as normal a life as possible.

Young children usually grow to accept the idiosyncrasies of their own bodies through the acceptance shown by their parents and other adults they trust, as well as the reactions of peers. In adolescence, the desire or ability to accept parental attitudes or advice is considerably less, so that having a familiar and trusted physician continue to accept one and one's disability is a supportive experience. This is true especially if the doctor makes it clear that he is "working for the patient" as well as for the parents (who are paying the bill). If the patient's diabetes, for instance, remains out of control (because of the severity of the illness, his emotional turmoil, and his reluctance to participate in the management of his illness) the possibility of hospitalization may have to be considered and discussed with the patient. Before resorting to hospitalization, however, the physician should first offer the patient a mutually agreeable medication and treatment plan, outside the hospital if at all possible.

Sexual Concerns in Adolescence

Although some additional information regarding sexuality and adolescent patients will be discussed in Chapter 23, a few words at this point about the concerns of adolescents about sexual matters seem appropriate. As a corollary to the bodily preoccupations shown by many adolescents, patients in this age group are also very concerned about their own sexuality and sexual practices. If statistics are to be believed, a very large number of adolescents have certainly had experience with masturbation, a fairly large number have had overt homosexual experiences, and a gradually increasing number are having overt heterosexual experiences (i.e., intercourse) during the adolescent years. Each of these types of experiences carries with it not only the chance of some personal growth, but also the possibility of guilt and shame. Especially in the case of homosexual experiences, acute distress, depression, and sometimes panic may emerge in response to what the adolescent sometimes considers "weakness" in betraying his basic moral values. The physican's role in these situations is to help resolve this. This help can consist of providing information:

> "A very large number of adolescents masturbate. It's a perfectly ordinary and normal thing to do, and it can't harm you physically."

or making an appropriate referral:

> "You've been saying that you believe you're homosexual, because you've had a number of homosexual experiences with one person and you feel deeply attached to that person. Since you've also had a lot of experience with girls and seem to enjoy this, I'm not at all sure that your current involvement means much one way or another in terms of what your sex life is or will be ten years from now. I'd like to schedule some additional time to talk with you about this, if you're willing. I could also arrange for you to see a counselor, if you want to spend some time looking at your feelings in depth...."

Peter and Barbara Wyden, in their excellent book, *Growing Up Straight: What Every Thoughtful Parent Should Know About Homosexuality* (18), discuss how the person who is homosexually inclined is often in a great state of anxiety and indecision, and is seeking desperately for a source of help, as he struggles with a decision about whether to become overtly homosexual or not. The Wydens suggest that at the very least, such a person have the benefit of a psychiatrist or other professional counselor experienced with homosexual problems and with a sympathetic attitude toward homosexual patients. They point out that many physicians often play ostrich to the possible homosexual conflicts of their patients, give them unhelpful advice to "pull themselves together," and that many physicians, like the population at large, have some feelings of revulsion toward homosexuality. In order for the counseling intervention to be successful, a physician at the very least must be comfortable enough with homosexuality to make an appropriate referral to a counselor who is neither naive, hopeless, nor defeated by the subject. Of course, a great deal of homosexual experimentation in adolescence comes within the range of "normal," so that the physician evaluating the problem must be very sensitive to normal sex play, "crushes," and other homosexual fantasies which are a normal part of preteen and early teenage fantasy life, and the "situational homosexuality" of boarding schools, summer camps, and military service (activity which by itself does not "produce" homosexuals).

In conclusion, in all situations involving sexuality and the adolescent, the physician must be empathic and understanding; he should be able to recognize and, if necessary, compensate for his own hang-ups; he needs to be well informed, but should not jump prematurely into giving advice; and if his own expertise and emotional comfort do not permit him to do appropriate counseling, he should be able to make a wise referral.

Identity Crises, Acute Psychoses, and Schizophrenia in Adolescent Patients

Occasionally a teenager appears to be decompensating or presents an acute or gradual behavioral change involving bizarre behavior, disorganized thinking, and subjective distress and turmoil. In this situation, the physician is likely to be consulted for either a diagnosis or a referral. The differential diagnosis lies between an identity crisis, an acute or brief psychotic episode triggered by environmental stress, and a schizophrenic disorder.

The term "identity crisis" is often bandied about these days, and is a reflection of the enormous influence of the work of Erik H. Erikson, a psychoanalyst whose writings and ideas about the formation of identity during the adolescent period have greatly influenced psychological thinking for the past thirty years (19). Clinically, it is only when the adolescent experiences severe problems in "putting it all together" and developing a coherent sense of self that the physician is consulted. Severe subjective distress regarding the integration of issues relating to identity—long term goals, career choice, friendship patterns, sexual orientation and behavior, religious identification, moral value systems, group loyalties, and a secondary impairment in social or occupational functioning for more than 3 months—justify the diagnosis, of Identity Disorder (20). The distress may in some individuals take a mild form, but in others appears with sufficient intensity and behavioral disorganization that observers, especially family members, wonder if the person is "going crazy." A detailed history often reveals the areas of identity conflict as well as mild anxiety and depression, self-doubt, doubts about the future, and difficulty making decisions or making decisions through impulsive experimentation. The history sometimes reveals negative or oppositional behavior as an attempt to define one's self as "different" from one's family or origin. Despite such conflicts, the individual does not show delusional thinking, hallucinatory activity, or a pervasive impairment in reality testing that interferes with the individual's ability to make appropriate decisions on a daily basis.

Management of Identity Crisis

If a physician has a good relationship with the patient, he may be able to help the patient get into a professional counseling or therapy relationship which generally is the treatment of choice. Therapy may be on an individual basis, but often goes faster if the patient may be seen with other peers who may be experiencing similar problems. College counseling services often have groups in which individuals experiencing identity problems explore the conflicts and issues with other individuals. A psychologically sophisticated primary physician or one especially trained to deal with such issues (through experience, reading, training, and supervision) may certainly be appropriate to deal with many of these issues, but rarely has the time required, which may be considerable, to give the patient and his problems an adequate hearing. Over a period of time, individuals usually resolve these problems, but experience enormous subjective distress while they are doing so. Medications are rarely useful, unless the patient has full-blown symptoms of another disorder, such as a major depression.

Brief Reactive Psychoses, Schizophreniform Disorder, and Schizophrenia

A second category of severe decompensation, which may sometimes occur with adolescent patients, is that of a brief reactive psychosis. A brief reactive psychosis occurs when, following a severe environmental stressor, an individual develops at least one of the following symptoms: incoherence or loosening of associations (thoughts or ideas strung together in a nonlogical or nonsequential way), delusions (false ideas), hallucinations (false perceptions, usually auditory), and disorganized behavior. Technically (according to DSM III criteria) (21), such a disorder may be diagnosed shortly after the onset of the psychotic symptoms.

If the psychotic disorder lasts more than 2 weeks (but less than 6 months) it is called a *schizophreniform disorder*. The implications of diagnosing both of these disorders is that the prognosis is far more favorable than if a schizophrenic disorder is diagnosed. A schizophreniform disorder has identical features with schizophrenia—a prodromal phase with some aspects of social isolation, impairment of role functioning, peculiar behavior, odd, magical thinking, and peculiar speech—an active phase with at least one of the following: bizarre, somatic, grandiose, nihilistic or other delusions; persecutory delusions; auditory hallucinations; incoherence and loosening of associations, and illogical thinking. The clinical picture is also accompanied by deterioration of functioning in work, social relations, or self-care. A residual phase following recovery from the illness is often accompanied by several symptoms characteristic of the prodromal phase.

With a brief *reactive psychosis*, many clinicians believe that one should hold off, at least for several days, before treating the patient with antipsychotic medication, and that the clear, precipitating stressor, combined with an adequate level of functioning prior to the psychotic episode, suggests that the patient does not have schizophrenia and should not be treated as if he does. The treatment of a brief psychotic episode involves mobilizing the patient's support system, keeping the patient in a place that is safe, clarifying reality, and maintaining as much contact as possible with the people with whom the patient is close. If the patient is violent, destructive, or self-destructive, medication is, of course, appropriate. The major differential diagnostic alternative to a brief reactive psychosis is a psychotic state precipitated by a drug intoxication [such as LSD, phencyclidine (PCP), or an amphetamine]. With any acute psychotic state, the most important thing is to be able to: (1) observe the patient in a quiet and safe place, (2) provide reassurance and reality clarification ("I'm Dr. Jones, and this is St. Ann's Hospital"), and (3) obtain a history from friends, family, and the patient, himself. The history should include information about drugs (known or unknown), which the patient may have ingested, as well as about possible environmental stressors (e.g., a house fire, following which the patient has not been able to sleep for several days).

The diagnosis of the adolescent with a schizophreniform disorder rests on the clinical observation that patients with this disorder have a more acute onset and resolution of their illness than do people with schizophrenia, and that the clinical picture more often involves "emotional turmoil, fear, confusion, and particularly vivid hallucinations" (22). Treatment involves medication, and if facilities are available, often involves the use of "rapid tranquilization" in which symptom control is achieved through the intensive use of tranquilizing medications such as haloperidol or navane during the first 24 hours (W. Dubin, *private communication*). (Other aspects of treatment of the adolescent with schizophreniform disorder will be discussed under the treatment of the adolescent with schizophrenia.)

Schizophrenia, as a diagnosis, carries with it a more ominous prognosis, with the expectation that a patient will rarely recover full functioning to his previous level. Although many diagnostic schemes have been proposed for the diagnosis of schizophrenia, current diagnostic criteria include the following (23).

1. Deterioration from a previous level of functioning, usually in the areas of work, social relations, and self-care.
2. Characteristic symptoms, involving multiple psychological areas, including several of the following.
   a. Thought content disturbance (delusions) of a bizarre, persecutory, or somatic variety. Common delusions include thought broadcasting (one's thoughts are broadcast to the world); thought insertion (other's thoughts are inserted into one's own mind); thought withdrawal (thoughts have been removed from one's mind); and delusions of being controlled by some external force.
   b. Formal thought disorder (thoughts are incoherent, disconnected, or tangentially related, and associations of thought are said to be "loose," without the patient being aware of the lack of connection).
   c. Perceptual disturbances, the most common of which are hallucinations, especially auditory, in which voices are perceived as coming from outside

one's head. (If visual, taste, or olfactory hallucinations are present without auditory hallucinations, the possibility of an organic or toxic psychosis must be considered.)
   d. Affect disturbance, especially blunted, flattened, or inappropriate affect. (Reduced or absent intensity of affective expression; or with affect discordant with what the patient is saying.)
   e. Self/identity disturbance, often taking the form of a patient being unable to tell where his beliefs, ideas, or feelings end and another person's begin (loss of ego boundaries).
   f. Volition disturbance, in which the person has trouble initiating or setting goals for himself regarding work or other role functioning.
   g. Withdrawal from the external world and preoccupation with one's own egocentric, illogical ideas and fantasies (autism).
   h. Psychomotor change (usually a decrease in reactivity to the environment, but occasionally the appearance of bizarre, stereotyped, or excited motor movements or postures).
3. Impairment in several areas of daily routine, often requiring supervision around nutrition and hygiene.

Management of the Adolescent Schizophrenic Patient

When an adolescent patient with a possible psychosis is referred for management to a primary physician, the first step is to obtain a detailed consultation with a psychiatrist regarding medical and environmental management. Often, the decision is very difficult about whether to keep the disturbed child at home in the community or to place him in the psychiatric ward of a general or mental hospital. At times, removing the child from his home can lead to rapid improvement. At the same time, separating him from family, friends, interests, and his usual social identity can itself be a disruptive and disorganizing experience. The decision about whether or not to hospitalize the adolescent patient depends on: (1) the severity of the disturbance (how agitated, wild, or unreachable the patient is); (2) the response to antipsychotic medication, and the willingness of the patient to take such medication; and (3) the availability of supportive resources outside the hospital, including the availability of people to work intensively with the patient (ideally, in a therapeutic day care setting combined with a school program), the availability of support from peers and the school system, and the level of tolerance to disruptiveness and regressive behavior which the family can stand and deal with.

Antipsychotic medication (as will be elaborated in Chapter 16) can be helpful in deferring hospitalization or even making it unnecessary. Adolescent patients are often resistant to taking medications regularly. Medication compliance depends both on a strong alliance with the patient, reinforcement of the need for medication by important persons in the patient's life (e.g., family, counselors, teachers), and an assessment by the treating physician about whether a long-acting injectable medication, such as fluphreazine decanoate, may be preferable to the struggle with the patient to take daily medication. [Unfortunately, long-acting injectable antipsychotic medications appear to have a high incidence of tardive dyskinesia as a side effect, so that the decision merits considerable thought (and explanation to the family and patient).] Avoidance of hospitalization may also be aided by seeing the patient frequently on an individual basis to provide support and an opportunity to ventilate current concerns. Although the adolescent patient may have to be hospitalized acutely for several days to develop a subsequent treatment plan as well as stabilize on medication, seeing him on a daily outpatient basis for support and medication may be equally efficacious.

It is important that despite his illness, the adolescent maintain those social contacts which he has and that the family continue to give as much support as possible. The interactions within the family should be assessed, however, to determine what existing familial factors may be contributing to the patient's psychosis. If the physician feels unable to deal with the family itself, a trained mental health professional should sit in as a consultant to a family interview to help decide whether the primary physician can continue to manage the patient with occasional advice from the mental health professional, or that the patient should be transferred for management to a psychiatrist or other mental health specialist. As noted earlier, those patients in whom a psychotic illness emerged relatively acutely in response to an environmental stressor, and following a history of reasonably intact and normal social functioning, have a much more hopeful prognosis than those patients in whom the onset of the illness has been very gradual, insidious, and especially where the patient, even from early childhood, was "peculiar," withdrawn, or socially very isolated.

A physician may periodically encounter an adolescent who has become, or is becoming, psychotic almost with the blessing of the parents. The family does not seek help until the child is so withdrawn, destructive, or bizarre, that it is quite clear that his removal from the home is obligatory. Studies suggest that in some families one child may be treated in such contradictory and confusing ways that the one solution open to him is to "go crazy," particularly when any other solution such as rebelling or running away is for some reason unacceptable (24). In most cases, however, there is strong evidence to suggest that the psychosis in an adolescent has many determinants and causes in addition to the "family system." It may be far more productive to view the psychosis as being like a suicide attempt or a run-away—a crisis which perhaps can be managed if quick countermeasures are taken. (This is not to imply that a schizophrenic disorder is like tonsillitis, which can be cured rapidly by penicillin.) Even if a cure for schizophrenia is beyond the current state of psychiatric knowledge (in ensuring prevention of future episodes), the effective management of any specific episode is often within the physician's power, particularly if the illness is caught early. Hallucinations, delusions, and garbled thinking can often respond dramatically to prompt support and pharmacotherapy.

There are several theories about the occurrence of schizophrenia in adolescents: (a) there are indications that there is a genetic predisposition to some kinds of schizophrenia (25,26); (b) schizophrenia may flourish in certain families because of peculiar family power structures (e.g., where parents have a great emotional distance from each other and from their children, but pretend they are a very close family, and where the children must deal with the disparity between what they are told and what they feel); (c) "crazy" symptomatology is a method the child has seized upon to prevent other family members from fighting with each other or the family from falling apart; (d) a child who is excessively dependent, particularly if the dependence was mixed with hostility, may fall apart when he is separated from the people he formerly relied upon (such as his parents).

An implication of these theories (all of which may be valid) is that even when an adolescent has developed a schizophrenic illness then recompensates and resumes a level of functioning not too dissimilar from the previous level, he may still be more vulnerable than other individuals for a recurrence of a similar illness. Such a youth requires long-term psychotherapy, at least of a supportive kind, and may continue to need antipsychotic medication to maintain his emotional equilibrium. The author believes strongly that many primary physicians, with periodic consultation from their psychiatric conferences, can provide excellent long-term supportive psychotherapy, as well as management of medication. In addition, an adolescent who has had a schizophrenic breakdown will continue to need "objective" and supportive persons (such as a physician), although his adolescent peers, despite any emotional upheaval of their own, will not require such special treatment. A physician should regard the adolescent patient who has had a schizophrenic illness as a person whose psychological diet must be monitored in the same way that a juvenile diabetic's actual diet needs special monitoring. Both patient and physician can and should remain emotionally involved long after the time necessary for other adolescents.

Psychotic adolescents, like psychotic adults (see Chapter 16), often respond well to the establishment of limits and a well-defined structure. The practicing physician might consider the following approaches.

1. Try to isolate the precipitating factors in the psychotic decompensation [drugs, separation from home, the loss of an important person (e.g., boyfriend), feelings of enormous guilt over sexual experimentation, etc.].

2. Clarify what rules, both explicit and implicit, have developed in the family for dealing with the adolescent's peculiar or crazy symptomatology. Does the patient get a great deal of affection or attention only when he is acting weird, or do the parents overlook the crazy behavior and respond more to the child's healthier communications? If the former situation exists, it will be necessary to work with the parents on responding to the clearer, more "normal" messages.

3. Other peculiar or conflicting stances of family members may contribute to the current behavior of the patient. For instance, do the parents say things like, "Stay out as late as you want—you're old enough to make your own decisions. But if you're not in by 11:00, you know how we'll worry!" Such a mixed message ("You are independent, but your independence is making us suffer") is called a

"double-bind" (27). Experts studying communication patterns in dysfunctional families with schizophrenic members often find these kinds of messages. Even in "normal" families, much covert anxiety is communicated from parents to children when the adolescent children experiment with behavior (such as sexual) about which the parents have mixed feelings. (The parents want their children to grow up, and know that sexual involvement is necessary and inevitable, and yet they worry about pregnancy, may feel jealous, and are reminded that they, themselves, are growing old.) If the doctor has sufficient rapport with the patient and his family, he may point out communications in the family which give this double-binding message. Once such a pattern is known to the family, the doctor might establish, possibly in writing, what rules or messages between parents and adolescent would be most productive. Consultation with a psychiatric colleague may be helpful to develop a strategy with such a family.

4. Many adolescents resist taking medications. They see this as setting them apart from their peers and reinforcing the ties of dependency and hostility between them and their parents. As a result, adolescents who need medications to prevent further psychotic decompensation present management difficulties to their doctors and don't comply with medication regimes, even though regular doses of antipsychotic medication are essential to maintain the patient. The physician should explain alternative possibilities (such as injectable medication every few weeks), and the consequences of missed doses should be clarified. Above all, it is crucial that the "contract" for medication, if at all possible, be made between the doctor and the patient, rather than through an intermediary, such as the parents. In this way, the patient is responsible for taking his own medication. To act through the parents supports the adolescent's suspicions that the "neutral doctor" is really an agent for the parents, rather than, as one would hope, an ally of both.

5. If, in the physician's judgment, the family situation is extremely unhealthy and is actively contributing to the adolescent's personality disintegration, temporary hospitalization may be necessary simply to separate the child and his family. Subsequent placement in a foster home, a group home, or with friends or relatives may enable the child to recompensate more rapidly if the setting is structured and the physician maintains close follow-up. Usually an optimal program includes educational, vocational, socializing, and psychotherapeutic components. Many day-treatment programs for adolescents and young adults which incorporate these ingredients are now a part of community mental health centers, particularly in urban areas. Checking out what is already available may save you a lot of time and vastly increase your effectiveness.

REFERENCES

1. Gardner, R. A. (1971): *Therapeutic Communication with Children: The Mutual Storytelling Technique*. Jason Aronson. New York.
2. Gardner, R. A. The Talking, Feeling, and Doing Game. Manufactured by Creative Therapeutics, 155 County Road, Creskill, New Jersey, 07626.
3. Burns, R., and Kaufman, S. H. (1970): *Kinetic Family Drawings*. Brunner/Mazel. New York.
4. *House, Tree, Person Manual*: Administration of the HTP Test. Buck, J., Consultant. Western

Psychological Services, Beverly Hills, California. 1964; and *House, Tree, Person Research Manual*, Hammer, E. F., Western Psychological Services, Los Angeles, 1955.
5. *Diagnostic and Statistical Manual* (1980): third edition, pp. 41–45. American Psychiatric Association. Washington, D.C.
6. Connors, C. K. (1965): A teacher rating scale for use in drug studies with children. *Am. J. Psychiatry*, 126:884.
7. Abbott Laboratories, North Chicago, Illinois 60064.
8. Trupin, E., Gilchrist, L., Mairo, R., and Faye, G.: Social skills training for learning disabled children. In: *Behavioral Programs for the Developmentally Disabled. (in press)*.
9. Trupin, E., Ph.D., Division of Child Psychiatry (GI-80), University of Washington, Seattle, Washington 98105.
10. Lewis, M., and Lewis, D. O. (1973): The crisis of death: A child dies. In: *Pediatric Management of Psychologic Crises*, pp. 5–13. Current Problems in Pediatrics, vol. 3. Year Book Medical Publishers, Chicago.
11. Lewis, M., and Lewis, D. O. (1973): In: *Pediatric Management of Psychologic Crises*, p. 12. Current Problems in Pediatrics, vol. 3. Year Book Medical Publishers, Chicago.
12. Kempe, C. H., and Helfer, R. E. (1972): *Helping the Battered Child and His Family*. Lippincott, Philadelphia.
13. Sexual Assault Center, Harborview Medical Center, Seattle, Washington. 1980 Client Characteristics.
14. This information was provided through the courtesy of the Sexual Assault Center, Harborview Medical Center, 329 Ninth Avenue, Seattle, Washington 98104. The material was originally prepared with support from grant no. 77-DF-10-0016 awarded to the Sexual Assault Center by the Law Enforcement Assistance Administration, U.S. Department of Justice.
15. Offer, D., Marcus, D., and Offer, J. L. (1970): A longitudinal study of normal adolescent boys. *Am. J. Psychiatry*, 126:917–924.
16. Pomeroy, W. (1968): *Boys and Sex*. Dell, New York.
17. Pomeroy, W. (1968): *Girls and Sex*. Dell, New York.
18. Wyden, P., and Wyden, B. (1968): *Growing Up Straight: What Every Thoughtful Parent Should Know About Homosexuality*. Stein and Day, New York. [Also published by Signet Books (paperback), New York, 1969.]
19. Erikson, E. H. (1971): *Identity: Youth and Crisis*. Faber and Faber, London.
20. *Diagnostic and Statistical Manual*, third edition. American Psychiatric Association, Washington, D.C., 1980. pp.65–67.
21. *Diagnostic and Statistical Manual*, third edition. American Psychiatric Association, Washington, D.C., 1980. pp. 200–202.
22. *Diagnostic and Statistical Manual*, third edition. American Psychiatric Association, Washington, D.C., 1980. pp. 199–200.
23. *Diagnostic and Statistical Manual*, third edition. American Psychiatric Association, Washington, D.C., 1980. pp. 181–193.
24. Bateson, G., Jackson, D., Haley, J., and Weakland, J. (1956): Toward a theory of schizophrenia. *Behavioral Sciences*, 1:4.
25. Wender, P. H., Rosenthal, D., Kety, S. S., et al. (1974): Cross fostering: a research strategy for clarifying the role of genetic and experimental factors in the etiology of schizophrenia. *Arch. General Psychiatry*, 30:121.
26. Freeman, D. E., Kety, S. S., Rosenthal, D., et al. (1972): The significance of genetics in schizophrenia. *Am. J. Psychiatry*, 128:1464.
27. Berger, M. (ed.) (1978): *Beyond The Double Bind*. Brunner/Mazel, New York.

8

Adult Development and Its Implications for Primary Care

Until quite recently it was assumed by observers of psychological development throughout the life cycle that nothing much happened in the inner lives of adults between their early twenties, when they had launched their careers, and retirement age, when they began preparing for the losses associated with aging and impending death. Erik Erickson, who had done so much to translate the stages of childhood psychological development as proposed by Freud into a more comprehensive, useful, and lively model for the mid-twentieth century, was vague about the adult life cycle (1). He implied that young adults were concerned about and had to master issues related to intimacy, which adults in their forties, if they were healthy, had achieved generatively, including a focus on leadership and the well-being of other people. Erickson believed that nothing much happened until old age, when issues of integrity would be paramount.

During the 1970s, a number of observers began to look in a much more systematic way at what happens to adults. To their surprise, they learned that a great deal happens. Workers who were especially concerned with adult male development include Levinson et al. (2,3), Gould (4,5), and Valliant (6). Fewer studies are available about women's development throughout the life cycle; major investigators in this area include Seiden (7,8), Miller (9), and Neugarten (10,11) (who has written about both men and women). The findings of these investigators have major significance and implications for the delivery of primary medical care.

All workers appear to agree that changes occur throughout the adult years far more frequently than was once thought. Furthermore, these changes, and the struggles and pain attendant on them, are normal and not necessarily a signal of pathology (unless, of course, someone gets bogged down during one of these changes). Most patients, along with their physicians, are relatively unaware of the existence of these predictable changes and life crises, and so everyone involved assumes the worst when they occur.

A mid-life crisis means a mid-life depression and is seen as indicating serious psychopathology, rather than a painful but necessary opportunity for growth and change. A physician may be particularly useful to his patient during these periods of transition by sharing information about the normality of such life changes and crises. The doctor also can act as a counselor and facilitator of the growth process during such transition periods. An adult experiencing such a life change almost invariably feels unsettled as well as anxious. Counseling, life planning, and support may all be called for; seeking out and treating such discomfiture as character weakness or incipient mental disorder is not.

NAIVE ASSUMPTIONS ABOUT ADULT LIFE

Gould, a psychiatrist who has extensively investigated the adult life cycle, cites a number of false assumptions which many persons acquire while growing up (5). They must then struggle with and divest themselves of these assumptions in order to grow and become persons in their own right, rather than extensions of their original families. Such assumptions include the following:

1. "You always belong to your parents." If you become too independent, some sort of disaster will strike. Obviously, such an assumption can be particularly disastrous for a person seeking a career or life-style very different from that of their original families or, for some women, any career at all.

2. "If I do things my parents' way, everything will turn out all right." This presupposes that some other person knows the "right" way for the person in question to live. Implicit in this assumption is that "respectability" and "doing the right thing" will answer the invariable questions of intimacy, renewal, self-fulfillment, and changing needs and values throughout the life cycle. This kind of attitude is seen in the often-overheard comment, "My mother said that being a mother would be the most fulfilling and satisfying thing of my life. But sometimes I'm depressed and hate it. There must be something wrong with me."

3. "There is no complicated inner life." This implies that things are fixed, simple, and what they seem—not complex, subtle, evolving, and ambivalent. Successful people are therefore surprised when they question if they really want the success they have worked for. One question seems to arise quite often: "Is this all there is?"

4. "There is no death or separation." This implies an illusion of safety and invulnerability forever. For males this may take the belief that, if successful, one is somehow protected from danger and separation, regardless of how one lives. For females this may take the form of believing that one requires a male around as a "protector" and to make decisions, the idea of "separateness" being only an abstraction.

When a patient indicates such assumptions about living, it may be important for the physician to question them: Does a woman need permission and a "protector" to make decisions or learn about balancing her own checkbook? Is a successful executive or doctor "safe" when he drives or flies recklessly? If one works long, exhausting hours but is paid well, is it surprising that one feels tired? What is success, and does it always mean the same thing?

ADULTHOOD AND LIFE STRUCTURE

Levinson, studying adult men throughout their lives (2), discovered that most men went through alternating periods of stability, punctuated every 7 years or so by a period of instability that usually lasted approximately 3 years. This series of stable and unstable periods occurs throughout the entire life cycle, even though some of the transitions may be more dramatic or have more anguish. The periods may be broken down this way.

Early adult transition (ages 17 to 22). The tasks of this period involve pulling up roots from one's original family, moving out into the world, and making preliminary sorties into the adult world of job, relationships and intimacy, identity, and life-style.

Entering the adult world (ages 22 to 28). This period involves shifting one's focus from being a child in one's family of origin to becoming a novice adult with a home base of one's own. It involves making and testing a variety of initial choices regarding job, love relationships, peers, values, and life-style. While making the beginnings of a stable life structure, the novice adult must "keep his options open."

Age 30 transition (ages 28 to 33). During this phase the adult looks back on the commitments and structure he has developed and wonders, "Is this all there is; is it worth it?" Life-style, occupation, and commitments are re-evaluated, sometimes with a great deal of emotional upset; this period is sometimes experienced as a crisis.

Settling down (ages 33 to 40). During this period a man's major preoccupation is usually "making it" in the adult world, especially as defined by work or occupation. The focus is usually to realize one's youthful goals and aspirations, and to establish a niche in society. Advancement and progress are often seen in terms of a timetable, with the imagery being that of "climbing a ladder." A distinct subphase during this period is from approximately age 36 to 40, which Levinson called "becoming one's own man." The major developmental task is that of becoming a "senior member" of one's own world, with a greater sense of self and greater authority.

Mid-life transition (ages 40 to 45). During this period, men again question their life structure and commitments. They often wonder, "What do I get? What do I give? What do I want?" Every aspect of their lives comes into question. It has been entitled the "Now that I've worked so hard to get where I am, is this all there is" blues.

Middle adulthood (ages 45 to 60). During this period men re-establish and reorder their priorities. The character of their life structure accomodates their unfulfilled dreams, their awareness of death, and their realization that they are aging. The sense of immortality and omnipotence is often given up during this phase.

Age 50 transition (ages 50 to 55). Modifications and reworking of the life structure occur during this period. This transition is sometimes, although not invariably, experienced as a crisis.

Second middle adult structure (ages 55 to 60). For many men this second period of adulthood assumes an increasingly nurturing quality. For men it includes taking on "fathering" and teaching roles, with transmission of important personal and cultural values to younger persons. This activation of nurturing roles has been seen as developing the "feminine side of a male's identity."

Late adult transition (ages 60 to 65). During this period the efforts of middle adulthood begin to be concluded, and the preparation of subsequent stages of aging, loss, and career diminution begins.

As can be seen from this extremely abbreviated outline, at many periods—especially during transition or crisis—the role of the primary physician as a counselor and listener, or as a facilitator of planning and life change, can be crucial. It is important, of course, that the physician himself not be so overwhelmed by his own or the patient's transitions or struggles that the physician responds with alarm, denial, or avoidance rather than acceptance and empathy.

DEFENSES THROUGHOUT THE LIFE CYCLE

Valliant, in his longitudinal studies of men beginning during the college years and continuing throughout their life cycle, concluded that both physical and mental health can be linked to the defense mechanisms which evolve during the person's life (6). Although Valliant does not imply that persons can easily change themselves or quickly modify their characteristic ways of handling conflict and anxiety, some of these ways of coping can be cultivated and nurtured.

Using a developmental perspective, Valliant found that those individuals who in mid- and late life were happier, achieved more, and had better physical health increasingly during their middle years began to use mature defense mechanisms. During adolescence, most men use immature coping defenses against anxiety. These include projection (blaming things on others), hypochondriasis, acting out, being passive-aggressive, intellectualizing and rationalizing, and having reaction formation [behaving in a way totally opposite to the (unacceptable) way one would really like to behave]. By the time mid-life is reached, healthier, more successful men were using fewer of the immature defenses. These men had developed much more capacity to use (1) humor, (2) suppression (the conscious decision to postpone paying attention to an area of conflict), (3) altruism (vicarious but constructive and gratifying service to others), (4) anticipation (realistic anticipation and planning for future crises or discomfort), and (5) sublimation (indirect expressions of drives or instincts without adverse effects or loss of pleasure; e.g., competitive sports as an expression of aggression and competitive wishes).

Clearly, suggesting to a patient that some things are best dealt with by ignoring them, accepting them, laughing about them, or perhaps focusing on other things raises new possibilities for some individuals who feel "hung up" or incapable of dealing with life issues which make them uncomfortable but which cannot easily be changed. (This statement does not, of course, do justice to Valliant's detailed research and writings.)

LIFE CYCLE OF MARRIAGE

Berman and Leif (12) studied the life cycle of marriage in much the way Levinson studied the life cycle of individual men. They concluded that many marriages echoed the life stages of individuals, with the issues at stake being power, intimacy, and inclusion-exclusion (including fulfillment of personal needs within the relationship). They found the following stages:

Pulling up roots (ages 18 to 21). Whereas the individual task at this age is to develop autonomy, the marital task is to shift from family or origin to a new commitment. Marital conflicts center around original family ties versus new commitments. There is fragile intimacy, a testing of power, and, on the inclusion-exclusion axis, conflicts over in-laws.

Provisional adulthood (ages 22 to 28). The individual task at this age is getting into the adult world, whereas the marital task is provisional marital commitment. Marital conflict centers around uncertainty of the marriage partner and stress over parenthood. There is deepening but ambivalent intimacy. Conflict resolution patterns are developed to deal with power issues, and boundary issues center around friends, potential lovers, and work versus the family.

Age 30 transition (ages 28 to 33). During this period of individual reappraisal of work, there is a similar marital commitment crisis as well as a feeling of restlessness. Marital conflicts center around doubts about the marital choice. During this transition there is greater distance while partners make up their minds about each other. There is sharp vying for power and dominance. Boundary issues may include temporary disruptions including extramarital sex or a reactive distancing ("fortress building").

Settling down (ages 32 to 39). The individual's task during this period is deepening commitment to and pursuance of long-range goals. The marital task focuses on productivity, which includes children, work, friends, and marriage. Marital conflict centers around the different ways in which the husband and wife achieve productivity. In good marriages intimacy is increased, whereas in bad marriages there is a gradual distancing. Definite patterns of decision-making and dominance are established. Boundary issues include the nuclear family closing boundaries.

Mid-life transition (ages 40 to 42). During this period, in which the individual task is characterized by Berman and Leif as searching for a "fit" between aspirations and environment, the marital task involves a summing up, in which success and failure are evaluated and future goals are sought. Marital conflict centers on the different perceptions of success by husband and wife, and the conflict that is felt between choosing individual success and/or remaining in the marriage. Intimacy is tenuous, as fantasies about other individuals increase. In the power dimension, power in the outside world is tested vis-à-vis power in the marriage. Boundaries are disrupted due to re-evaluation and the conflict between drives outside the relationship versus the desire to restabilize.

Middle adulthood (ages 43 to 59). Whereas the individual task is to restabilize and reorder priorities, the marital task is to resolve conflicts and stabilize the marriage for the remaining years. Marital conflict centers on conflicting rates and directions of emotional growth as well as concerns about losing youthfulness (which may lead to depression or acting out). Intimacy is threatened by aging and boredom within a secure, stable relationship. Children departing may increase or decrease intimacy. Power conflicts increase when children leave and security seems threatened. Marital boundaries are usually fixed except during crises, e.g., illness, death, or job change.

Older age (ages 60+). The individual task at this age is to retain zest for life while simultaneously dealing with aging, illness, and death. The marital task is to support and enhance each partner's struggle for productivity and fulfillment despite aging. Marital conflicts arise because of re-emerging fears of desertion, loneliness, and sexual failure. There is a struggle to maintain intimacy in the face of eventual separation; usually intimacy achieves some stability. Survival fears stir up some needs for control and dominance. Marital boundary issues focus on the closing in of boundaries in relation to loss of family and friends. The physical environment determines the degree to which outside ties are maintained with the outside world.

Having a knowledge of the marital as well as the individual life cycles can be very useful to the primary physician for anticipating predictable life crises within relationships. Having and sharing the knowledge with the patients normalizes some of their crises and feelings, rather than their believing that their feelings, and even their actions, are pathological or bad.

WOMEN'S ISSUES

The development of women throughout the life cycle has not been studied as thoroughly as that of men. Clouding the issues are marked changes in the ways in which women are viewed and view themselves, the increasing emphasis on "personhood" rather than the "woman's role" (e.g., mother), and the contentions of more militant feminists that differences between men and women are entirely environmentally induced rather than biologically based.

One empirical observation about the development of women, noted by Moris (13), is that the development of personal identity may be quite different. Whereas men often focus on career and work, and define themselves at least until mid-life in terms of their careers, women often define themselves by the multiple strands of emotional attachments and connections to specific individuals. Moris believes that, in contrast with men, whose identity is often solid and focused because of the career orientation, women in early adulthood may have a much more diffuse identity and define themselves as X's daughter, Y's wife, and Z's mother, rather than in terms of what they do. Whereas men often expand their identity with added dimensions of nurturing and emotionality during mid-life, women often solidify their identity by focusing, sometimes for the first time, on something they themselves want, rather than something other people want for them. Whether this is true for women who have had a career is unknown, although at thirty, women without children often experience a crisis of "this will be my last opportunity to be a mother." Women who are successful in careers often have a male mentor during their twenties and thirties who can help "show them the ropes" as well as support their abilities to negotiate and deal with men in an effective and assertive way, even while remaining very feminine; by the time they reach their forties, the need for such a mentor is usually much less crucial and the mentor may even be resented (14).

Other studies have outlined the conflicts experienced by women who are in the process of developing a sense of self. They must struggle with their distaste for "traditional" (now seen as inferior) roles while still valuing the role that constitutes their unique fulfillment.

Review articles by Seiden (7,8), although not providing specific details about the development of women throughout the life cycle, do provide a summary of current research studies about women which have extremely important clinical implications. These data are particularly useful in helping the clinician decide whether a complaint is more likely to be normative for women in general or a particular, idiosyncratic indication of individual pathology. Some of the generalizations abstracted from the articles include the following.

1. Young, married, childless women have a significantly higher level of satisfaction than married women with young children.

2. Married women are more likely than unmarried women to seek psychiatric help, attempt suicide, and report somatic symptoms indicative of psychological distress.

3. "It is likely that some of the toll exerted by child rearing and perhaps marriage as well arises from intrinsic stress and lack of adequate anticipatory information . . . it is important for clinicians . . . to have a realistic appraisal of the occupational hazards of child rearing and the need for adequate support and backup. . . ."

4. "Studies suggest that achieving women have learned to fear that society might punish them for that achievement, particularly if it is perceived as deviant, while achieving men have learned to expect societal reward to maintain their behavior."

5. Therapeutic theories have not questioned stereotyped assumptions about sex roles. There are thus different standards of mental health for women and men, based on the assumptions that dependency, masochism, and passivity are normal for women.

6. "There has been a kind of (often unconscious) arrogance in the willingness of male professionals to tell women how to define their problems and lead their lives and, in parallel, a curious willingness of women to accept male definitions of women's needs."

7. Although as a group more women than men report life satisfaction, this difference drops precipitously if the woman is married and has young children. The life satisfaction of women with young children is insignificantly greater in the childbearing years than that of men.

In view of these data, it becomes extremely important that primary care physicians, especially male physicians, thoroughly evaluate the situation of a woman coming to treatment, for example, because of depression. A partial respite from nonstop motherhood may often be as valuable as antidepressant medication and/or psychotherapy to help the patient work through conflicts about being a mother.

IMPLICATIONS OF LIFE CYCLE RESEARCH

Research into the life cycles of both men and women is a growing, exciting field. The more informed the primary physician becomes about predictable crises, stages, and conflicts throughout the adult life cycle, the stronger position he will be in to offer help to his adult patients.

REFERENCES

1. Erickson, E. H. (1963): *Childhood and Society.* Norton, New York.
2. Levinson, D. J. (1978): *The Seasons of a Man's Life.* Ballantine, New York.
3. Levinson, D. J., Darrow, C. M., et al. (1974): The psychosocial development of men in early adulthood and the mid-life transition. In: *Life History Research in Psychopathology,* Vol. 3, pp. 243–258, edited by R. Merrill. University of Minnesota Press, Minneapolis.
4. Gould, R. L. (1972): The phases of adult life: a study of developmental psychology. *Am. J. Psychiatry,* 129:521–531.
5. Gould, R. L. (1978): Evolution of adult consciousness. *Audiodigest Psychiatry,* 7:1.
6. Valliant, G. (1977): *Adaptation to Life.* Little, Brown, Boston.
7. Seiden, A. M. (1976): Overview: research on the psychology of women. I. Gender differences and sexual and reproductive life. *Am. J. Psychiatry,* 133:995–1007.
8. Seiden, A. M. (1976): Overview: research on the psychology of women. II. Women in families, work, and psychotherapy. *Am. J. Psychiatry,* 133:1111–1123.
9. Miller, J. B. (1976): *Toward a New Psychology of Women.* Beacon Press, Boston.
10. Neugarten, B. L. (1975): Adult personality: toward a psychology of the life cycle. In: *The Human Life Cycle,* edited by W. C. Sze. Jason Aronson, New York.
11. Neugarten, B. L. (1963): Women's attitudes toward the menopause. *Vita Humana,* 6:140–151.
12. Berman, E. M., and Leif, H. I. (1975): Marital therapy from a psychiatric perspective: an overview. *Am. J. Psychiatry,* 132:583-592.
13. Moris, A. H. (1981): *Male and female created.* Puget Soundings, Seattle.
14. Adams, J. (1981): Personal communication.

9

The Aging Patient and Primary Care

Aging may be seen as a series of significant losses: loss of income; loss of friends and relatives; loss of status as a worker, parent, and active member of the community; and loss of self-esteem simply because one is old in a country in which youth is glorified. There is also a loss of mobility and physical independence through disability and loss of cognitive abilities (e.g., memory loss, slowed ability to learn, decreased response speed, and poorer integrative functioning) (1). Of course these statements present both an overgeneralization and a mythology about aging.

The geriatric population of the United States (arbitrarily defined as those individuals 65 years and older) now comprises 10% of the population, or about 20 million people; by the year 2020 this age group is expected to make up 25% of the population. These people form a vastly underrepresented minority in terms of the preventive and health maintenance medical and mental health care they receive (although their medical and mental problems keep many hospitals and convalescent beds occupied).

Because of the special and severe problems of aging, both emotional and physical, and because much of the current treatment of the elderly is based on personal biases and cultural myths about aging, it seems important to include some recent data on aging, much of which challenges the hopelessness with which the elderly are regarded.

1. The new retiree is not "about to die." A 65-year-old man can expect to live 13 more years, and a 65-year-old woman can expect to live 16 more years (2).

2. Only 5% of the elderly live in institutions or nursing homes (despite the great visibility of such facilities).

3. Old people can learn new information, although they learn at a slower pace and have a much greater fear of failing to perform adequately than those who are

younger. The elderly therefore often "omit" information when they are unsure, preferring to appear uninformed or forgetful rather than foolish (3).

4. A mild increase in blood pressure in older people is often necessary to maintain near-normal intellectual functioning, and those individuals with marked hypertension show a severe decline in intellectual functioning (4).

5. Eighty-six percent of those 65 years of age and over in the United States have one or more chronic ailments, and 42% of the elderly find that this chronic ailment limits their activity. The degree of disability, however, may depend as much on the personal perception by the elderly person that he is "sick" and should protect himself from further illness by avoiding activity as it does on the nature of the disability itself.

Juxtaposed with these "facts" are the fictions and mythology of aging, which Butler has called "myths and stereotypes about the old" (5). To paraphrase Butler:

1. *The myth of aging.* The assumption is that all elderly people are as old as their chronological age, whereas in fact there are greater physiological and personality differences among the elderly than among any other age group.

2. *The myth of unproductivity.* Despite the belief that the old are unproductive, old people tend to be productive and actively involved in life, except when affected by disease or social adversity.

3. *The myth of disengagement.* Despite the myth that older people prefer to disengage from life, there is no evidence that this is so.

4. *The myth of inflexibility.* The belief that old people are less responsive to innovation and change because of age is not supported by studies of people living in the community or by clinical observations.

5. *The myth of senility.* That the elderly are "senile," with forgetfulness, confusion, and reduced attention, is often untrue. Such manifestations may actually conceal anxiety, depression, drug tranquilization, physical illnesses, malnutrition, and alcoholism—all reversible conditions—as well as irreversible organic brain changes. This myth accounts for the underdiagnosis and undertreatment of reversible conditions, which account for 50% of what is labeled "senile."

TREATMENT TECHNIQUES WITH THE ELDERLY PATIENT

Given the realities and the mythology of aging, physicians must modify their usual counseling techniques to be of help to the elderly patient. Pfeiffer (6) has suggested specific modifications applicable to primary care settings:

1. *Increased interactional activity on the part of the physician.* The doctor should not leave the responsibility for defining the problem up to the patient ("How are you today?") but should take the initiative by inquiring in detail about a number of areas of the patient's life which might be troubling him. These areas include his physical health, economic status, living arrangements, current social contacts, the

use of his time, the meaningfulness of his activities, and whether he has had any losses—recent, impending, or feared. In effect, Pfeiffer suggests that the doctor develop a problem-oriented approach so that specific treatment may be mapped out for each problem and specific goals set. (See also item 3, below.)

2. *Symbolic giving*. Pfeiffer suggests that a visit to a doctor can have increased therapeutic value if the doctor can make a long-term commitment to the patient for continued care. Each visit can then be planned to be something of an event for the patient, and specific small tasks which he has been asked to do between visits emphasize the continuity of the relationship. Such a task might be asking the patient to bring flowers he has grown in his own garden to the doctor's office. In this way he can show that he still has something of value to contribute and share with other people (other patients and office staff). Another symbolic way of giving to the elderly patient involves spending a portion of the interview in social conversation, including such topics as the weather, the season, and even the doctor's own family and his minor worries. This increases the personal meaning of the visits for the patient and renders them more supportive. This does not mean that the doctor-patient relationship becomes a social rather than professional one; what it does mean, however, is that the patient can feel that his doctor has a real and personal interest in him and values his perspective on various topics.

3. *Limited goals*. Pfeiffer urges that the doctor define specific goals, paying particular attention to ones which have a reasonable chance for achievement. Psychotherapeutic goals might include symptom relief, better adaptation to changed life situations (e.g., widowhood), acceptance of a somewhat more dependent status, and renewed or continued active involvement in a broad range of activities.

Pfeiffer also remarks that an elderly patient may often treat her (relatively) younger doctor as if he were her parent or one of her adult children. This might take the form of the patient expressing criticism, pride, or jealousy. Sometimes elderly patients act seductively with their physicians, which may evoke disapproving feelings in the doctor. Understanding these phenomena as something that the patient may need to go through will help the doctor tolerate this behavior. Finally, Pfeiffer advises that it is not advisable to call an elderly patient "Mom" or "Pop" or to use his first name unless a first-name-basis relationship already exists between them. Such forms of address create an atmosphere that robs the patient of dignity, conveys contempt, and overall is likely to be resented (6).

Other physicians working with elderly patients have changed their offices to some extent to make the patients feel more comfortable and welcome. Because of the impairment of vision and hearing in a large number of elderly patients, office signs are in LARGE TYPE which are easily read. This prevents confusion and preserves dignity in the elderly patient. If such a patient is directed to "Room 3" in a doctor's office, but the sign is so small that the patient cannot read it, he will be forced to ask a member of the office staff for help (when he would prefer to be independent), or he may simply "stumble" into an office he thinks (and hopes) is number 3. Large type also prevents embarrassing confusion about where to put the urine specimen, etc. Elderly patients with visual impairment are also forced to sit "twiddling their thumbs" if the print of the office magazines is too small to read. This is certainly not necessary when the "large print" version of magazines such as the *Reader's Digest* is available.

Similarly, a patient who has a hearing problem may become embarrassed and angry at having to ask an office staff member to repeat what he just said, and the staff member in turn is liable to become angry at the patient and "raise his voice" to him. In such a situation, it is all too easy for the staff member to begin to treat the patient as if he were not only partly deaf but stupid or senile as well. It is helpful to prepare the office staff for handling patients with hearing difficulties by teaching them to give instructions slowly and clearly.

MENTAL STATUS ASSESSMENT

Because of the cultural mythology of senility in the elderly, it is important to have some objective measures of intellectual functioning, so that an evaluation of any particular patient can assess whether intellectual functioning is constant, increasing, or declining. One easy test, the Goldfarb 10-point scale to estimate organic impairment (7), may be applied readily by a physician in his office or while making hospital rounds (assuming that the patient's hearing is intact). In this test, 0 to 2 errors mean no or mild impairment, 3 to 8 errors mean moderately advanced impairment, and 9 or 10 errors imply severe brain dysfunction:

1. Where are we now? (place orientation)
2. Where is this place located? (place orientation)
3. What month is it? (time orientation)
4. What day of the month is it? (time)
5. What year is it? (time)
6. How old are you? (memory)
7. When is your birthday? (memory)
8. Where were you born? (memory)
9. Who is the President of the United States? (general information and memory)
10. Who was the President before him? (general information and memory)

A clear scale on which to chart the fluctuations and the improving or deteriorating mental status of an elderly patient is often useful for determining whether the patient needs nursing care or should be transferred to some kind of residential facility. A deteriorating performance may suggest a vigorous work-up for a concurrent physical illness or a more structured program which might decrease the mental confusion experienced by the patient. Occasionally such a decline suggests a process different from an organic brain syndrome, e.g., a severe depressive illness or a schizophrenic process. In this situation, of course, an appropriate antidepressant or antipsychotic medication may be indicated.

ORIENTATION

Sometimes an elderly patient appears to be gradually "losing contact" or is becoming more forgetful, confused, and disoriented. In these cases a structured program for decreasing the confusion and "reorienting" the patient to everyday realities may be helpful. Folsom developed a technique for dealing with disoriented patients at the Tuscaloosa State Hospital: it is entitled "Reality Orientation" (8). Other programs (e.g., "Orientation and Motivational Programs for the Elderly") have been described by Bier (9). Each of these methods embodies a specific, yet simple, scheme for rehabilitation of patients with moderate confusion, disorientation, and memory loss. Although these techniques are usually applied to elderly patients in a hospital or nursing home, they are also useful with mildly disoriented persons living at home with a companion or family members.

The methods are based on the recognition that the person with brain damage, because he is confused or disoriented, may progressively lose interest in his surroundings and over time will withdraw and gradually become even more disoriented, confused, and isolated. The specific methodology, which can be employed by a nurse, aide, or family member, involves approaching the patient many times during the day with a statement such as, "Mrs. Jones, I'm your nurse, Betty Smith. Today is Tuesday, April 2, 1981, and this is the Mt. Rainier Nursing Home in Seattle. It's 8 o'clock in the morning, and it's raining outside. Perhaps you can see the rain if you get near the window. It's time to get up now, so you can go down with me to have breakfast in the dining room." The verbal message should be accompanied by eye contact, touching the patient, holding the patient's hand, etc.

When staff in nursing homes (or relatives if the patient is at home) have been trained to use these relatively simple techniques, patients who have been withdrawn for years often become interested in their environment again. This reaction lends credence to the theory that much of what is labeled as "senility" does not involve irreversible organic changes. Reality orientation in a nursing home or extended care facility is often done with a group of elderly people so they will start to interact and relate to each other. This is done by asking a question such as, "What does this picture remind you of?" while showing a farming picture (which often acts as a stimulus to reminiscences about earlier parts of their lives). In addition, group reality orientation may involve asking more structured, "standard" questions, e.g., "Who is the President?" Like any technique, reality orientation must be done with tact, sensitivity, and competence, and is only one part of a total rehabilitation program. As Busse remarks (10): "Reality orientation deals with the restoration of information. But it can only be successfully implemented if confusing elements in the environment and in the routine of the hospital are reduced to a minimum so that communications become consistent, clear, and non-threatening. Such principles are not easy to establish and maintain. To assume otherwise is a fallacy which will lead to failure in the program."

Reality orientation should be combined with various other programs: occupational therapy, appropriate exercises, encouraging the hospitalized elderly to work with each other, and maximal social interaction of staff and patients or patient and patient (eating, doing crafts or projects together, playing checkers or cards, etc.). The physician-consultant can be the catalyst of these activities for the institution. He must also continue to coordinate and support the activities after they have begun (11,12). Such programs often cost little money, as in nursing homes much of the "structure" which would allow staff to interact therapeutically with patients is already present. What the program does require, however, is the belief that talking and working actively with elderly patients is humane, desirable, and to be encouraged; they must also have the ingenuity to establish a structure which permits these goals to be implemented.

PLANNING AND PREVENTION FOR THE LATER YEARS: THE PHYSICIAN'S ROLE

Although in America the expectation of growing old is something with which doctors and patients must eventually contend, both groups avoid grappling with the issue as long as possible. Old age is seen as invariably "bad," and denial of the painful prospect that "it will happen to me" is maintained for as long as possible and usually too long to allow adequate anticipation and planning for this period of one's life. Even psychiatrists and primary care physicians who espouse humanistic values often view the elderly as problem patients whose difficulties with health, living, and coping are to be addressed only after they become manifest. This seems particularly unfortunate, as clinical and research observations about people who have remained psychologically, and to a large extent physically, healthy suggest that those individuals prepare for and cope with being old in a somewhat different way than do others (13). Some of these ingredients include the following:

1. Maintenance of adequate health care.

2. Continued involvement throughout life not only with specific individuals but also with activities and processes which are renewing and helping to maintain an individual's sense of integrity and identity. These may include hobbies (painting, music, reading), as well as writing, taking continuing education courses, gardening, cooking, and traveling. Participation in such activities often begins during the early or middle years of a person's life and so is simply a continuation during the later years.

3. Deliberately being involved in activities in which a continued altruistic role may be maintained, particularly where young people in some way receive nurturing from the older person. Such continued giving helps maintain a positive self-image, a continued view of oneself as a person who can contribute to others and society;

it preserves the sense of oneself as an individual and not simply as a member of a group (e.g., "senior citizen"). Activities such as tutoring or volunteering for "a good cause" (e.g., typing, helping with accounting, telephoning) are examples of this kind of activity.

4. Demythologizing and confronting one's own prejudices about aging a decade or two before one is planning to retire, as well as gradually making a conscious change of focus from a future orientation to a present orientation. This can make a partial (although not total) difference in how one approaches this period of life. Feelings about aging, however, like the feelings when one is dying, can never be totally anticipated or controlled.

5. Developing and maintaining relationships in which there are shared tasks (e.g., altar guilds and organizational fund raising) and not just leisure time activities.

Many of the attitudes and activities which can maintain psychological health must be developed long before one becomes chronologically old. A primary physician is often in a pivotal position to present issues of aging to a person who, within a few years or decades, may face or seek retirement. Anticipating and choosing how one is to deal with old age can be a deliberate action. The primary physician, depending on his understanding and his approach to his patients, can be an unwitting enemy or a valiant ally.

THE PHYSICIAN AS CONSULTANT AND TEACHER IN THE NURSING HOME

Having specific guidelines which can be taught and discussed with personnel in a nursing home or extended care facility whose clientele are primarily elderly can be useful to the primary physician. The following is a brief topical list of diagnostic and treatment issues which arise in nursing home care with the elderly and which can be part of a curriculum for in-service education. [The list was originally to accompany a teaching videotape, "The Disturbed Patient in the Nursing Home" (14).]

I. Depression (withdrawn, apathetic patient).
   A. Diagnostic issues.
      1. Depressed mood.
      2. Apathy and withdrawal.
      3. Sleep disturbances (especially early morning awakening).
      4. Eating disturbances (usually decreased appetite).
      5. Fatigue.
      6. Constipation.
      7. Slowed movements and speech.
      8. Reduced eye contact.
      9. Occasionally agitation, paranoid ideas, and somatic delusions.
      10. Avoidance of social and recreational activities.
      11. Fear of new activities.

12. Hopelessness and helplessness.
B. Rehabilitation issues and suggestions.
    1. Frequent contact with staff and familiar staff members. Members of the staff can reach out without expecting the patient to respond immediately while daily chores are taking place (e.g., making the bed). Patient contacts do not have to be limited to planned interviews.
    2. Staff attention to the personal and physical needs of patients (e.g., grooming). Depressed and withdrawn elderly patients often respond to touch or to someone demonstrating a caring attitude in other nonverbal ways. Verbalization of this attitude may not be necessary initially.
    3. Familiar objects. Keeping alive the memories and symbols of independence and life outside the institution through familiar clothes, pictures, and personal mementos.
    4. Assessing cultural isolation. Are there significant racial, religious, or cultural differences between the patient and the other residents and staff? Do these differences contribute to the patient's depression?
    5. Antidepressant medications. Such medications, usually tricyclic antidepressants, are often useful for alleviating severe symptomatology. Cardiac status and appropriate dosage must be carefully assessed as these drugs can alter cardiac and urinary functioning, etc.
    6. Medical assessment. Some illnesses (e.g., congestive heart failure or hepatitis) and medications (e.g., reserpine) may produce or mimic a profound psychological depression.
    7. Gradual re-entry into social and recreational activities, including contact with friends and family.
    8. Depressed patients as helpers. One way to feel useful, even when depressed, is to help other people who need physical or emotional help or support. Such intervention may simultaneously begin to alleviate the patient's depression.
    9. Enough time to talk. A person grieving over the loss of friends, family, job, or home needs sufficient time to talk about his feelings and about the losses. Talking, rather than medications, is needed to work through these feelings.
    10. Assessment of patient capacities and specific program planning. A detailed and accurate assessment of the depressed patient's former and current capacities should be made and a specific program developed to promote gradual and increasing accomplishment by the patient, with positive reinforcement for each achievement. An unrealistic program will lead to failure and more depression.
    11. Furniture arrangement to encourage communication. Arrangements of chairs, tables, and other furniture should be made to encourage conversation and social contact during meals, game playing, and

times of relaxation. Chairs lined against the wall should be discouraged.
   12. Acknowledging the feelings of the staff. Depressed patients are sometimes ignored because they evoke feelings of discomfort, guilt, or inadequacy. These feelings should be brought into the open, discussed, and shared, with the hope that the feelings will then become less intense and immobilizing.
   13. Sensory losses. Depression may certainly be aggravated when hearing and sight are not optimal, especially if they can be improved with new glasses or a new hearing aid. Vision and hearing should be tested routinely for all patients.
II. Forgetfulness (the senile patient with mild organic brain syndrome).
   A. Diagnostic issues.
      1. Memory impairment, especially for recent events.
      2. Misperception of events and disorientation for time, place, and person.
      3. Poor judgment in social and interpersonal situations.
      4. Changed emotional expression: lability or flattened affect.
      5. Impaired intellectual abilities, as with arithmetic.
      6. Impaired abstract thinking, including shades of meaning, subtleties of language, and symbolic expression (such patients often become extremely concrete in their language usage and interpretation).
      7. Disorders of thinking and feeling may be added to the basic disorder of organic impairment, giving rise to such symptoms as paranoia, depression, and anxiety.
   B. Rehabilitation issues.
      1. Consistent and regular staff contact.
      2. Familiar and predictable routines with reminders by staff.
      3. Visual reminders of names, dates, activities, and settings.
      4. Reality orientation group programs.
      5. Adequate lighting at all times. Such patients become disoriented at night without familiar objects to see.
      6. Appropriate limits for safety. With disoriented patients, doors occasionally need to be locked to provide adequate safety.
      7. Familiar objects. A personal orientation, as well as memories and symbols of independent living, may be maintained through familiar clothes, pictures, and personal mementos.
      8. Sensory losses. Disorientation may be severely aggravated by hearing and visual losses. Vision and hearing should be tested routinely for all patients, as well as attention paid to glasses and hearing aid batteries.
      9. Stimulating personal and intellectual activities to maintain optimal intellectual functioning.

THE AGING PATIENT AND PRIMARY CARE

    10. Consistent limit-setting through tactful reminders rather than coercion.
    11. Monitoring of physical health. Patients with compromised intellectual functioning may become severely disoriented even with mild physical illnesses, high blood pressure, or fever. Any change in intellectual functioning should immediately alert the staff for some change in physical status.

III. The abusive, combative patient.
  A. Diagnostic issues.
    1. Justified irritation. Has the patient been waiting 2 hours for breakfast?
    2. Defensive behavior. Does the behavior of the patient conceal depression or an avoidance of acknowledging dependence on others?
    3. Specific staff-patient conflicts. If difficulties occur with only one staff member, that particular staff member may be contributing to the conflict in some way.
    4. Contributing medical problems. Some medical conditions (e.g., anemias, thyroid problems, depression, or hypoglycemia) may make a
    5. Taking patient cues about the relationship. Paranoid patients may become extremely anxious or even panicky when they perceive the relationship between themselves and a staff member to be excessively close. Patients often indicate their degree of tolerance for closeness.
    6. Clarification of male-female patient-staff relationships. If the patient-staff relationship is between a male and a female, it may be necessary to emphasize the professional rather than the sexual nature of the relationship.
    patient irritable. Regular physical assessment should be routine.
  B. Rehabilitation issues.
    1. Firm, consistent limit-setting. Physical restraints are rarely necessary and should be used only as the last resort.
    2. Staff empathy. Listening and trying to clarify the basis for the hostility are more effective than defensive or hostile staff responses; re-establishing "human" communication should be done if possible.
    3. Medications. Occasionally tranquilizers in low doses and for brief periods of time are useful for decreasing anxiety, irritability, or impulsive rage. Medical or psychiatric consultation may be useful in this situation.
    4. Sensory losses. Patients with visual or hearing impairments may become more paranoid, misinterpret data, or become more combative or abusive because of not understanding the instructions or requests of staff members. Vision and hearing should be tested routinely for all patients, and attention paid to glasses and hearing aids.

IV. The disturbed (psychotic) patient.
  A. Diagnostic issues.
    1. Bizarre thinking. Such thinking may be overtly delusional and in-

clude hallucinations, or it may take the form of consistent paranoid ideas about other patients or staff. Such patients frequently have been hospitalized previously for schizophrenia.
  2. Mistrust of close relationships. Such patients usually have a reduced capacity to trust other patients or staff and thus may have difficulty maintaining predictable or close relationships.
  3. Intrusive or personalized thinking. If delusions or hallucinations intrude into a patient's usual thinking processes, the patient may be unable to converse rationally or make decisions necessary for daily living.
B. Rehabilitation issues.
  1. Clarification and explanation of staff role.
  2. Conflict avoidance. Paranoid delusions cannot be dispelled by arguments, but staff should clarify how they see the situation.
  3. Evaluation of paranoid ideas. Some paranoid ideas may be justified or based on insufficient explanations. Such situations, whenever possible, should be corrected.
  4. Regular and predictable staff contact.
  7. Antipsychotic medication. With very paranoid, excited, panicky, or agitated patients, antipsychotic medications may be helpful for maintaining control and usual functioning. Nonsedating major tranquilizers (e.g., thioridazine, haloperidol, or trifluoperazine) in low doses may be particularly useful. Careful monitoring for side effects (e.g., orthostatic hypotension or dyskinesias) is essential, however.
  8. Expectation of healthy functioning. Despite psychological disabilities, such disturbed patients need activities, warmth, and social relationships, like everyone else. They also need a sense of personal competence and an opportunity to manage as many facets of their daily lives as possible.
  9. Sensory losses. Patients with visual or hearing impairments may become more paranoid or delusional because of their increasing misinterpretation of data or expectations. Vision and hearing should be tested routinely in all patients, as well as attention paid to glasses and hearing aids.

REFERENCES

1. Palmore, E. G. (1973): Social factors in mental illness of the aged. In: *Mental Illness in Later Life*, edited by E. Busse and E. Pfeiffer, pp. 41–48. American Psychiatric Association, Washington, D.C.
2. Brotman, H. B. (1973): Who are the aging? In: *Mental Illness in Later Life*, edited by E. Busse and E. Pfeiffer, p. 19. American Psychiatric Association, Washington, D.C.
3. Eisdorder, C. (1968): Arousal and performance: experiments in verbal learning and a tentative theory. In: *Human Aging and Behavior*, edited by G. A. Tolland, p. 189. Academic Press, New York.
4. Wilkie, F., and Eisdorfer, C. (1971): Intelligence and blood pressure. *Science*, 172:959.

5. Butler, R. N. (1975): *Why Survive: Being Old in America*, pp. 6–11, Harper & Row, New York.
6. Pfeiffer, E. (1973): Affective disorders. In: *Mental Illness in Later Life*, edited by E. Busse and E. Pfeiffer, p. 110. American Psychiatric Association, Washington, D.C.
7. Kahn, R. L., Goldfarb, A. I., Pollack, M., et al. (1960): Brief objective measures for the determination of mental status in the aged. *Am. J. Psychiatry*, 111:326.
8. Folsom, J. C. (1960): Reality orientation for the elderly mental patient. *J. Geriatr. Psychiatry*, 111:326.
9. Bier, R. (1965): The nurse's management of the aged dependent patient. In: *Exploring Progress in Geriatric Nursing Practice*. American Nursing Association, New York..
10. Busse, E. (1973): Reality orientation. In: *Mental Illness in Later Life*, edited by E. Busse and E. Pfeiffer, p. 75. American Psychiatric Association, Washington, D.C.
11. Metzelaar, L. (1973): *Social Interaction Groups in a Therapeutic Community: Some Principles and Guidelines*. Institute of Gerontology, The University of Michigan–Wayne State University, Ann Arbor, Michigan.
12. Stotsky, B. A. (1970): *The Nursing Home and the Aged Psychiatric Patient*. Appleton-Century-Crofts, New York.
13. Suggested by (1) observations of A. Moris of the Individual Development Center, Seattle (personal communication); (2) research compiled by the Duke University Center for the Study of Aging and Human Development (cited by E. Busse in a continuing education conference on aging at the University of Washington School of Medicine in 1973); (3) studies by Valliant (*Adaptation to Life*, Little-Brown, Boston, 1977); and (4) clinical observations by the author.
14. Lurie, H. J., producer and scriptwriter (1981): *The Disturbed Patient in the Nursing Home* (videotape). Developed for the Office On Aging, Department of Social and Health Services, State of Washington, Olympia, Washington. Distributed through University of Washington Press, Seattle.

10

The Doctor and the Dying Patient

Discussion and examination of the attitudes and practices surrounding death and dying have recently become more open and tolerable for the medical community. Until recently, doctors were notoriously reluctant to talk much about death and dying, either with patients or with each other. Part of the reason for this is that death and dying were depressing topics about which one did not usually have much to say. Another reason is that, for those of us with backgrounds in medicine who have been trained to save lives and cure people, it is almost a personal failure when we find we are not able to save someone from dying.

The new willingness to look at reactions to death has been triggered by a number of factors. These include a growing interest in the expanding geriatric population by medical personnel, the increasing assertiveness by the elderly about the right to die with dignity, and the widespread popularity of a book which made acceptable the notion that one should talk with dying patients about death.

This book, *On Death and Dying* (1), not only illuminates the process of dying but shows how this process can be discussed with patients. The author of the book, Kubler-Ross, is a Chicago psychiatrist who discovered, as she talked with large numbers of patients who were dying, that the dying person tends to pass through distinct and usually sequential stages of dying. According to Kubler-Ross, the patient initially reacts with (1) *shock, denial,* and *disbelief* when he learns that he is dying. (2) *Anger* is the next reaction, which is often displaced and deflected onto physicians, nurses, and family members, in part for their still being healthy and active. (3) A *bargaining phase* is often next, during which the patient makes a magical "bargain" in exchange for a respite in the illness: "If I can go to my son's graduation, I'll be a model patient after this." (4) A *depression phase* follows, during which the patient struggles with giving up everything he has ever loved and goes through a preparatory grieving over his own death. This phase is often accompanied by feelings of hopelessness, helplessness, despair, and at times suicidal feelings. (5) *Acceptance* is the final phase, when the patient comes to terms with his own death.

On Death and Dying has been an extremely important and influential book in the whole field of thanatology and an excellent starting place for anyone who is going to counsel a dying patient. Since the book was written, a number of other books and articles have appeared, some of which suggest that the process of dying may not be nearly as orderly and sequential as Kubler-Ross suggests. It is possible for some of the stages of dying to occur simultaneously or in different sequences in any particular patient. The use of chemotherapeutic agents, for example, which produce significant remissions in leukemic patients, have been shown to reverse psychological stages, and the patient who has "accepted" his death returns to a stage of "denial" (2). White and Epstein (3), in their videotaped studies of dying patients, suggest that the previous life-style of the patient and his attitude about living determine the patient's attitude about his death: Neurotic, complaining persons continue their complaints during the dying process; optimistic, active persons often continue to confront their death in an active, even positive, way as one more aspect of living. White and Epstein also object to Kubler-Ross's implicit assumption that the physician's or counselor's role is to help the patient move smoothly through the early stages of dying to the final acceptance of death. They feel that if the patient is "stuck" at a particular stage, this stage is probably adaptive for him and that it is impertinent and probably destructive to "push" the patient or challenge the adaptation.

The management of children who are dying takes a particular toll on staff, families, and the child himself. Kubler-Ross and many other experts who have studied dying children are convinced that children know if they are dying. As mentioned elsewhere (Chapter 7), the questions which most concern very ill children are, "Will I be safe? Will someone I trust be near me? Will I be abandoned?" Because medical personnel and the families of the patient are usually very upset when a child is dying, elaborate ruses are often used to try to save children from the "pain" of knowing how ill they are. In fact, the strategy is more to help the physician, other caretakers, and the family feel less guilty; unfortunately, it often results in the child feeling isolated and alone, sensing that it is not permissible to talk about dying.

Comprehensive teaching about death and dying is slowly entering the curricula of paraprofessional, professional, and nursing education (4). *Life and Death and Medicine* (5) describes the ways in which health manpower training programs can include topics such as caring for the elderly and dying patient. In addition to basic didactic material, audiovisual materials are extremely useful for sensitizing viewers about their own feelings and those of the patients, demonstrating interviews with dying patients, and serving as a stimulus for discussion of the material (which usually provokes strong feelings in the viewers). Role playing between simulated dying patients and those counseling them is also very instructive. This is one of the few training strategies which allows feedback to the interviewer about "how he/she comes across" as well as a chance to critique the overall approach to the dying patient. Interviewing strategies with dying patients (using the Kubler-Ross schema) must include the following:

Denial phase: The patient, after hearing the "bad news" or inquiring how ill he is, may not be able to focus on what the physician is saying, may deny it, or may "forget it." Follow-up interviews with the patient and family must be scheduled for a specific date in the near future. At this phase of struggling with the dying process, the patient is as concerned with the precise details of "what will happen to me" as he is with an empathic and supportive approach from the doctor (these two, of course, are not mutually exclusive). Being given details about chemotherapy, radiation, and a hopeful explanation of the ways in which symptoms (e.g., pain) may be managed offers considerable relief at this point. The patient may also be seeking advice about statistics of the illness, in terms of longevity, although he rarely wishes to be told a chilling, "You have 6 months to live."

Anger phase: As with any angry patient, the patient should be accepted and the anger understood as an adaptive response to a personal catastrophe. If the anger is directed toward the nursing staff, the physician or chief nurse may have to set limits on the extent to which the patient may "abuse" the staff. The patient may empathically be requested to alter his behavior somewhat. Isolation of the patient or retaliation toward him should be avoided, and a continued, accepting relationship should be maintained.

Depression phase: Caregivers have particular difficulty dealing with the depressed, dying patient. Physicians often feel guilty, do not know what to say, and feel they should "do something." Letting the patient know that he will "leave something of himself with us" and that he will continue to have control over how he deals, negotiates, and talks with the persons he sees even as he is dying restores a considerable measure of hope and dignity to a person who may feel hopeless and helpless.

THE HOSPICE MOVEMENT AND ITS RELEVANCE TO PRIMARY CARE

The hospice movement, which began in England during the 1960s, has had a significant influence on the care of the terminally ill patient in England, Europe, and more recently, the United States. Hospice care is active care, which may be given a patient in his home, at a hospital, or in a hospice setting. Spearheaded by the founder of St. Christopher's Hospice in South London, Dr. Cecily Saunders, hospice care has focused on effective pain management, control of nausea, and developing an attitude which meets the patient's emotional and spiritual needs. Some of their conclusions are discussed in the following sections.

Chronic Pain

Physicians working at St. Christopher's Hospice make a sophisticated assessment of the components of a patient's pain and then develop a treatment plan accordingly.

They find that there are many causes of pain in the patient with an advanced malignancy in addition to pain caused by the malignant process: (1) fear, anxiety, depression; (2) constipation, hemorrhoids; (3) musculoskeletal pains; (4) bedsores; (5) infection; (6) venous thrombosis; and (7) pulmonary embolism (ref. 6). (They note that with the anxious patient, for example, frank discussion about the patient's concerns often significantly reduces the degree of pain complaints.) However, Twycross notes that "When pain is of such a degree that the synthetic drugs fail to provide adequate relief, the doctor should not hesitate to turn to morphine.... When other drugs have failed you are failing in your duty as a doctor if you do not give morphine or diamorphine" (6).

In England heroin is sometimes used along with other ingredients for the management of severe terminal pain. Heroin is not available in the United States; methadone is used instead. The physicians at St. Christopher's Hospice note that when patients truly have pain relieved effectively, they do not crave additional medication, nor does the effective dose escalate (e.g., tolerance does not develop). They insist that "The right dose of any analgesic is that dose which brings about adequate pain relief for a reasonable period of time. Patients do not want to be constantly swallowing tablets or receiving injections. A 4-hour interval between doses should be regarded as the norm.... Once a drug has been shown to be ineffectual, the patient must be transferred to an alternative" (6).

In addition to specific medications, they consider that additional analgesic measures may be effective, including antidepressants, tranquilizers, steroids, specific "physical" analgesics (refrigerant spray, local heat, fixation, joint decompression, sensory blockade), as well as various kinds of nerve blocks, neurosurgical procedures, and hypnosis (6,7).

According to Levy (8), the following schema is often useful when determining drug usage for severe pain with hospice patients:

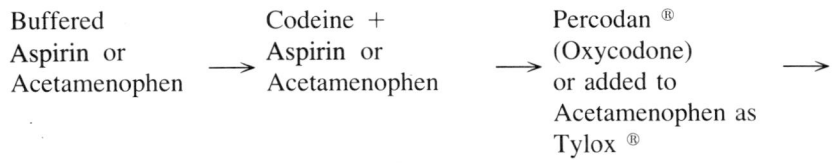

Buffered Aspirin or Acetamenophen $\rightarrow$ Codeine + Aspirin or Acetamenophen $\rightarrow$ Percodan® (Oxycodone) or added to Acetamenophen as Tylox® $\rightarrow$

Liquid Morphine (probably the treatment of choice) or if not tolerated, Methadone

or, if severe bone pain: Dilaudid® or Levodromeran®

Hospices also use steroids at times for their "nonspecific" effects which pragmatically have been observed to include decreased nausea, decreased anorexia, and increased mood. Specifically, Decadron®, 2 to 4 mg b.i.d., is usually used, although Medrol® or Solu-medrol® is also used.

Nausea

When the relief of symptoms and improvement of physical and psychological functioning were assessed at St. Christopher's Hospice, it was concluded that controling nausea made a tremendous difference in the way patients responded to treatment, how they felt, and if they were able to eat. Because the integrative vomiting center of the mid-brain may be stimulated in four ways—from the gut, the vestibular apparatus, through raised intracranial pressure, and from a chemoreceptor trigger zone—patients may need different medications to control their specific type of nausea.

Of the first 100 patients with pain studied at St. Christopher's during 1980, 35 also had a vomiting problem. Of these, 12 had obstruction; metoclorpamide (Reglan®) was effective if the obstruction was in the pylorus or duodenum, and antihistamine antiemetics (e.g., Marezine®, Cyclizine) were effective if the obstruction was in the ileum or large bowel (although such antiemetics produce severe sedation). Thirteen patients had biochemical changes that produced nausea (e.g., hypercalcemia, liver failure, uremia); antiemetics (e.g., haloperidol) acting on the chemoreceptor trigger zones were the effective treatment of choice. For gastric irritation, antiemetics acting on the gut or vomiting center were indicated (e.g., Compazine®, prochlorperazine); 'whereas in cases of raised intracranial pressure, antiemetics acting centrally on the vomiting center were indicated. Vestibular nausea responded to Droperidol (Inapsine®). A summary of these findings may be obtained from St. Christopher's Hospice (9).

According to Levy (10), THC, the active ingredient of marijuana, is now becoming available. For younger patients, especially those experienced in marijuana smoking, THC appears to be as effective as, or better than, Compazine in controlling nausea.

Quiet Confidence and Cautious Optimism

Another very important tenet of hospice care is the explicit reassurance that you, the doctor, are going to stand by the patient and "give him your best" (6). Other aspects specifically addressed by physicians trained in hospice care are mental or emotional pain, social pain, and spiritual pain (11,12).

Twycross, a former research fellow at St. Christopher's, recommends that "we must forget about the disease process and think of the symptoms as diseases in their own right. We are then fighting such things as the diseases of weakness, nausea, vomiting, anorexia, and pain, rather than an incurable cancer. It is important, therefore, to have more than just one treatment for any particular symptom. 'If this doesn't suit you, we have plenty of alternatives that we can try until we find the right one for you'" (6,13).

The notion that the physician will stick with the patient, not give up, and remain confident makes a tremendous difference. Although workers in St. Christopher's Hospice are also aided by their religious faith, their optimism and confidence are part of their medical and professional demeanor.

CONTINUITY OF CARE

As has been known in the medical setting in the United States for years, optimal medical management of a seriously ill patient depends on one physician assuming responsibility over a long period of time. In teaching hospitals this may be particularly difficult because of the rapid turnover of house staff, attending staff, etc. In the hospice concept of providing optimal care for the dying patient, this sense of personal involvement and personal responsibility, especially by the primary physician, is paramount:

> "The first fact for the GP to realize is that the number of patients in an average practice likely to need such care is very small, so that although it may involve extra time for each case, the total workload is not greatly affected. The second fact is that, once the GP has divested himself of the feeling that the whole exercise is one of failure, this kind of care can become immensely rewarding. The perennial anxieties over what to tell the patient and how to handle the relatives' wishes or how to conduct the management wither away, provided the doctor can allow them to talk out their anxieties and can assure them that the control of pain will be maintained"(14).

To be available as counselor, manager, and the person doing major liaison work with other services or service providers, orchestrating the demands of the relatives, and being available to consult with nursing personnel and other doctors about his patient affords a unique opportunity in medicine:

> "To be with another person by turns frightened, angry, fighting, and denying reality is a training process in itself. The doctor needs to identify with the patient, and then stand back professionally.... Paradoxically, the certainty of losing the battle allows the GP the greatest possible freedom in being the patient's personal doctor" (14).

More information about the hospice movement in the United States may be obtained from the first American Hospice, Hospice, Inc., 765 Prospect Street, New Haven, Conn., or from Dr. John Fryer, Temple University Medical Center, Philadelphia, who has consulted with the hospice movement in the United States and internationally.

REFERENCES

1. Kubler-Ross, E. (1970): *On Death and Dying*. Macmillan, New York.
2. Hertzberg, L. J. (1972): Cancer and the dying patient. *Am. J. Psychiatry*, 128:806.
3. White, L., and Epstein, L. (1973): Aspects of death and dying. Address given at a conference on Depression and Aging, Continuing Medical Education, University of Washington, Seattle.
4. *Until I Die* (film). Video Nursing, Inc., 2645 Girard Ave., Evanston, Ill. 60201 (description of Kubler-Ross teaching program and philosophy).
5. *Life and Death and Medicine* (1973): Scientific American Books. Freeman Press, San Francisco.
6. Twycross, R. G. (1972): *Principles and Practice of the Relief of Pain in Terminal Cancer*. Update (England).
7. Twycross, R. G. (1978): Pain and analgesics. *Curr. Med. Res. Opin.*, 5:497–505.
8. Levy, D. (1980): Department of Oncology, University of Pennsylvania. Personal communication. Also see, Narcotic analgesics in terminal cancer. *Drugs Bull.*, 18:69–72.
9. *How Does Cancer Cause Pain* (1979): St. Christopher's Hospice, 51–53 Lorie Park Rd., Sydenham SE 266DZ, England.

10. Levy, D. (1980): Department of Oncology, University of Pennsylvania. Personal communication.
11. Saunders, C. M. (1976): The challenge of terminal care. In: *Scientific Foundations of Oncology*, edited by T. Symington and R. L. Carter, pp. 673–679. Heinemann, London.
12. Saunders, C. M. (1965): Watch with me. *Nursing Times (Lond.)*, Nov. 26.
13. Twycross, R. G. (1978): The assessment of pain in advanced cancer. *J. Med. Ethics*, 4:112–116.
14. Courtenay, M. J. F. (1978): A comment: the general practitioner and the dying patient. In: *The Management of Terminal Disease*, edited by C. M. Saunders, pp. 166–168. Edward Arnold, London.

11

The Depressed Patient

Depression is a pervasive human malady that most individuals, including physicians, experience at one time or another. Fatigue, disappointment, overwork, the loss of a valued friend or possession: all of these can be associated with a change of mood we call depression. When this mood change becomes combined with an inability to experience pleasure, a sleep disturbance, an eating disturbance, a change in motor activity and similar complaints, the *symptom* of depression may be replaced by the *syndrome* of depression. When this syndrome, in turn, assumes a life and intensity of its own and shows no indications that it will easily or quickly change its course, it has become a major *depressive disorder*. With the new *Diagnostic and Statistical Manual of Mental Disorders* (DSM III), published by the American Psychiatric Association (1), the classification and interpretation of depression have become much more lucid and comprehensible than was possible with earlier classification schemes. This chapter will look both at the more serious depressive illnesses in which the intensity and duration of the depression and vegetative symptoms seriously interfere with the ability of the patient to function, make decisions, carry out normal activities, work, or relate to other people in a satisfying way, as well as look at the more "garden variety" depressions requiring specific, but less acute, interventions. Depressions are a very common problem in primary care, and their early diagnosis and treatment are critical.

It is estimated that 5–6% of the population at any one time is suffering from a depressive disorder, that 18–23% of the females and 8–11% of the males in the population have at some time had a major depressive illness (although only a third of these have required hospitalization). Thus, females are 3 times as susceptible as males to this disorder. Men who are married are less likely to get depressed, whereas

---

Special thanks go to Professor Nick Ward, whose detailed criticism and suggestions on this chapter have been invaluable.

women who are married, especially with young children, are more likely to get depressed (2,3). Adult patients, both male and female, with depression are estimated to seek medical help 6–8 times more frequently than patients without depression, although females may be more overt in presenting with a mood disorder compared with males who are more likely to present with a somatic complaint. Among hospitalized pediatric patients, approximately 38% exhibited dysphoric mood, while 7% were classified as having a major depression (4).

THE CLASSIFICATION OF DEPRESSION

In recent years it has become clear that two different kinds of major affective (mood disorder) illnesses may present initially with serious depressive symptoms: major depression (unipolar), and manic-depressive (bipolar) disorder. The genetics, the natural course of the illness, and the treatment of the two disorders are different, although with the initial illness, it is frequently difficult to predict, other than by inference, which is the most likely diagnosis. The diagnostic criteria for a major (unipolar) depressive episode include the following:

1. A dysphoric mood or loss of pleasure in most activities
   —not caring anymore
   —more noticeable to friends and relatives
2. Four of the following symptoms present almost every day for at least two weeks:
   —reduced appetite or weight loss
   —increased appetite or weight gain
   —insomnia or hypersomnia
   —psychomotor agitation or retardation
   —loss of interest or pleasure in usual activities
   —decrease in sexual drive or interest
   —fatigue and loss of energy
   —feelings of worthlessness, self-reproach, or guilt
   —problems in concentration
   —recurrent thoughts of death or suicide
3. Subtle symptoms of depression (often presenting as "masked depression")
   —changes in sexual patterns: impotence or 2° frigidity
   —subtle dysphoric mood
      unable to feel good
      greater irritability
   —hypochondriacal symptoms
   —chronic pain complaints (2/3 of patients with depression present with pain, most frequently headache and backache) (5)
   —history of recent exploratory laparotomies or dental extractions, without the presence of pathology
   —increased anxiety, tension, irritability
   —increased use of alcohol/marijuana/coffee

—hyperphagia, especially with sweets
—sleep disturbance
  early morning awakening, especially
—diurnal fluctuation in fatigue (usually worse in morning, better by afternoon)

A bipolar illness characteristically occurs for the first time before the age of 30. Approximately half of persons with unipolar depression have their first illness in their late 30s and early 40s, with the rest distributed throughout the life cycle. An untreated major depression may last from 3 months to a year, whereas a bipolar depression is usually shorter for any specific episode. Recurrences of both types of depression are reasonably common: bipolar illnesses tend to recur from several times a decade to several times a year; 50% of unipolar depressions occur at least twice (6).

As mentioned, the principal illness from which major depression must be distinguished is *Bipolar Illness* (manic-depressive disorder). The urgency of this distinction lies in the fact that manic-depressive illness can often be controlled in an extremely effective way by using lithium, whereas major depression requires treatment with a variety of modalities, most of which have significant drawbacks. The diagnosis of manic episodes is often not especially difficult, and involves hyperactivity, pressure of speech, flight of ideas, inflated self-esteem, decreased need for sleep, distractibility, and an excessive involvement in activities which may, if not stopped, lead to painful consequences (e.g., wildly investing one's life savings in risky ventures) (7). The depressive episodes of a manic-depressive illness are diagnostically indistinguishable from a major depressive episode. Looking for a family history of bipolar illness is often the principal clue to help decide the most likely diagnosis.

Affective disorders other than major depression or manic-depressive illness include several conditions in which a long-standing illness of at least 2 years' duration is present, with either sustained or intermittent disturbance in mood and associated symptoms. Unlike the major affective disorders, a full affective syndrome is not present, and there are no psychotic features. These disorders, cyclothymic disorder and dysthymic disorder, usually begin in early adult life, without a clear onset.

In patients with cyclothymic disorders there have been numerous periods (over the previous 2 years) during which some symptoms of both depressive and manic syndromes were present, but without sufficient severity and duration to be considered a major depressive or manic episode. In addition, the depressive or hypomanic periods may be separated by periods of normal mood. During the depressive period of cyclothymic disorder, symptoms including three of the following are present:

insomnia or hypersomnia
low energy or chronic fatigue
feelings of inadequacy
decreased effectiveness or productivity at school, work, or home
decreased attention or concentration
social withdrawal

loss of interest in or enjoyment of sex
decreased involvement in pleasurable activities or guilt over past activities
feeling slowed down
less talkative than usual
pessimistic attitude
tearfulness or crying

During a hypomanic period, a person with cyclothymic disorder experiences an elevated, expansive, or irritable mood, and at least three of the following:

decreased need for sleep
more energy than usual
inflated self-esteen
increased productivity; often associated with unusual and self-imposed working hours
sharpened and unusually creative thinking
extreme gregariousness
hypersexuality
excessive risk taking, without insight to possible consequences (e.g., buying sprees, reckless driving)
physical restlessness
excessive talkativeness
excessive optimism
inappropriate laughing, joking, punning

A dysthymic disorder (previously called depressive neurosis) is a chronic disturbance of mood involving either depressed mood or loss of interest or pleasure in most or usual activities, but not of sufficient severity or duration to meet the criteria for a major depressive episode. The depressed mood/loss of interest may either be persistent or intermittent, and separated by periods of normal mood.

The importance of recognizing dysthymic disorder and cyclothymic disorder in contrast with major affective disorder is that the latter illness is more likely to respond to pharmacologic interventions, especially if vegetative symptoms (e.g., sleep, eating disturbance, weight loss, etc.) are present, whereas the former two conditions are less likely to respond to medical interventions.

DIFFERENTIAL DIAGNOSIS OF DEPRESSION

In addition to the possibilities already mentioned, depression must be considered as a secondary effect or a concealed condition in a variety of other primary care situations:

Physical illnesses often mimic depressive illness. Hepatitis, infectious mononucleosis, and pancreatic tumor often show psychological manifestations of depression (including vegetative symptoms) even before the physical symptoms appear. Fatigue and depressed mood may appear with anemias, endocrine abnormalities (hypothyroidism, adrenal insufficiency). With depression, the patient usually feels worse in the morning and better later in the day. The reverse is true of physical illness.

Drugs which are commonly prescribed may produce depression as a side effect. Most notorious for this are the rauwolfia alkaloids (e.g., reserpine) used for hypertension. Propranolol, indomethacin, levodopa, methyldopa, isoniazid, and diazepam are other commonly prescribed medications with which depression may occur (8). Approximately 15% of women taking birth control pills have a depression, half of this being specifically related to the medication (9). Withdrawal from a prolonged intake of alcohol or an extensive intake of amphetamine-like drugs is also often accompanied by marked depressive mood, sleep disturbance, fatigue. (Heavy alcohol usage over a prolonged time can produce symptoms of depression, as well.)

DEPRESSION IN CHILDHOOD

In the diagnosis of major depressive disorder in children and adolescents, somewhat different criteria must be used than with adults. Although adolescents usually show the clinical picture associated with adult depressive illness, approximately one-quarter of adolescents remanded to the juvenile justice system for delinquency have been shown (in addition to antisocial behavior) to have a significant depressive illness which responds to antidepressant medication (10). With children, definite symptoms are present, although not always volunteered. To make a diagnosis involves asking the children in a systematic way about their symptoms rather than relying on them to tell you about the symptoms. The Bellevue Index of Depression (BID) (11) includes the following ten items, each of which should be inquired about to establish the diagnosis of depression:

Dysphoric mood
Self-deprecatory ideation
Aggressive behavior
Sleep disturbance
Change in school performance
Diminished socialization
Change in attitude toward school
Somatic complaints
Loss of usual energy
Change in appetite or weight

Each of these items is scored from 0 (absent) to 3 (severe); a total score of 20 is needed for a child to be considered to have a depressive disorder.

Normal Grief (uncomplicated bereavement): With the death of a loved one, many persons experience a full depressive syndrome, including depressed mood, poor appetite and weight loss, and insomnia. If morbid preoccupation with worthlessness, a fixed anhedonia, a prolonged and marked functional impairment, and marked psychomotor retardation are present, grief may have become a major depressive episode. Guilt, which is sometimes present both in normal grief and major depression, usually in the former takes the form of obsessing about what should or should not have been done by the survivor at the time of the death; with depressive disorders, the guilt and sense of worthlessness may assume enormous, delusional proportions.

Schizophrenia: Many individuals with schizophrenia have depressive symptomatology as part of this disease. Individuals with catatonic schizophrenia may be withdrawn and depressed, and the diagnosis may be hard to make. Some persons with schizophrenia may appear agitated, "hyper," have pressure of speech, loose associations, and appear delusional. It may be difficult to distinguish these individuals from those with mania, although the delusions of the latter are usually less bizarre and "mood congruent."

Intoxications with Drugs, especially those with atropine-containing substances, may produce a clinical picture of agitation, depression, and delusional thinking, which may be hard to distinguish from an agitated depression, although in drug intoxications, the onset of these symptoms is usually more abrupt.

Dementias of Degenerative or Multi-Infarct Types: These may include such depressive symptoms as disorientation, apathy, and complaints of difficulty concentrating, which are difficult to distinguish from a major depressive episode.

CAUSES OF DEPRESSION

There are many theories about the causes of depression, without any absolutely clear-cut explanation, in any particular case. However, many of these hypotheses are particularly useful in helping define the problem and plan for effective solutions.

Psychodynamic Explanations: Many articles, particularly in early psychoanalytic literature, focus on the role of loss—either fantasied or real—of significant persons in the evolution of the clinical picture of depression in an individual (12,13). Losses which are perceived ambivalently (e.g., the person in part wished for the death of the person who died) are more likely to become pathological. Approximately 10% of normal grief reactions change into pathological mourning accompanied by a clinical picture of a major depression.

With studies of depressed children, there is considerable literature suggesting the role of separation and attachment disorders as the precursor of clinical depressive disorders (14,15). The role of parental depression in the development of depression in children has also been observed (16,17).

Life Stress: Work by Holmes, Rahe (18), and others suggests that an individual's response to a great many life changes of any kind coming at once can produce rather marked emotional problems, including a clinical depression. Paykel (19) found that depressed adults reported stressful life events at a frequency 3 times that of control patients. (Also, see Chapter 21.)

Learned Helplessness: In research with animals, dogs exposed to inescapable shocks developed a clinical picture suggestive of hopelessness and passivity, which did not change even when the animals later could escape from the shocks (20). This model has been applied to human behavior and implies that the depressed patient sees his behavior as being independent of the reinforcements he receives, and subsequently leads to a hopeless position. Correcting this misperception is the crux of treatment.

Genetics: Twin and adoption studies have clearly demonstrated a genetic predisposition for both major depressive illness and manic-depressive (bipolar) illness. There is uncertainty about the precise mechanisms of genetic linkage, but approximately 30% of those with a major depression have relatives with a similar illness, and approximately twice that number with a bipolar illness have relatives with a similar illness (21). There is also increasing evidence that a "depressive spectrum disorder" may exist that includes alcoholism in the fathers and "hysteria" in the mothers of children who subsequently develop a depressive disorder.

Cognitive Distortion: Beck and Kovacs studied a large number of depressed adults, and concluded that disturbances in affect and motivation are the result of negative conceptualizations—"cognitive distortions"—resulting in an outlook which emphasizes and exaggerates the negative aspects of life (22). Their therapeutic work involves correcting these distortions through talking with the patients and encouraging them to try out new ways of acting.

Lack of Positive Reinforcement: Lewinsohn (23) has studied depressed individuals and shown that these patients elicit fewer behaviors, less positive reinforcement, have fewer social skills, and are involved in fewer activities than other people. In addition, the environment sympathetically reinforces the depressive behavior (i.e., responds to the depressive complaints).

Biochemical Disorder: For the past twenty years, systematic research has produced an abundance of somewhat contradictory data, most of which relates biochemical data to affective disorders. Although the research is in a state of tremendous flux, the predominant theories are that there is a predisposition or disorder of catecholamine metabolism in some patients, and a disorder of serotonin metabolism in other patients (24,25). The fact that increasingly new numbers of neurotransmitters are being discovered makes a definitive statement about the biochemical mechanisms extremely hazardous at this point.

TREATMENT ALTERNATIVES, STRATEGIES, AND OBJECTIVES

Psychotherapy and Other "Talking" Interventions

Particularly with the milder forms of depression, and with uncomplicated bereavement, the chance for a person to express feelings to someone who will actively and empathically listen is often very useful. If a depression has been caused by a loss or traumatic event, talking with a person able to tolerate depressed feelings (with their components of anger and demandingness) may be enough to begin to facilitate a change in the clinical picture—from that of depressed mood, discouragement, and loss of pleasure, to the gradual emergence of something more positive. In this case, the depression is being "worked through," and the function of the intervention is to facilitate this natural process.

Disadvantages: With major affective disorders [major (unipolar) depression and bipolar disorder], talking simply is not enough, and is helpful primarily as an adjunct to other forms of treatment, particularly drug therapy. Many experienced clinicians feel that illnesses in which psychotic symptoms (depressive or manic delusions) are present, are simply immune to "talking treatment" at least during the delusional phase.

Strengthening the Patient's Support System: Although a severe or psychotic depression may require drug therapy or other relatively heroic measures to deal with the disorder, the course of an escalating depression may often be interrupted or shortened if the patient has a sufficiently strong support system. Such a support system may be found in the patient's family, his friends, his place of work, or in his physician's office. Since people with even minor forms of depression suffer cognitive disturbances of a greater or lesser degree (everything looks black/people look uninterested/a person feels unloved and unwanted), mobilizing the important people in the depressed person's life (or making other people temporarily important to that person) may be lifesaving. Specific strategies to strengthen the depressed patient's support system include the following.

In the Doctor's Office

The key ingredient for the medical office to be a source of genuine support to the depressed patient is the development of an explicit collaboration and a desire by the whole staff to help the patient in somewhat less traditional ways. The staff in helping the physician must be able to view their professional roles and activities as active, flexible, and responsive to the patient's unique and changing needs, rather than as the usual stereotyped roles in which most serious or difficult questions are answered by, "Ask your doctor." With such collaboration and flexibility by the staff, the patient often will become attached to and trust one staff person rather than the entire group. When this occurs, the staff member "chosen" by the patient should be encouraged to make positive overtures to the depressed patient. This might include telephoning the patient if an appointment is missed, inquiring about his health, and expressing disappointment at his absence. The staff member can also arrange specific times during the week when the patient can drop in to chat, or, if the patient needs a "medical" reason for an office visit, arrange to take the patient's blood pressure or weight on a regular basis.

In addition to providing support and expressing interest in the depressed person, the designated "key member" of the support team should also attempt other approaches such as encouraging the patient to take the prescribed medication, learning about specific activities the patient once enjoyed, and encouraging—but not demanding—that he resume some of these activities. The key staff person can also facilitate communication between the patient and his family, the patient and his friends, or the patient and other patients who come regularly to the physician's office. For instance, if a depressed patient who comes to see a doctor regularly is permitted and encouraged to form a relationship with other regular patients who are also in the waiting room, this contact may give a great deal of comfort to all of them. The topics of their conversation are immaterial—and may even take the form of griping and bitching about how misunderstood they are—but meeting regularly in a doctor's office for purposes of ventilation and mutual comfort may significantly decrease the depressive symptomatology.

In some offices, particularly those located in remote or rural areas, a member of the office staff may be designated a "visiting nurse" to make regular visits to the patient in his or her home. This might include dropping by to see the patient; bringing the patient to the office; stopping by to administer medications; and establishing a close and supportive relationship. The nurse would become someone to lean on as the patient makes the transition back from a depressed state into a more positive and active role in the community and family. The physician may also use regular community health nurses or other outreach teams (such as those associated with mental health clinics) if they are available. It is extremely important, however, that the referring physician describe the patient's problem and the behavior he wants observed, and/or the necessary interventions in detail, and specify the frequency of the visiting team's observations and reports. Turning the treatment of a depressed patient over to a community health nurse or even a mental health team, without specifying the doctor's continuing role in treatment and his persistent concern for the patient, may lead to disaster. The patient may conclude that he has been "dumped" by the doctor because he is so depressed, nagging, no good, or impossible to get along with. If the role of the visiting team is not explained to the patient and the continuing role of the physician clarified, the patient may not feel positive about receiving more intensive, ongoing care, but instead conclude that he is indeed "hopeless" and that the doctor simply is not telling him the truth.

Working with the Family

Although details of family therapy with a depressed person and his family are beyond the scope of this monograph, it is important to mention that the physician who knows the family of the depressed person must be able to talk with them, either together or individually. The purpose is both to provide support and encouragement during the patient's depression, as well as to assess the degree to which the interaction of the family with the depressed individual reinforces either movement toward more depression or toward recovery.

Living with a depressed person is often wearing, frustrating, and eventually provokes anger and rejection. Thus, physician support for an exhausted family member can take the form of encouraging some time away to recuperate from the patient's demands. At the same time, the family could be asked to break the cycle of negative, debilitating interaction by trying activities which might be positive experiences for the whole family (going to a movie, joining in cooking a meal, taking a short trip, etc.). The family may also need to be encouraged to set reasonable limits on the depressed patient's behavior and to establish some expectations. For instance, in the case of a depressed elderly patient, the family could insist that the patient join a therapy group for older people or spend some time with friends of his own age. The patient will doubtless resist such suggestions, and even use hostile, guilt-provoking tactics, such as accusing his family of simply wanting to be rid of him and wanting him to die. Ultimately, once the patient is more involved with therapy or friends, a positive step toward improvement has been made. Resumed social contact with peers and support from them (even if it takes them from their mutual agreement that their families are ungrateful, rejecting, and odious) will go a long way toward lifting the depression.

For the patient as a family member, support may take the form of the doctor explaining to the rest of the family that the individual "has an illness that we don't fully understand" and encouraging the family to be easy on the patient, not nag him too much, and if possible, find some other way to deal with the demanding aspects of the patient's depression other than fighting with him. The doctor might also explain to the family that even when the patient complies bitterly and is hostilely demanding, the very relationships within the family unit (whether overtly positive or negative) have a supportive aspect (Someone to fight with is better than no one at all!). If the family can adopt this point of view, they will be able to accept the personal accusations and criticisms with less rancor.

The goal of mobilizing the family as a support system for the depressed patient is not just to promote positive feelings between the patient and the family, but also to develop a system through which both patient and family can stand to spend time together—a system in which personal needs and feelings can be expressed and met without anyone feeling so angry that withdrawal is the only option.

The Scandinavian System of Dealing with Depression

A. J. Mandell has recently described experimental methodology in Scandinavia for treating depression (26). These new techniques must clearly be viewed as experimental at the present time, but may eventually be incorporated into more conventional treatment plans for depressed persons (although not proven or recommended at the present time). For persons who have a severe depressive illness, a four-stage program is implemented in some treatment centers: (1) a very hot sauna for 20 minutes twice a day; (2) enforced exercise for up to an hour a day (both to increase the patient's anger and his level of activity); (3) enforced social interaction and group discussion several times a day (again, possibly against the natural inclinations of the patient, but since all patients are in the same boat, they will at least have a common focus for their wrath—the prescribing physician); and (4) monitoring of sleep so that hypersomaniac patients have their sleep cut down to "reasonable amounts" (Mandell and others have cited research studies that suggest that when depressed patients sleep for longer and longer periods, they become more, rather than less, depressed) (27,28).

No-Suicide Contracts

Drye (29) has described "no-suicide decisions," in which a patient makes an explicit decision for himself with a therapist's urging: for a specified period of time not to attempt any suicidal activity (see Chapter 13 on Psychiatric Emergencies). The contract is very specific, and practitioners using such contracts have had the experience of being confronted by renewed suicidal intent once the specified period of the contract has expired. It is essential that the patient (and not just the hopeful physician) agree clearly and definitely to the terms of the contract. At the expiration of the contract (e.g., seven days), the contract should be reviewed, and, hopefully, if the patient still has no suicidal feelings, renewed.

Behavioral-Contractual Approaches to Depression

This somewhat unfelicitous title describes a situation in which a physician makes a contract with a depressed patient in order that the patient carry out some specific behavior which he knows the patient is capable of but which the patient himself fears he cannot perform. Such a contract is a variety of a behavior modification strategy. The assumption behind such a contract is that future behavior is shaped or modified by the consequences of present behavior. One of the regular occurrences in depression is a cognitive distortion in which the patient becomes convinced not only that he is "no good," but that he is incompetent, and never was competent, and never will be again. Believing this distortion then leads to his trying fewer activities, withdrawing more, and reconfirming his prophecy of incompetence and worthlessness. A behavioral contract with a written agreement to accomplish specific small tasks between office visits produces a visible sign of competence, which can then be used to challenge in a concrete way the patient's cognitive distortion.

It is very important that the specific tasks chosen by the physician or the person he designates to work with the depressed person be tasks which have personal relevance for the patient. Making a contract with a depressed retired man who used to enjoy woodworking to "go to the hardware store today to buy a can of paint remover and tomorrow begin refinishing an old table" will be far more relevant than encouraging him to weave baskets, try a "paint by number" kit, or the even more vague, "take up a hobby."

A woman who has a severe depressive disorder with retardation of energy and activities, stops cooking and does no housework, even though she previously prided herself on her abilities as a housekeeper. If a physician made a contract with this woman, the initial item might be an agreement that she go home that day and boil some water. The next day she would return to the doctor's office to report how this went. The next day the contract would call for boiling an egg in water; the third day, boiling an egg for her husband, etc.

Thus, by being able to observe and record directly his own activities, the patient's sense of competence is modified, and his positive activities are noticed, reinforced, and recognized by another person.

Sometimes a behavioral contract can be constructed utilizing community needs and resources. For example, the depressed person can agree to spend some time each week helping a person who needs him, such as an elderly lady in a nursing home or hospital, a retarded child who needs a "visiting parent or grandparent," or a third-grader who needs tutoring in arithmetic. The focus of such contracts is, once again, to change small amounts of the patient's behavior so that the patient can become convinced of his own competence. A bonus to a contract that involves a "volunteer" activity is that the patient may become much more aware of his own present or future usefulness (despite his current depression), as well as gratify vicariously his own needs to be noticed and nurtured.

Advantages of Behavioral Contracts

Specific behavioral and attitudinal objectives can be set between the physician and patient, and some definable aspects of the depressed patient's progress may be charted.

Disadvantages of Behavioral Contracts

A contract between patient and physician—even when the patient agrees to it—may be seen as a rebuff. The patient may view it as the doctor's way to avoid dealing with the patient on a feeling level of pain and suffering. This treatment model also has the disadvantage of being slow, requiring meticulous and persistent follow-up of the patient. Frequent reassessment of the patient's progress also requires extra time: time to add tasks of increasing difficulty until the patient has recovered his vanished social functioning and self-esteem.

Crisis Intervention in Depression: The Physician's Role

A number of studies (30,31) have shown that a prompt intervention at the time of an acute depressive or psychotic crisis may prevent hospitalization of the patient or residual psychological disability. Some principles of crisis treatment include (1) identifying the sources of stress which have precipitated the crisis; (2) identifying and choosing which options are available to relieve the crisis; (3) mobilizing the supportive people—the "support system" of the patient—who may provide emotional, physical, and financial relief; and (4) implementing a specific plan designed to restore the person to the previous level of functioning. With a depressed patient, the "crisis team" is often specifically trained individuals at a mental health center or agency. In many rural communities, the luxury of such a designated crisis team is not available. A physician, utilizing his knowledge of the community and its resources, may be able to construct his own crisis intervention team, using his office staff, himself, community health nurses, and those persons in the community skilled in counseling (such as clergymen). Confronted with a severely depressed individual (whom the physician is often the first to see), the crisis team may mobilize friends, family, social and financial community resources, or whatever is needed. Coordination of efforts and follow-up may rest with the physician, his office staff, or another member on the team. This kind of approach might find special relevance with a depressed or suicidal adolescent: resources might include school personnel, relatives, friends, and medical personnel (hopefully choosing specific individuals with whom the adolescent formerly had rapport). A similar approach might apply to a depressed and distraught young mother no longer able to cope with her children, considering suicide, and very anxious: a crisis team might provide temporary care for the children in a foster home or with relatives; arrange financial assistance to provide partial day care services for the children when they return home; prescribe antidepressants and possibly antianxiety agents for the patient; and mobilize a support system of friends and relatives. Brief hospitalization in a general hospital may occasionally be necessary to relieve the patient of outside responsibilities, to begin medications (if necessary), and to mobilize the relatives for the time when the patient leaves the hospital. The physician's office personnel may also serve as back-up in long-term treatment of the seriously depressed patient. The length of each interview may not always be as important as the frequency of contact between the patient and the helping person(s).

Day care or day hospital programs for adults with serious emotional problems including depression are part of the services offered by many community mental health centers. The purpose of such day care programs is to provide some place for the disturbed patient to go to talk with someone about his problems, receive medications, participate in a group with other patients who are also having troubles, and perhaps join in some "structured" activity such as an arts and crafts project. Some day care programs may be an adjunct or an alternative to some of the treatment strategies discussed earlier. If none exists, and the physician is aware of particularly talented personnnel in a nursing home, he might collaborate in designing a day care program for emotionally disturbed individuals, which might have its headquarters in that nursing home. It would, however, be irresponsible to establish a program as a "dumping ground" for depressed patients, if neither skilled personnel nor adequate medical supervision were available. (Sometimes, no treatment is preferable to bad treatment.)

Group Counseling

A somewhat uncommon but feasible method to increase the support and social contact of a depressed patient reluctant or unmotivated to initiate socialization himself is to establish and run "depression" groups within the physician's office. Such groups can be run by the physician himself, by an outside mental health professional, or by a member of the office team with special counseling skills, such as a nurse or physician's assistant. Groups within an office have the advantage of seeming medically "legitimate," and avoid the need for referral to a mental health clinic or a psychiatrist (a referral which many patients might resent or resist). It further simplifies the massive logistical problems of several people in different settings treating different aspects of the same condition (e.g., the physician prescribing antidepressant drugs, and the psychiatrist doing psychotherapy). The group setting is attractive for both patient and physician, since the small amount one patient pays for a group session is balanced by the number being treated. Such a program of group therapy in a primary physician's office has been described by N.I.H. as efficient and effective (32).

Less conventional treatment groups for individuals whose depression in part reflects difficult life circumstances or conflicts relating to their current life situation utilize life planning skills, activities, and strategies (see Chapter 21). As with ordinary group counseling, such techniques may also be employed within an office setting. Like all therapeutic techniques, competence and experience in facilitating such exercises and activities are important.

Prescribing a Homogeneous Group or "A Cause"

Sometimes a physician finds that his patient is depressed because he needs specific support from others who have experienced a similar situation, an awareness of specific community resources, including "unconventional" ones, may often be useful. For example, in the case of a homosexual patient depressed after being left by his/her lover or conscious of growing old, a homophile group could provide considerable support, either formally if the group has regular meetings, or informally if the community has a "gay bar." For many homosexuals, seeing their friends regularly in a bar or in similarly relaxed surroundings may be a major source of support and satisfaction and provide the sense that the patient is "not alone." A gay bar, of course, may be a destructive, predatory place, so the physician should "choose his resources" before prescribing.

Similarly, women's groups—for consciousness raising, mutual support, and problem solving—can be of great use to women "traditionally raised" but now wishing, or being forced, to reenter and compete in the job market, or who find themselves suddenly single or widowed. A patient experiencing the depression related to the loss or dysfunction of a body part—loss of a breast, dealing with an ileostomy, a patient after amputation—often gets considerable relief and support from talking with others who have been through similar situations. Such groups exist in many communities; physicians are often instrumental in their creation, if they are needed.

Patients of retarded children, deaf children, children with learning disabilities, or of children who have died of crib deaths [sudden infant death syndrome (SIDS)], often organize, both to "do something" about the prevention or treatment of the condition, but also to provide mutual support and to work through much of the sadness, depression, and grief that such situations invariably entail. When a physician wants to refer a patient to such a group, having a specific person—preferably known to the physician—to call rather than just a telephone number is often likely to make the referral more successful. With other kinds of people experiencing a situational depression—e.g., a black college student leaving home to go to a predominantly white college—prescribing a specific social group (in this case, a black college organization) may simultaneously offer support, direction, and help the student "snap out" of his depression. In this kind of situation the physician acts as a social sanctioner—one who gives permission to the patient to do some of the things the patient wanted to do, but was afraid or hesitant about. To be comfortable making such a prescription, the doctor must be comfortable separating his own values and needs (and what he, personally, would find supportive) from what his patients need.

Finally, at this time it is critical that the physician be aware of the special support groups available for the veterans of Vietnam who are experiencing depression and other symptoms of posttraumatic stress disorder (depression, rage, nightmares, obsessive ruminations about their experiences in the war, reliving particular events, etc.). A number of these groups have been formed under the auspices of the Disabled American Veterans (33), and often offer support to both veterans and families of veterans. In order for such a group to work effectively, it must be led predominantly by trained Vietnam veterans themselves, since anecdotal reports (34) suggest that many depressed veterans fear both lack of comprehension, rejection, and exploitation from nonveteran health professionals. An interested physician may certainly facilitate the formation of such a group, and often offer medical backup, when medication is needed. The dimensions of this specific syndrome are vast, since one-half to one million Vietnam-era veterans are affected; the suicide rate among the group is 23% higher than among Americans, generally, and 60% have stress symptoms (35).

Medications for Depression

In discussing medications for depression, it is well to keep in mind that although the last ten years have seen an explosion of information relating to therapeutic drug usage, a considerable amount of information is yet to be discovered, and recommendations for antidepressant therapy are a combination of research data, clinical experience, and speculation.

Bielsky and Friedel (36) have pointed out that the more closely the patient's symptoms fit formal diagnostic criteria of depression, especially with vegetative symptoms, the more likely the patient will respond to specific antidepressant medication. When the symptoms are not so clear or specific, the probability of successful drug treatment diminishes (37). Particularly when the depressive picture is complicated by anxiety (a subjective feeling of restlessness, shakiness, irritability, and anger), the clinical decision of whether to administer an antidepressant alone, or in combination with an antianxiety agent, is unclear. Some experts recommend treating most of these with a sedating tricyclic antidepressant, and increasing the dose more rapidly than usual (38). Similarly, patients with severe medical illnesses (e.g., cancer) or patients with major addictive problems (opiates, alcohol) may also have symptoms strongly suggestive of a depressive disorder: anorexia, sleep disturbance, sad affect, irritability. The decision about whether a depressive disorder exists apart from the primary disorder, and hence should be treated with antidepressants, calls for a minute history-taking, and at times, initiating treatment when significant depression exists (39). All patients must be warned about the dangers of drinking and taking antidepressants at the same time—a combination which could produce uncoordination and drowsiness.

Medications which are currently used to treat depression include primarily tricyclic and tetracyclic antidepressants [imipramine, desipramine, amitriptyline, nortriptyline, amoxapine, protriptyline, doxepin, and maprotiline (40)], and monoamine oxidase inhibitors (tranylcypromine, phenelzine). Tricyclic antidepressants have a number of pharmacological effects, especially blocking synaptic reuptake of norepinephrine and serotonin. Tertiary tricyclic amines (imipramine, amitriptyline, doxepin) are more active with serotonin reuptake, whereas secondary amines are more active with norepinephrine reuptake. Since all tertiary amines are metabolized to secondary amines, however, it is often a pragmatic rather than rational decision about which drug to start with. (If, however, a patient begun on a tertiary amine does not respond, a trial with a secondary amine may be indicated, and vice versa). Clinically, the decision about which specific tricyclic medication to try depends on the following factors: (1) the potency of the medication itself; (2) the sedating effects of the medication; (3) the degree to which the anticholinergic side-effects affect the particular patient; and (4) the amount of anxiety present with the depression.

Regarding the first of these factors, there appear to be clinical and research data supporting the conclusion that all tricyclics, given in adequate dosages for long enough periods with a particular patient, are equivalent in their antidepressant effects. Some work faster, and the newer antidepressants, such as maprotiline (41) and amoxapine, may be recommended for patients who have not responded to other antidepressants. As mentioned previously, clinicians often begin with a secondary tricyclic, and then switch to a tertiary tricyclic, and vice versa, if there has not been an adequate response. As Shader (42) remarks, however, fixed dose responses are usually inappropriate for most patients. He recommends increasing the dose gradually until the desired effects occur or side-effects intervene, and then reducing the dosage slightly for maintenance therapy. He mentions that 30-fold variations in plasma concentrations can occur with 150 mg of desipramine a day, but also that treatment failures may occur with plasma concentrations above or below the therapeutic range, so that a blood level determination may not always be helpful in making a clinical decision about dosage. He also reiterates, however, that with adequate blood levels, very high response rates can be obtained with patients who have nondelusional major depressive episodes of a recurrent unipolar type. Clinically, it is often necessary for the physician to raise dosage levels in a particular patient and maintain them for a sufficiently long period (3–6 weeks) before deciding that a particular patient is unresponsive to the medication.

The second of these critical factors, *sedation*, is a critical variable in patient compliance. Tertiary tricyclics (imipramine, amitriptyline, and doxepin), are notorious for producing sedation in many patients, which may be very desirable if the patient is agitated, feels anxious, or has insomnia. (In most tricyclics there is a brief 24–48 hr intense sedation period which then ends; the drugs mentioned have a longer lasting sedative effect.) It is a disaster if the patient has to work during the daytime. Even if the medication is administered in a single dose only at night—which is usually adequate for maintaining therapeutic blood levels—many patients taking these drugs experience debilitating hangovers the next day, and stop taking the drug. Warning the patient, and also considering if the patient *must* get up as usual in the morning, may aid in the selection of the right antidepressant. Other patients who value their alertness and "can't stand" being sedated under any circumstances, will also stop their antidepressant, rather than tolerate "feeling dopey," "in a straight jacket," or "spacey." Many patients stop the medication without telling the physician first, so warning about side-effects and contracting about what to do will pay off in patient compliance.

The third factor, *anticholinergic side-effects*, may be experienced in different degrees by different patients and also tolerated in different ways, depending upon the physical and psychological condition of the patient. Common anticholinergic effects include dry mouth and generally decreased secretions, blurred vision, constipation, and urinary retention. Postural hypotension is also a frequent side-effect, especially with amitriptyline and doxepine. If warned, otherwise healthy patients may tolerate these side-effects; if unwarned, many patients will stop their medications. The true problems occur with drug–drug interactions, such as when a person taking a tricyclic antidepressant is taking another drug also with anticholinergic side-effects, such as a phenothiazine tranquilizer: the combination may result in constipation, paralytic ileus, or urinary retention. Even when used alone some tricyclics may cause sufficient urinary retention in an elderly person with prostatic hypertrophy that the patient may decide that his depression is not as bad as the effects of the medication. Sack and Shore (43) describe in detail drug–drug and drug–disease interactions of potential concern to the primary physician. Another common side-effect of tricyclics is their cardiac effects. In general tricyclics slow conduction time, which would help those patients with myocardial irritability, but could lead to complications in those patients who already have conduction defects. Doxepin or amoxapine has the least effect on conduction time and may be the drug of choice if the patient has a conduction defect. (When in doubt, call your cardiac consultant!) Table 1 (see p. 126) reprinted from Sack and Shore (44), gives a pharmacological profile of factors which may influence drug selection of an antidepressant drug.

The other major consideration in choosing a tricyclic antidepressant for a particular patient is the level of *anxiety* present along with the depressive symptoms. As noted earlier, irritability and agitation may be symptoms of the depressive disorder itself; anxiety by itself is not, although clinicians often encounter patients with both depression and anxiety. Many experienced clinicians feel that when anxiety occurs with a depressive disorder, it should be considered part of the depressive picture, and a more "sedating" tricyclic prescribed (45). On the other hand, studies by Raskin (46) from the National Institutes of Mental Health show the following:

1. For hospitalized patients with depression who were not psychotic and whose depression appeared to be related primarily to a specific precipitating event, a high spontaneous recovery rate occurred, and these patients often did as well without any drug treatment as those patients treated with medications. These patients often had the poorest tolerance for the side-effects of medications, as well.

2. For the 60% of hospitalized patients who are both anxious and depressed, one of the major tranquilizers such as thioridazine or chlorpromazine may be the best treatment. Other possibilities include the use of diazepam; a combination tranquilizer/antidepressant, such as amitriptyline and perphenazine; and a tricyclic antidepressant alone.

3. With patients with major vegetative symptoms, especially those of being severely slowed down and with little interest in the environment, tricyclics are the treatment of choice. (Some tricyclics, such as protriptyline, which has no sedating qualities, and nortriptyline and desipramine, which have minimal sedating qualities, are considered "energizing.")

4. When hostility, restlessness, agitation, paranoid ideation, and irritability are prominent in the depressive picture, there is little consensus on a truly effective regime. A number of drugs appear to aggravate the condition: these include diazepam and chlorodiazepoxide and often tricyclic antidepressants as well. These reactions appear somewhat paradoxical, since diazepam, chlorodiazepoxide, and tricyclic antidepressants often are helpful in anxious depressions.

Studies by Weissman and Klerman (47) suggest that with reactive depressions, patients respond as well to tricyclic antidepressants as to psychotherapy, and that the combination of drugs and therapy is the most effective regime. Studies by Schatzberg and Cole (48) suggest that while benzodiazepines may help significantly with the anxiety associated with depressive illnesses, they exert "limited effect on the core symptoms of endogenous depression."

Klein (49) has recommended the use of monoamine oxidase inhibitors (MAOI) for atypical depressions which he has called "hysteroid dysphorias." While there has been a great deal of concern in the American literature about the extreme dangerousness of monoamine oxidase inhibitors, their use has continued in Britain and in some research settings in the United States, and side-effects have been very rare (50). The depressions for which monoamine oxidase inhibitors seem most effective (in addition to those situations where patients did not respond to tricyclics) include depressions in which there are much chronic dysphoria, somatic complaints and preoccupations, and hostility. Shader (51) has also suggested the use of monoamine oxidase inhibitors to stabilize those "characterologic depressions" he labels "rejection-sensitive dysphorics" who become extremely upset at a social or occupational setback or rejection other people would easily shrug off. Patients, of course, must be warned of specific foods and medications to be avoided (tyramine-containing foods, such as blue cheese, salami, and red wine, often referred to as the delicatessen syndrome). Usually, a product insert is available for the MAOI listing such foods. Hypertensive crises still can occur, but are much more rare than previously believed.

Experts (52) in the treatment of psychotic depressions have also noted that for depressed patients with delusions, that treatment should involve antipsychotic medication alone or in combination with a tricyclic antidepressant. ECT is also a treatment with considerable efficacy in patients with these severe symptoms.

Treatment of Recurrent Depression

In contrast with a chronic depression which tends to be characterologic and have very prolonged periods of dysphoric mood, recurrent depressive disorders are discrete episodes of illnesses which appear to remit almost totally between the episodes. Shader (53) suggests that with the natural history of depressive disorders, after three episodes of unipolar depression, recurrences are likely to be 2–5 years apart, with the duration of 3–9 months per episode. He recommends maintenance therapy following the third episode of depressive illness and also suggests that once therapy is begun, it should continue for at least as long as the untreated episode would have been (e.g., 6 months).

Prediction of Response to Tricyclic Medication

Although used primarily as research tools at research centers at the present time, two significant tests to help predict response to tricyclic antidepressant medications are presently available. The first, the dexamethasone suppression test, distinguishes a biological (endogenous) depression from a secondary depression (e.g., a depression secondary to alcoholism or carcinoma). With a true primary depressive disorder, endogenous cortisol production is not suppressed after administration of the steroid, dexamethasone; patients with secondary depressions and normal persons do have their endogenous cortisol production suppressed (54). Patients with a primary depression (who do not suppress cortisol production—dexamethasone) are much more likely to respond to tricyclic antidepressants or other "biological" therapies. Patients who do suppress cortisol production after receiving dexamethasone may or may not respond to biological interventions.

Another tool, the sleep EEG, has recently been used to predict response to tricyclic antidepressants. Following the administration of a test dose of amitriptyline (50 mg), the REM percent of sleep decreased by 44%, the REM activity by a third, and the REM latency period increased by almost double (the number of minutes of sleep until the onset of the first REM period). Those patients showing such initial responses were the ones to show continued significant clinical and symptomatic responses to additional tricyclic antidepressant treatment (55). (Although still a research tool, sleep laboratories are becoming an increasing part of many major medical centers.)

Treatment of Manic Depressive Illness

Once a manic or hypomanic episode has occurred in a patient who has had a previous episode of depression, the diagnosis of bipolar affective disorder can be made with some assurance. If the initial episode or two has been depression, the diagnosis remains in doubt (even though later, the patient may develop manic-depressive illness). Suggestive evidence is a family history of mania or hypomania; a family history of bankruptcy; and a personal history of hypersomnia. Current prescribing suggestions suggest that once the diagnosis of manic-depressive illness has been made, lithium should be used on a regular basis to prevent the recurrence of both manic and depressive episodes. Shader (54) notes that side-effects of lithium, such as tremor and gastrointestinal disturbances, are related to surges in concentration of lithium, and suggests slow-release lithium or lithium tablets given in six divided daily doses to avoid such peak surges. Thyroid and renal functioning must be monitored on a regular basis, however, and precautions taken if the patient should coincidentally be prescribed a diuretic or become dehydrated for some other reason. Lithium has also been recommended (56) for "labile borderline patients" with severe, disabling mood swings: lithium appears to stabilize the mood, even though a manic-depressive disorder, or even a cyclothymic disorder by DSM III criteria does not exist.

Electroconvulsive Treatment (ECT)

Electroconvulsive treatment has appeared as a major treatment sporadically over the past 15 years, especially since other treatments, such as tricyclic antidepressants, became available for major depressive disorders. In addition, there has been a tremendous emotional reaction to the use of ECT, in which it has been seen as a "punishment" imposed by the diabolical physician upon his helpless patient. Films, and popular literature, such as *One Flew Over the Cuckoo's Nest* by Ken Keasey, helped maintain the notion that ECT was an agent of punishment used by "bad" physicians, rather than a legitimate medical intervention. It is true that in the early days of its use, ECT was often accompanied by severe side-effects, such as broken bones, because knowledge of the muscle relaxants and anesthesia that should be used with ECT was less sophisticated. All of this has changed, and the usage of ECT is far more specific, cautious, and "scientific" than previously, and can be a life-saving intervention (57). ECT therapy is indicated in severe depressions, particularly those with psychotic features (delusions or hallucinations), especially when the severity of such depressions is either immediately life-threatening because of suicidal potential, or the patients have been resistant to other forms of treatment (58). Previous suicide attempts, suicidal preoccupations, or severe agitation are obvious indicators of greater suicidal risk: these may make the decision for ECT justifiable. In the elderly in whom a depressive picture includes confusion, agitation, hostility, and paranoid ideation, or where severe anorexia makes a rapid amelioration of symptoms critical, ECT therapy may be the treatment of choice. It is critical that ECT be avoided with those patients who have an acute or chronic brain syndrome, or where a brain tumor is suspected. ECT in these cases may severely compromise the already limited intellectual functioning. Recent literature (59) has suggested that ECT is extremely effective with seriously depressed patients who did not respond to a variety of pharmacological treatments, and that improvement was rapid, dramatic, and sustained (all ECT responders were free of depression for at least one year after treatment).

Those clinicians advocating the use of ECT vary in their recommended dosages. These recommendations range from low convulsive voltages to multiple high-dosage treatments over a short period of time. Some clinicians who work primarily with the elderly recommend unilateral ECT on the nondominant hemisphere, since it decreases the postconvulsive memory loss. A minimum of four such treatments is usually required. However, there is usually a less spectacular amelioration of the depressive symptoms than in the case of bilateral ECT (60). In general, bilateral ECT is administered after the patient has been prepared with succinylcholine and has also been anesthetized with sodium pentothal (61). With nonelderly severely depressed patients, refractory to other treatments, a usual course of from four to eight treatments is suggested.

DEPRESSION AND THE LIFE CYCLE

Studies by Holmes, Rahe, and others have shown correlations between the appearance of illness and a number of "life stresses" and life changes (62). Depending on the culture, certain social changes are more likely to produce stresses than are others, and if a sufficient number of these stress-producing changes occur during a particular year, the statistical possibility of physical or psychological illness is strikingly increased. The "vulnerability level" of a particular individual cannot always be predicted, regardless of the number of stressful events; given adequate social support and effective problem-anticipation and problem-solving (63), the debilitating effects of specific stressful events may be significantly reduced. At the same time, the fundamental observation is that change itself, whether positive or negative, forces a person to modify his usual mechanisms of adaption and coping, and this modification takes its toll.

Another way to view these phenomena is in relation to the development stages within a person's life. From birth through death, an individual passes through many stages, each of which may produce unique stress which may be experienced clinically as medical or emotional illness.

Childhood

Erik Erikson, the noted child psychoanalyst and writer, has described various stages of maturation and development throughout the life cycle, implying that each is accompanied by its own stress as the developmental "task" is either successfully or unsuccessfully resolved (64). Some of these tasks—particularly if they are not being solved—produce in the child symptoms of depression. For instance, a child who is not receiving adequate stimulation and "mothering" in the first few weeks and months of life may withdraw, refuse to eat, and may die (65,66). [These phenomena are not simple: they may result from an inattentive or depressed mother, a feeble or weak infant, a lack of attachment (between a premature infant in an incubator and a mother who has no opportunity to hold or feed her child), and a severely damaged or retarded child whose special needs cannot be responded to by any "ordinary" mother.] A child who loses a parent through death or divorce, or who "loses a mother" through the birth of a sibling, may express depression by regressing to an earlier stage of development. For example, a toddler who was toilet trained may suddenly lose this skill and start whining: a preschooler who was speaking fluently and clearly may begin to speak in baby talk, and a first grader who seemed to be assertive and aggressive may suddenly become rather withdrawn and begin sucking his thumb, have nightmares, or possibly become hyperactive. In addition, children express true depressive symptoms: withdrawal, eating disturbance, detachment. Because symptoms in children are often so nonspecific, it is very important that when a child begins to develop a problem like those outlined above, the physician be alerted by parents and his own observation to the possibility that the problem is not a "disciplinary" one, but is instead a manifestation of depression or some other emotional problem.

If the child is depressed, he does not need greater discipline and firmer limits. What is indicated in this case is a greater effort on the part of the parent to understand what the child is experiencing, to get closer to and spend more time with the child, and to encourage him to play out symbolically—with toys, coloring, clay, etc.—what he is experiencing. Although there are specific diagnostic criteria for uncovering major depressive disorder in children (see this Chapter, p. 103), most children have an intermittent alteration of mood, a sense of discouragement, and many protean symptoms which, while not "masking" a depression, are more visible and noticeable to observers than is a mood disorder. Depression in the young school-age child often finds expression in a sudden withdrawal from both academic and social school activities, and the emergence of a petulant and whining relationship with both peers and adults. Depression in this age group is often related to feelings of low self-esteem. This may be due to a move from a familiar neighborhood, the loss of a friend, or to academic difficulties which lead the child to conclude that he is dumb or "retarded." For example, children with attention deficit disorder (formerly called minimal brain dysfunction) are notorious for developing secondary depression and behavior disorders. They conclude they are stupid since they cannot do the work. Depression may also coincide with a growing recognition on the part of the child of his own physical or intellectual limitations and his "differentness" from those children he wishes to emulate and be admired by. This "differentness" may be due to a physical defect, a difference in physical appearance, or a realization that he requires "special classes." It may simply be an awareness that he is not as bright as his brothers and sisters and that his parents are disappointed in him.

As in younger children, manifestations and symptoms of the depression may be nonspecific. They may range from hyperactivity and "clownishness" through apathy, refusal to eat, withdrawal, and development of school phobias, up to, on rare occasions, self-destructive gestures. As Weinberg et al. (67) have demonstrated, depression meeting the diagnostic criteria of major depressive disorder can be found, even in young children, provided the interviewer inquires about specific symptoms. It is relatively rare, however, that a child below the age of mid-adolescence will complain of depression and depressive symptoms as would an adult.

Adolescence

The preadolescent and early adolescent may express depression in similar ways: being turned off by school, withdrawing from friends and family, finding everything "boring." In addition, many adolescents experience a "normal depression." The child feels impulses of both child and adult. He wants to be independent but at the same time to be taken care of. He wishes to be free of parental authority, but has fears about being on his own. The close feelings and wishes to be dependent, which younger children experience toward their parents, are often transferred in adolescence to either another adult (neighbor, teacher) or to a member of the child's peer group—a girl friend or boy friend or even a "gang." Thus, losing a boy or girl friend, being "jilted," or being excluded by a "clique" can be a devastating experience for a teenager because the emotional involvement with the friend or group may have been terribly intense.

Many more suicidal attempts occur at mid-adolescence than at earlier ages. It becomes the physician's task to sort out "gestures" that are pleas for help (but which also may have a highly manipulative component to them) from true suicide attempts in which the adolescent imagines himself dead, wishes to die, sees no alternative except death, and has a specific, well-formulated suicide plan. The distinction between suicidal gestures and bona fide attempts is often difficult, but depends on the clinician's judgment about the severity of the depressive symptoms, whether the incident was a sudden, impulsive action (which might still be lethal), or had been premeditated and carefully planned. Above all, what is the *current* state of the patient? Does the only "way out" still appear to be a self-destructive gesture or do more positive options come to the patient's mind? As in the evaluation of suicidal attempts in general, the presence of a previous history of similar incidents, any suggestion of psychotic thinking, or any history of a family member who has used suicide as a solution should raise the physician's anxiety and suggest to him that such a "gesture" be viewed extremely seriously.

Treatment for a suicidal adolescent should offer the adolescent a relationship with either the doctor or someone he designates from his office, who has both empathy and counseling skills (such as a nurse or physician assistant). The "treater" should be someone with whom the young person can easily relate but also transfer some of his feelings of dependency; a person who is available to give support; and a person who can help with constructive problem solving. Such a patient may also be referred to a mental health or child guidance clinic for additional support or counseling (although the physician must make extra efforts to make sure that the referral "takes"). Seeing the family of the adolescent with the adolescent present may often not only reveal important information necessary to work out a treatment plan for the patient, but may assume the aspect of a "crisis intervention," which may convince the adolescent that someone does indeed care. Of note is that whether an adolescent has made a self-destructive attempt that the physician considers either a "genuine attempt" or a "gesture," the patient needs help, understanding, support, and a treatment plan. "Teaching the kid a lesson" through painful lavage or humiliating lectures is cruel, ineffective, and unprofessional.

Many physicians are reluctant to give antidepressant medication to children before mid-adolescence. For true depression in this age group, however, antidepressant medication is certainly indicated, although dosage limits based on weight must be strictly followed. Whereas both amitriptyline and imipramine have been used with success in depressed children (68–70), studies have used variable criteria for diagnosis, or open trial rather than double-blind designs. In prescribing medication to an adolescent, it is extremely helpful if the physician, after evaluating suicide risk and impulsivity, can make a "contract" with the adolescent to take the medication himself rather than asking the parents to supervise its administration. Adolescents often are very suspicious of whether the doctor is "on their side" or simply an agent for the parents. If this issue does not get clarified, the adolescent patient may well refuse to take the pills "which his mother wants to give him."

Group or family therapy, as opposed to individual therapy, is often the most effective treatment modality for an adolescent patient. Many teenagers are uncomfortable at being "singled out" and feel less constrained when revealing their troubles in the presence of peers who "feel the same way themselves." In family therapy responsibility and blame are often shared, although a high level of skill on the part of the therapist is necessary to prevent the family from labeling the adolescent as "the problem."

Early Adulthood

When young persons reach their late teens, things may go smoothly until it becomes necessary to choose a career. Although some upheaval is a normal part of this phase of young adult life (see Chapter 8), the need to make specific choices and preliminary commitments at this time may cause depression to strike. Some young adults and adolescents from minority groups—blacks, chicanos, native Americans—may experience a more intense depression at this time because of a heightened realization of the limited career opportunities open to them. This type of depression may be expressed by withdrawal, the abuse of drugs or alcohol, flurries of sexual activity without much enjoyment or satisfaction, or self-destructive activities ranging from delinquency when the person knows he will be caught or hurt, to suicide attempts. In some groups, such as native American adolescents, suicide at this age is the leading cause of death.

Although there is considerable disagreement about this, the author frankly feels that black, native American, and chicano teenagers relate best to counselors with whom they share a racial or cultural background. Obviously, it may be impractical to refer all such youths to facilities which have such counselors, and indeed such counselors may not be available in many communities. Nonetheless, depressive problems in adolescence which a caucasian doctor would be able to treat comfortably and effectively in a caucasian adolescent or young adult may not respond to the same treatment if the patient is from a racial or cultural minority. If a counselor from such a minority group is not available, the physician or those members of his staff who will be treating the patient should at least try to understand "where the patient is coming from." Some of this information can be gained by talking with the patient himself, and some is available in the literature (71–73).

Getting married, after the first enthusiasm and excitement, can often turn into a stressful, anxiety provoking, and depressing experience, particularly if the newlyweds have had relatively little experience in compromising with other persons in regard to money, schedules, responsibilities, and shared expectations. (Living together—an increasingly popular alternative to matrimony—may offer both less commitment and less sense of entrapment; it does not avoid, however, the issues of having to compromise and evolve mutual decision-making patterns.)

Frequently, a primary physician can play an "uncle" role to a couple who have suddenly discovered that marriage is not only very demanding, but in some ways disappointing. More teenagers appear to be experimenting with a number of aspects of marriage prior to marriage itself, and more school systems are requiring courses on family life, so that perhaps this specific stress and their accompanying depression regarding marriage, per se, may decrease in time. A marriage which begins as the result of an unwanted pregnancy gets off to a bad start, especially if the families are unsupportive or hostile, and either member of the couple has to drop out of school because of the pregnancy. The physician can play a useful role as a consultant to schools which offer family life courses—either providing information about birth control (if this is consistent with his own and the school's philosophies)—or by providing backup and counseling to an unmarried and pregnant girl trying to decide whether to marry, give the child up for adoption, have an abortion, etc. (Also, see Chapter 7.)

It is clear that the primary physician needs to be well informed about most of the options regarding both contraception and pregnancy and be able to share this knowledge with teenagers and young adults who need advice. Being informed and knowledgeable about different alternatives does not mean having to advocate them indiscriminately. The doctor may wish to share his personal beliefs and values with his patients, but the decisions must ultimately rest with the patients.

The birth of the first child is often a distressing and depressing experience for young couples. The new parent finds that the spouse has less time for him. There is now a third member of the family—one who demands a lot and gives relatively little. The unromantic body changes or pregnancy may persist, and being a good mother and glamorous wife are frequently impossible simultaneously. Seiden (3) documents that women with young children are often much less happy than they were previously, despite the popular mythology that "this should be the culmination of a woman's life." A physician should look for and anticipate depression at this stage. He should urge the new parents not to get too caught up in the parent as opposed to the person role, and he should be prepared to refer these parents for counseling if their problems seem beyond the scope of his brief intervention.

Middle Age

Episodes of depression often appear for the first time in women in the late 30s and for men in their mid-40s. Although again a predictable crisis of mid-life (see Chapter 8), the subjective experience of such a crisis may be considerable and at times overwhelming. The causes of the depression may be a combination of physiological changes, changes in the life situation leading to role and intimacy changes (children leaving home to go to college or work; the couple being *alone* together for the first time in years); and a total reassessment by the individual of the past and the recognition that the choices for the future—vocationally, emotionally, and creatively—may be limited or more circumscribed than formerly (74,75).

Typically, women in this age group, especially those without jobs, avocations, or outside interests, present to the physician as depressed, having feelings of no longer being useful to their families, and with a sense of frustration about their own personal directions and goals. This cluster of symptoms is often termed the "empty nest syndrome." If the depression is severe and incapacitating (and meets the criteria for a major depressive disorder), medication may be warranted. More often, provided the symptoms are less severe, the most useful strategy for relieving the depression may be to get her involved in new activities, to help her do some life planning and assessment for second career; and to assist her in investigating additional education possibilities. A reassessment at this stage of life, triggered by the depression, offers an opportunity for personal growth and reordering of life goals; these opportunities should be encouraged.

Men in their mid-40s (give or take 10 years) are forced to come to terms with the fact that they are getting older, that their looks and physical and sexual vigor may be decreasing (aided by the cultural expectation that they *will* decrease). Although they have been successful in their careers, to which they have devoted so much time and energy, they may feel a lack of personal intimacy in their lives and a sense that career options are rapidly decreasing. Because our culture (aided strenuously by the media) is so youth-oriented, middle-aged men (and women) often compare themselves with the dazzling TV stars, and sometimes their own children, and feel envious, depressed, and highly competitive. Growing old suddenly seems a catastrophe, and the advice of Mickey Spillane's hero to "live dangerously, die young, and have a beautiful corpse" becomes appealing.

Under these biological, psychological, and cultural pressures, the middle-aged man may suddenly plunge into sexual escapades with younger women or make a desperate change of life style because of the feeling that "life should have more meaning than it does." Increased drinking, divorce, or loss of enthusiasm for many of his former interests is not uncommon. Aided by systematic research (58), we are coming to realize that, as women go through a physiological menopause, men may experience at approximately the same age a psychological "male menopause" marked by depression, a sense of frustration, disillusionment with old goals, and a sudden awareness that "time is running out." These feelings, if recognized and understood, may serve as useful motivational forces to lead a man in mid-life to adopt new, productive, and more creative and satisfying living patterns. Without such recognition, the individual may deal with this crisis by changing everything about him—through new wives, new values, cosmetic surgery, and drugs or experiences—to help forget, deny, or ignore what he is actually experiencing.

If a physician has come to terms with his own life patterns, he can often be extremely helpful to individuals in their middle years by steering them toward vocational or other counseling to re-establish viable life goals. When marital difficulties are part of the pattern, the physician may also refer the patient for marital counseling. He can undertake couple therapy himself if he feels comfortable acting as a negotiating and bargaining agent between the partners, one or both of whom may be experiencing a sense of constriction and a desire for openness and freedom.

For any of the middle-age troubles mentioned above, the most productive role of the physician (rather than condemning or moralizing) is to try to understand the behavior, be supportive, and help the individual come to terms with the turmoil and struggles within him. It is obviously important for the doctor to have an awareness of where he himself "is at," so his advice to patients and his own actions lead to productive new solutions and understanding. If the physician is not clear about himself, his work with patients may reflect the physician's own personal struggles.

Both male and female patients in the middle years have a rapid increase in psychosomatic complaints, many of which have been interpreted as depressive equivalents (77). Such complaints may be of sufficient intensity that needless medical and dental surgery are performed before it becomes apparent that no surgical problem exists. An increase in pain and somatic complaints often indicate severe psychological distress and depression: the physician needs to inspect what is going on at the moment within the person or his environment that could account for the appearance of such symptoms.

Physicians are by no means immune to the ills which plague their middle-aged patients (78). If anything, they seem to be even more susceptible to feelings of middle-age malaise, and they deal with these feelings in much the same way their patients do—by denial, drinking too much, using drugs, acquiring new spouses, etc. (Chapter 24). This series of defenses may make them less adept at recognizing and dealing with these issues when they arise in patients. A person experiencing a life crisis is usually unaware of what to do about it. It is crucial that the physician devise as adequate a treatment plan for himself as he would for his patients, and not simply hope to "work it out" alone. A physician in a middle-age slump cannot be very objective about his options and alternatives. He, at least, needs consultation with a colleague or friend who is interested but not personally involved in the situation.

TABLE 11-1. *Antidepressant drugs: pharmacological profile of factors that influence drug selection in medically ill patients*

Drug	Sedation	Anti-cholinergic activity	Slowed cardiac conduction	Postural hypotension	Elimination half-life	Type of amine	Metabolism	Representative brands
Tricyclic antidepressants								
Imipramine	2	2	3	2	8 hr	3°		Tofranil
Desipramine	1	1	3	1	17 hr	2°	→	Norpramin, Pertofrane
Amitriptyline	3	3	2	3	15 hr	3°	→	Elavil, Endep
Nortriptyline	1	1	2	2	27 hr	2°		Aventyl, Pamelor
Protriptyline	0	2	2	1	78 hr	2°		Vivactil
Doxepin	3	3	1	3	17 hr	3°	→	Sinequan, Adapin
Desmethyldoxepin	—	—	—	—	51 hr	2°		(not marketed)
MAO inhibitors								
Tranylcypromine	0	1	0	1	1–2 wk[a]	—		Parnate
Phenelzine	0	1	0	1	1–2 wk[a]	—		Nardil

From ref. 35.
Rating when compared to other drugs of the same class: 1 = least, 2 = intermediate or average, 3 = most.
[a]Time needed for MAO activity to be restored.

Old Age

Depression is an extremely common phenomenon during both pre- and post-retirement periods. The suicide rate for white males (an index of depression) shows a steady increase with age (this rate levels off for women during their later years) (79). The increasing and relentless losses of old age—visual, auditory, economic, and social—mean that the older person will probably experience periodic episodes of reactive depression. Of all age groups, the elderly are the most in need of ongoing and continued support from a primary physician. Fear and concern about death and illness, pain, and loneliness, and the ever-present awareness that there are no more "expanding horizons" (so important to Americans), brings persistent depression and sometimes despair.

A primary physician who has known a patient over a period of time is in a unique position to evaluate the patient should he become withdrawn, apathetic, or forgetful. Although the patient may be developing an organic brain disorder, he may also have a "pseudodementia," a variation of a severe depression that is often triggered in an elderly person with marginal intellectual functioning by a fever, a change of residence, or unfamiliar surroundings (e.g., a hospital or nursing home). Pseudodementia is aggravated by sedatives or the side-effects of many medications. Treatment can reverse the pseudodementia: sometimes with antidepressants, but more often with medical treatment and the restoration of familiar surroundings and people. The primary physician can often identify which components of the present environment need to be changed, and which aspects of the previous environment (family, objects, activities) need to be reinstated.

In milder depressions in the elderly, symptoms are often expressed in somatic terms. However, in contrast with the treatment strategies for other age groups in which the goal may be symptom removal, in the elderly it may be best to tolerate the symptom and allow the patient to use it as a means of ventilating anger, rage, and dissatisfaction with the world. Studies by Busse (80) suggest that a deliberate decision by the physician to tolerate a hypochondriacal symptom may, in fact, have a definitely supportive effect on the patient. He found that hostility of a relative (particularly a hostile and critical daughter-in-law) was a key factor in the persistence of a psychosomatic symptom in one patient. In such a case the physician can work with the family, advising them that:

> "We don't know exactly what is wrong with your mother-in-law. We will have to continue our investigations, but we suggest that you try to be supportive to her while we make more tests."

According to Ward, (5) hypochondriacal patients often do well with "complaint sessions" scheduled in advance. Patients come in to review problems, but not necessarily to change their medications or for any more work-ups. This is a chance to ventilate, and the physician is providing the opportunity. When one is dealing with a depressed and hypochondriacal patient, it is important that the interviewer acknowledge the patient's feelings but not confirm his misperceptions. For example, "That must be a painful feeling that everybody has turned against you," rather than,

"So everybody has turned against you, huh?" In the same way, nodding agreement or saying "uh-huh" to a patient's complaints tends to inadvertently indicate agreement with his depressed symptoms.

Providing support to the family while they in turn provide support to the patient may allow an elderly person, whose sources of self-expression and self-esteem may be marginal, an adaptive way to deal with his environment. A depressive or hypochondriacal complaint may still be a way to say, "I'm still important; don't forget about me."

Depression and its relationships to death and dying is discussed elsewhere (Chapter 10). Although death is the "ultimate loss," a patient's reaction to dying is not necessarily depression. It involves a number of emotions at various times and depends on the person's past life style, his previous losses, his present support system, and the way in which he regards living as well as dying.

REFERENCES

1. *Diagnostic and Statistical Manual* (1980): third edition, pp. 205–224. American Psychiatric Association. Washington, D.C.
2. *Diagnostic and Statistical Manual* (1980): third edition, p. 217. American Psychiatric Association. Washington, D.C.
3. Seiden, A. M. (1976): Overview: research on the psychology of women. I. Gender differences and sexual and reproductive life. *Am. J. Psychiatry*, 133:995–1007.
4. Kashani, J. H., Barbero, G. J., and Bolander, F. D. (1981): Depression in hospitalized pediatric patients. *J. Am. Acad. Child Psychiatry*, 20:123–234.
5. Ward, N., Department of Psychiatry, University of Washington. Personal communication.
6. *Diagnostic and Statistical Manual* (1980): third edition, p. 216. American Psychiatric Association, Washington, D.C.
7. *Diagnostic and Statistical Manual* (1980): third edition, p. 206. American Psychiatric Association, Washington, D.C.
8. Drugs that cause psychiatric symptoms (1981): *Med. Lett. Drugs Ther.*, 23:9–12.
9. Ward, N., personal communication.
10. Chiles, J. (1978): Delinquency and Depression. Address before the Washington State Psychiatric Association and Washington State Medical Association, Spokane, Washington.
11. Petti, T. A. (1978): Depression in hospitalized child psychiatry patients. *J. Am. Acad. Child Psychiatry*, 17:49–59.
12. *Diagnostic and Statistical Manual* (1980): third edition, pp. 333. American Psychiatric Association. Washington, D.C.
13. Freud, S. (1917): Mourning and Melancholia. In: *Complete Psychological Works, Standard Edition*, vol. 14. Translated and edited by J. Strachey. Hogarth Press, London, 1957.
14. Freud, A., and Burlingham, D. (1944): *Infants Without Families*. International Universities Press, New York.
15. Bowlby, J. (1973): *Separation: Attachment and Loss*, vol. 2. Basic Books, New York.
16. Phillips, I. (1979): Childhood depression: interpersonal interactions and depressive phenomena. *Am. J. Psychiatry*, 136:511–515.
17. Poznanski, E., and Krull, J. P. (1970): Childhood depressions: clinical characteristics of overtly depressed children. *Arch. Gen. Psychiatry*, 23:8–15.
18. Holmes, T. H., and Rahe, R. H. (1967): The social readjustment rating scale. *J. Psychosomatic Research*, 11:213–218.
19. Paykel, E., Myers, J., et al. (1969): Life events and depression. *Arch. Gen. Psychiatry*, 21:753–760.
20. Seligman, M. E. P. (1975): *Helplessness: On Depression, Development, and Death*. W. H. Freeman and Company, San Francisco.

21. Mandell, A. J. (1972): An overview of depression. Address presented at a continuing medical education conference, University of Washington School of Medicine.
22. Kovacs, M., and Beck, A. T. (1975): Maladaptive cognitive structures in depression. *Am. J. Psychiatry*, 32:285–305.
23. Lewinsohn, P. M., Biglan, A., and Zeiss, A. M. (1967): Behavioral treatment of depression. In: *The Behavioral Management of Anxiety, Depression, and Pain*, edited by P. O. Davidson. Brunner/Mazel, New York.
24. Schildkraut, J. J., and Kety, S. S. (1976): Biogenic amines and emotions. *Science*, 156:21–30.
25. Schildkraut, J. J. (1965): The catecholamine hypothesis of affective disorders: a review of supporting evidence. *Am. J. Psychiatry*, 122:509–522.
26. Mandell, A. J. (1972): An overview of depression. Address presented at a continuing medical education conference, University of Washington School of Medicine.
27. Detre, T., Himmelhoch, J., Swartzburg, M., et al. (1972): Hypersomnia and manic-depressive disease. *Am. J. Psychiatry*, 128:1203.
28. Kupfer, D. (University of Pittsburgh School of Medicine), personal communication.
29. Drye, R. C., Goulding, R. L., and Goulding, M. E. (1973): No-suicide decisions: patient monitoring of suicidal risk. *Am. J. Psychiatry*, 130:171–174.
30. Fromenhaft, K., Kaplan, D., and Langley, D. (1968): Avoiding psychiatric hospitalization. *Social Work*, 38–45.
31. Caplan, G. (1981): Mastery of stress: psychosocial aspects. *Am. J. Psychiatry*, 138:413–420.
32. Group session techniques in medical practice, a practice profile. U.S. Dept. H.E.W., Public Health Service, N.I.H. Bureau of Health Professions, Education, and Manpower Training. July, 1970.
33. Disabled American Veterans. 807 Maine Ave., S.W., Washington, D.C., 20024.
34. Wilson, J. P. Toward an understanding of post-traumatic stress disorders among Vietnam veterans. Testimony before U.S. Senate Subcommittee on Vietnam Affairs, May 21, 1980, Washington, D.C. (Dr. Wilson is with the Department of Psychology, Cleveland State University, Cleveland, OH 44115).
35. Forgotten warriors: America's Vietnam-era veterans. *Disabled American Veterans Journal*, 807 Maine Ave., S.W., Washington, D.C., 20024. January, 1980.
36. Bielski, R. J., and Friedel, R. O. (1977): Subtypes of depression—diagnosis and medical management. *West. J. Med.*, 126:347–352.
37. Sack, R. L., and Shore, J. H. (1981): Psychopharmacology in medical practice—the benefits and the risks. Medical Progress. *West. J. Med.*, 134:223–233.
38. Ward, N., personal communication.
39. Sack, R. L., and Shore, J. H. (1981): Psychopharmacology in medical practice—the benefits and the risks. Medical Progress. *West. J. Med.*, 134:223–233.
40. Ayd, F. (1980): The first tetracyclic antidepressant. *Audiodigest Psychiatry*, 9:24.
41. Ayd, F. (1980): The first tetracyclic antidepressant. *Audiodigest Psychiatry*, 9:24.
42. Shader, R. (1980): Psychopharmacology for the 80's. *Audiodigest Psychiatry*. 9:24.
43. Sack, R. I., and Shore, J. H. (1981): Psychopharmacology in medical practice—the benefits and the risks. Medical Progress. *West. J. Med.*, 134:228–229, table 5.
44. Sack, R. I., and Shore, J. H. (1981): Psychopharmacology in medical practice—the benefits and the risks. Medical Progress. *West. J. Med.*, 134:225.
45. Ward, N., personal communication.
46. Raskin, A. (1974): A guide for drug use in depressive disorders. *Am. J. Psychiatry*, 131:181.
47. Klerman, G. L., DiMascio, A., Weissman, M. M., et al. (1974): Treatment of depression by drugs and psychotherapy. *Am. J. Psychiatry*, 131:186–191.
48. Schatzberg, A. F., and Cole, J. O. (1978): Benzodiazepines in depressive disorders. *Archives Gen. Psychiatry*, 35:1359–1365.
49. Klein, D. F., and Davis, J. M. (1969): *Diagnosis and Drug Treatment of Psychiatric Disorders*. Williams and Wilkins, Baltimore.
50. Sack, R. L., and Shore, J. H. (1981): Psychopharmacology in medical practice—the benefits and the risks. Medical Progress. *West. J. Med.*, 134:230.
51. Shader, R. (1980): Psychopharmacology for the 80's. *Audiodigest Psychiatry*. 9:24.
52. Sack, R. L., and Shore, J. H. (1981): Psychopharmacology in medical practice—the benefits and the risks. Medical Progress. *West J. Med.*, 134:226.
53. Shader, R. (1980): Psychopharmacology for the 80's. *Audiodigest Psychiatry*. 9:24.
54. Shader, R. (1980): Psychopharmacology for the 80's. *Audiodigest Psychiatry*. 9:24.

55. Kupfer, D. J., Spiker, D. G., Coble, P. A., et al. (1981): Sleep and treatment prediction in endogenous depression. *Am. J. Psychiatry*, 138:429–435.
56. Shader, R. (1980): Psychopharmacology for the 80's. *Audiodigest Psychiatry*. 9:24.
57. Fink, M. (1981): Random thoughts about ECT (editorial). *Am. J. Psychiatry*, 138:484–485.
58. Berezin, M. A., and Stotsky, B. A. (1970): The geriatric patient. In: *The Practice of Community Mental Health*, edited by H. Grunebaum, p. 234. Little, Brown and Co., Boston, p. 234.
59. Paul, S. M., Extein, I., Calil, H. M., et al. (1981): Use of ECT with treatment-resistant depressed patients at the National Institute of Mental Health. *Am. J. Psychiatry*, 138:486–489.
60. Cole, O. J., and Stotsky, B. A. (1973): Psychiatric drug therapy in the elderly. Unpublished paper given as part of a symposium on Depression and Aging, Continuing Medical Education, University of Washington School of Medicine, Seattle, Washington.
61. Kalinowsky, L. (1967): The convulsive therapies. In: *Comprehensive Textbook of Psychiatry*, edited by A. M. Friedman and H. I. Kaplan, p. 1279. Williams and Wilkins, Baltimore.
62. Holmes, T. H., and Rahe, R. H. (1967): The social readjustment rating scale. *J. Psychosomatic Research*, 11:213–218.
63. Caplan, G. (1981): Mastery of stress: psychosocial aspects. *Am. J. Psychiatry*, 138:413–420.
64. Erikson, E. H. (1963): *Childhood and Society*. Norton, New York.
65. Spitz, R. A. (1945): Hospitalism. *The Psychoanalytic Study of the Child*, Vol. 1, p. 53. International University Press, New York.
66. Bowlby, J. (1961): The Adolf Meyer Lecture: Childhood mourning and its implications for psychiatry. *Am. J. Psychiatry*, 118:481.
67. Weinberg, W. A., Rutman, J., Sullivan, L., et al. (1973): Depression in children referred to an educational diagnostic center. *J. Pediatrics*, 83:1065–1072.
68. Weinberg, W. A., Rutman, J., Sullivan, L., et al. (1973): Depression in children referred to an educational diagnostic center. *J. Pediatrics*, 83:1065–1072.
69. Lucas, A. R., Lockett, H. J., and Grimm, F. (1965): Amitriptyline in childhood depression. *Dis. Nerv. Syst.*, 26:105–110.
70. Spitzer, R. L., Endicott, J., and Robbins, E. (1975): *Research Diagnostic Criteria for a Selected Group of Functional Disorders*, 2nd ed. New York Psychiatric Institute, New York.
71. Carlson, G. A., and Cantwell, D. P. (1979): A survey of depressive symptoms in a child and adolescent psychiatric population. *J. Am. Acad. Child Psychiatry*, 18:587–599.
72. Lurie, H. J., and Lawrence, G. L. (1972): Communication problems between rural Mexican-American patients and their physicians: description of a solution. *Am. J. Orthopsychiatry*, 42:777.
73. Shore, J. H., Bopp, J. E., et al. (1972): A suicide prevention center on an Indian reservation. *Am. J. Psychiatry*, 128:1086.
74. Neugarten, B. (1968): *Middle Age and Aging*. University of Chicago Press, Chicago.
75. Levinson, D. J. (1978): *The Seasons of A Man's Life*. Ballantine, New York.
76. Levinson, D. J. (1978): *The Seasons of A Man's Life*. Ballantine, New York.
77. Ross, M. (1966): The practical recognition of depression and suicidal states. *Annals Int. Med.*, 64:1079.
78. Rose, K., et al. (1973): Physicians who kill themselves. *Arch. Gen. Psychiatry*, 29:800.
79. Pfeiffer, E., and Busse, E. (1973): Affective disorders. In: *Mental Illness in Later Life*, edited by E. Busse and E. Pfeiffer, p. 123, American Psychiatric Association, Washington, D.C.
80. Remarks made at a Continuing Medical Education Conference on Depression and Aging, at the University of Washington School of Medicine, October, 1973. (E. Busse).

12

The Anxious Patient

"Anxiety," like "depression," has a range of meanings, depending on whether the focus is physiological or psychological. It also depends on whether one is speaking of a person who has a lifelong history of disabling symptoms or one who has developed acute symptoms in reaction to a current or anticipated stressful event. Most people at one time or another feel anxious, with motor tension (jitteriness, inability to relax), autonomic hyperactivity (sweating, heart pounding, clammy hands), apprehension ("something bad will happen; I will lose control"), and apprehensive hyperattentiveness (irritability, trouble concentrating, trouble falling asleep). It is when such symptoms become chronic (for more than a month) that one becomes concerned, although symptomatic treatment may be indicated when symptoms are present for a much shorter period if they are severe. Anxiety may also be a prominent feature of posttraumatic stress disorder, e.g., following a combat situation or a natural disaster.

Generalized anxiety disorder and posttraumatic stress disorder occur commonly enough to justify the primary care physician acquiring expertise in their management. Two other variations of anxiety disorders, phobic disorders and obsessive-compulsive disorders, seem to the author to be beyond the realm of most primary care practices; they justify referral and/or consultation with a mental health expert for their management.

DIFFERENTIAL DIAGNOSIS

Overuse of caffeine: Many people, especially older individuals, have symptoms strongly mimicking anxiety symptoms when they drink more than five or six cups of coffee a day.

Withdrawal from heavy alcohol use: During the withdrawal phase, if there is either physiological or psychological dependency, anxiety symptoms of both a physiological and a psychological nature may be present.

Stimulant abuse: Dextroamphetamine or methylphenidate abuse may simulate anxiety symptoms.

Hyperthyroidism: Anxiety symptoms are present with hyperthyroidism, together with heat intolerance, fine tremor, brisk reflexes, and hyperphagia.

Hypoglycemia: Anxiety symptoms, together with sweating, flushing, and hunger cured by carbohydrate ingestion may be present. This usually occurs 2 to 3 hours after a meal.

Paroxysmal atrial tachycardia (PAT): Anxiety and a racing heart with sudden onset and sudden termination merit an electrocardiogram.

Organic brain syndrome: Either acute or chronic organic brain syndrome may be accompanied by symptoms of anxiety. A posttrauma syndrome which includes symptoms of anxiety is often present 3 to 4 weeks following a head injury.

MANAGEMENT OF ACUTE ANXIETY

Management of the acutely anxious patient often involves a combination of verbal reassurance (done with "authority" to minimize its placebo effect), an opportunity to talk with a sympathetic listener about the situation that is making the person anxious, and antianxiety agents in low dosages for a short period of time (see below). Patients often become obsessed with their own symptoms, especially insomnia, or a fear they will "lose control." An explanation that insomnia is not necessarily harmful and an exploration of the fantasies about losing control may relieve some of the symptoms.

PANIC ATTACKS

Recent research information has perceived that panic disorder/agoraphobia is not simply an extension or severe form of a generalized anxiety disorder but a separate entity (1). Data presented by Sheehan (2) at the 1982 American Psychiatric Association meeting suggests that for panic disorders "... a triazolo benzodiazepine called alprazolam has been shown to be effective in controlling panic attacks and phobic anxiety. Because of its rapid onset of action and safety it may become the drug of first choice in this disorder."

CHRONIC ANXIETY AND ITS MANAGEMENT

The management of chronic anxiety is more complex than the management of acute anxiety, as symptom relief may be unpredictable, on the one hand, and may respond to a variety of measures, including placebos, on the other. In general, the following approaches may be useful with the chronically anxious patient.

Medications

The only drugs in recent years that have been used significantly as antianxiety agents have been the benzodiazepines. All of these have a much greater margin of safety than barbiturates, although all of them have the capacity for psychological dependence and, in higher dosages, physiological dependence. A mild degree of sedation is common with two of the compounds, diazepam and clorazepate (Valium® and Tranxene®); another benzodiazepine, flurazepam (Dalmane®), may induce significant daytime sedation following nighttime use because of its prolonged half-life (2 to 5 days are needed for elimination). Apart from personal preference, many physicians find that the decision about using benzodiazepines for anxiety depends on whether one wants an acute effect which can be precisely titrated—in which case a short-acting drug such as oxazepam, chlordiazepoxide, or lorazepam (Serax®, Librium®, or Ativan®, respectively) is used—or a significant blood level of antianxiety agent so that the patient can be totally anxiety-free for a specified period of time (e.g., 2 weeks)—in which case diazepam, chlorazepate, or prazepam (Valium®, Tranxene®, or Verstran®, respectively) is prescribed.

The most effective way to avoid drug dependency is not to give the drug on a p.r.n. basis. It is best to administer a reasonably long-acting antianxiety agent such as diazepam once a day and then raise the dosage to the point that symptoms are relieved for an extended period of time. After several weeks, or when the stress abates, the dosage should then be gradually reduced.

Patients, of course, experience idiosyncratic responses to many medications, some patients becoming inordinately sleepy with one medication and intensely hostile with another (3). With sedative-hypnotics, both tolerance and psychological and physical dependence are possible. Physical addiction to chlordiazepoxide or diazepam can occur when amounts that are 10 to 20 times the usual daily dosage are consumed for more than 1 month. Meprobamate is physically addictive at an even lower dose. Diazepam, because of its rapid oral absorption and its tendency to produce euphoria, makes it a drug which can easily lead to psychological dependence. Table 12-1 outlines the pharmacological profiles of some common antianxiety agents.

Withdrawal reactions with the benzodiazepines are usually seen at 4 to 8 days, but sometimes they become apparent only at 2 weeks after withdrawal from the drug (3). Like barbiturate withdrawal, withdrawal from benzodiazepine may include agitation, hallucinations, and convulsions.

Major tranquilizers are occasionally useful for relieving chronic anxiety. These medications may be particularly effective in those patients whose reality testing becomes somewhat impaired when anxious (e.g., the secretary who becomes progressively harassed by the increasing amount of work and then starts to believe that people are talking about her). Major tranquilizers, unlike minor tranquilizers, have no physiological addictive potential and do not produce euphoria (as do some of the benzodiazepines). In fact, many patients experience an unpleasant "drugged" effect with major tranquilizers. For all these reasons, a p.r.n. utilization, even with chronic anxiety, seems justified.

For anxious children and adults whose anxiety is largely expressed through social phobias, the use of tricyclic antidepressants, especially imipramine, is often useful for relieving phobia symptoms and symptoms of anxiety. Tricyclic antidepressants have also been used for prevention of panic attacks.

TABLE 12-1. *Antianxiety agents: pharmacological profile of factors that may influence drug selection in medically ill patients*

Benzodiazepines	Sedation[a]	Elimination half-life (hr)	Intramuscular absorption	Active no. of metabolites	pH dependent intragastric conversion	Representative brands
Chlordiazepoxide	2	5–30	Variable	3	0	Librium
Diazepam	3	20–50	Variable	1	0	Valium
Oxazepam	2	5–20	Parenteral form not available	0	0	Serax
Clorazepate	3	30–60	Parenteral form not available	1	+	Tranxene, Azene
Prazepam	2	20–50	Parenteral form not available	2	+	Verstran
Lorazepam	2	10–15	Parenteral form not available	0	0	Ativan
Flurazepam	3	47–100	Parenteral form not available	1	0	Dalmane

From ref. 4.
[a]Rating when compared to other drugs of the same class: 1 = least, 2 = intermediate or average, 3 = most.

STRESS REDUCTION PROCEDURES

Relaxation training and various forms of meditation are being used increasingly in the treatment of chronic anxiety. For those who follow these procedures, relaxation training can be very effective. In order for the method to be successful, however, the patient must practice it continually, and only a limited number of patients are willing to do so. The meditation technique described by Benson (5), in use at some of the Harvard teaching hospitals, involves the following:

1. Sit quietly in a comfortable position.
2. Close your eyes.
3. Deeply relax all your muscles, beginning at your feet and progressing up to your face. Keep them relaxed.
4. Breathe through your nose. Become aware of your breathing. As you breathe out, say the word "one" silently to yourself. For example, breathe in . . . out, "one"; in . . . out, "one"; etc. Breathe easily and naturally.
5. Continue for 10 to 20 minutes. You may open your eyes to check the time but do not use an alarm. When you finish, sit quietly for several minutes, at first with your eyes closed and later with your eyes open. Do not stand up for a few minutes.
6. Do not worry about whether you are successful in achieving a deep level of relaxation. Maintain a passive attitude and permit relaxation to occur at its own pace. When distracting thoughts occur, try to ignore them by not dwelling upon them and return to repeating "one." With practice, the response should come with little effort. Practice the technique once or twice daily but not within 2 hours after any meal, as the digestive processes seem to interfere with the elicitation of the relaxation response.

Once a relaxation ritual is learned, patients can often relax their entire bodies in a matter of several seconds and achieve a relaxed state with little conscious effort (without using the relaxation procedure described here).

Other techniques may involve progressive relaxation (Chapter 20), biofeedback linked with relaxation, and specific meditation techniques, e.g., Transcendental Meditation.

STRUCTURED ACTIVITIES

For chronically anxious patients with a compulsive streak, doing activities which can be charted, counted, practiced, and changed may be a way to relieve anxiety. In such cases, asking patients to keep extensive logs of symptoms (or, preferably, symptom-free periods), mood, antecedent events, what appeared to relieve the anxiety, specific fears at the time, etc. may be useful. Having patients identify the specific components of their anxious state (e.g., motor restlessness) and then try to practice reproducing such symptoms is a way that some patients are able to get such symptoms under control.

REASSURANCE AND SUPPORT

Many patients respond to reassurance and support in the midst of a bout of acute anxiety. The "placebo effect" of reassurance may be enhanced if the physician makes strong, positive, reassuring statements (rather than settling for tepid, empathic statements alone). After listening to the patient, the physician might say, "You're doing remarkably well, considering all you've been through. I know you'll feel much better in 2 or 3 days." Reiterating that he will stick by the patient and will be available can also provide the support and structure the patient needs to calm down.

In a similar fashion, presentation of medication—placebo or benzodiazepine—to an anxious patient works best if, as Baldessarini (3) suggests, it is offered with an "enthusiastic, charismatic presentation."

COGNITIVE APPROACHES TO CATASTROPHIZING

As with the depressed patient, the anxious patient may obsess and brood over possible impending catastrophes and work himself into a frenzy. Exploring the fantasies of the patient can often diffuse some of the anxiety, as absurdities and contradictions become more apparent.

Question: "Could you explain why you are so worried about being on time?"
Answer: "Oh, if I'm late they'd fire me."
Question: "Oh, for being 15 minutes late?"
Answer: "They might not, but I'd feel very guilty."
Question: "What would that be like. Could you describe how quilty you would feel?"
And so on.

Exploring in an inquiring and interested way about the patient's fantasies, obsessions, and concerns, and even exaggerating them, will help him begin to look more objectively at his worries. This technique may somewhat desensitize the patient to his worries as well.

THERAPY GROUPS

For long-term anxious patients whose symptoms are chronic, a supportive psychotherapy group run either by the physician or a member of the staff with expertise in group therapy or counseling may help reduce the need for medications as well as the symptomatology. The focus of the group may range from a relatively unstructured approach ("How did it go this week?") to a structured, behaviorally oriented group approach that reinforces relaxation training, activity charting, and specific tension-reducing techniques.

Many special groups perform a major supportive function and, through their activities, focus, and structure, offer "moral support" through rules, ethics, codes of conduct, and meeting rituals (benedictions, organizational structure, planned group activities, oaths of allegiance, etc.). For the patient whose anxiety is relieved by such structure, a wide variety of groups ranging from fraternal organizations, service clubs, church groups, bridge clubs, and bowling leagues offer some relief. Goal-directed "work" groups are often useful for anxious patients by providing a clear structure and channel for energy and direction (planning a food drive for the poor, collecting eyeglasses for refugees, etc.).

Though the role of support groups has been emphasized here and elsewhere in this monograph, it cannot be emphasized too strongly that one person's stress-reducer is another's stress-intensifier. The anxious person who finds working with a church altar guild a supportive, relaxing, and rewarding experience may find himself "trapped" and anxious around the "overly friendly and supportive" physician. In such a relationship the patient may fear that he is surrendering his control to the physician, and certain feelings (e.g., erotic feelings) may become more pronounced and threatening. Conversely, some anxious patients may be too shy to share their intimate feelings with a group. The anxiety of such a patient may be relieved significantly by meeting regularly for 5 or 10 minutes with an interested and friendly physician who knows the patient well enough to offer support, reassurance, and, if necessary, medication.

ATHLETICS

Vigorous exercise offers tension relief to many people and, in fact, often produces a sense of invigoration as tension drops. If the activity is competitive, feelings of aggression and anger may be sublimated into it. Because of the tendency of exercise to produce insomnia in some patients, it should be done at least 4 hours before bedtime.

SEXUAL ACTIVITY

Overt sexual activity, ranging from masturbation to intercourse, if it is seen as "good" by the patient (positive, acceptable, pleasurable), often releases tension significantly. However, if the sexual activity engenders conflict, guilt, or worry, anxiety may be increased rather than decreased.

TOUCH

Many anxious patients are reassured by physical contact. People other than physicians can legitimately touch other individuals: hairdressers and sometimes barbers, a masseur, relatives, young children, occupational and physical therapists, etc. Many doctors have noted empirically that some patients become less anxious after being held by a spouse, after a massage, or after going to the hairdresser. Of course, some patients feel threatened by closeness and touch. Nevertheless, the "laying on of hands" by various types of professionals does, in fact, play a significant role in reducing anxiety for many people. Touch can be an enormous comfort, particularly for elderly people. Many patients derive as much support and anxiety reduction from the human touch and warmth of the physician as from the knowledge that the examination is thorough and the doctor competent.

SAUNAS, SPAS, AND HOT TUBS

As the Finns and Japanese have known for centuries, saunas, spas, and hot tubs can provide a way to unwind and relax, as well as a way to reduce anxiety in the susceptible. (It is well to remember, however, that some patients hate all of these!)

RELAXATION RITUALS

In the same way that anxiety and tension may be coupled with specific stressful events, so too may the reduction of tension be coupled with specific rituals. For many individuals this is the ceremonial martini and the evening paper or TV news program. Establishing time to "unwind" before tackling new responsibilities (e.g., having a "breathing space" after a day at the office before tackling domestic duties such as helping the kids with the homework) can be a way to relax and reduce anxiety when otherwise it is likely to escalate.

REFERENCES

1. Klein, D., Rabkin, J. G. (eds.) (1981): *Anxiety: New Research and Current Concepts.* Raven Press, New York.
2. Sheehan, D. (1982): Panic Disorders: A treatment overview lecture and written summary, Presented at the American Psychiatric Association, Toronto (The Tufts University School of Medicine/New England Medical Center Symposium on "Panic Disorders: Current Perspectives," Richard Shader, Chairman.)
3. Baldessarini, R. J. (1978): Chemotherapy. In: *Harvard Guide to Modern Psychiatry*, edited by A. M. Nicholi Jr., pp. 427–429. Belknap/Harvard, Cambridge, MA.
4. Sack, R. L., and Shore, J. H. (1981): Psychopharmacology in medical practice—the benefits and the risks. *West. J. Med.*, 134:223–234.
5. Benson, H. (1975): *The Relaxation Response*, pp. 114–115. William Morrow, New York.

13

Psychiatric Emergencies: The Physician's Role

There is usually unanimity about what constitutes a life-threatening illness or behavior within the realm of physical medicine. The definition of a psychiatric emergency, however, depends much more on the eye of the beholder. An "emergency," of course, means some situation which requires immediate action. This may range from a situation in which a patient is involved in life-threatening behavior (his own life or that of someone else) to a situation where the physician's anxiety level is raised high enough that some sort of immediate relief through action is necessary to decrease the doctor's anxiety. In the latter situation, the "emergency" nature of the situation may not be apparent to the patient himself.

Dealing with medical and psychiatric emergencies requires many of the same steps as crisis intervention: (1) diagnosis of the various components of the emergency; (2) development of a strategy for handling the situation acutely and restoring the patient to a previous equilibrium; (3) mobilizing friends, relatives, and community individuals as a support system to help the person resolve the crisis; and (4) using whatever medical, psychiatric, or community resources (institutional and personal) that may be required to reduce the acute nature of the crisis situation.

Psychiatric emergencies which are likely to come to the attention of the physician include acutely depressed patients who are suicidal, psychotic patients who become wilder in the hospital or "ordinary" patients who become disorganized or psychotic in response to medical or surgical procedures performed or contemplated; violent patients, potentially homicidal patients, persons who have been acutely abused or traumatized, and persons who have committed the abuse and trauma.

Two common examples of the psychiatric emergency are the patient who becomes agitated before surgery and one who becomes severely depressed after surgery.

> A 39-year-old woman who discovers a lump on her breast undergoes a biopsy which reveals a malignancy. She is scheduled for a radical mastectomy the next

day and seems quite stoic about the surgery but asks few questions about the possible outcome. Late that night the surgeon receives a frantic phone call from the charge nurse, who describes the patient as being extremely agitated, threatening suicide, and packing her clothes to leave against medical advice, saying that she would rather be dead than "cut up." After the surgeon talks with the patient for several hours, he learns that she is extremely concerned that her husband will leave her if she is "mutilated"; he also learns that her mother and an aunt died of cancer when they were in their forties. After postponing surgery for several days and having daily discussions with the patient, she calms down. She has received assurance from her husband that he will stick by her, and she has been visited by a woman who had a mastectomy and who is comfortable physically and psychologically with her prosthetic breast. The patient undergoes surgery and makes an uneventful recovery.

A 45-year-old man has a colostomy for cancer of the bowel. Several months following surgery the patient's wife phones the physician, saying that her husband has lost a lot of weight, refuses to eat, and will not discuss going back to work. He has become progressively quieter, and refuses to allow his wife to invite old friends or fellow employees over for a visit. When the doctor talks with the patient, the patient reveals the notion that he is now "terribly dirty" and that he supposes everyone will smell him if he considers returning to work. He says that he wants to diet, as he imagines that if he eats almost nothing people will not be able to smell him (the patient is meticulously clean and has no odor). A detailed evaluation reveals that the patient is not sleeping well, is depressed, and often ruminates about whether it would have been better to have died on the operating table rather than to have to continue to live such a "dirty," isolated life.

Over the next several weeks the physician arranges frequent visits with the patient and schedules joint conferences with the patient and his wife, and the patient and his employer; they develop a plan acceptable to the patient of gradually returning to work for several hours a day. After several months the patient is back at work full time and no longer has his morbid preoccupations.

The doctor who is aware that a patient may have these reactions and fears related to a disease process or surgery should take time to talk them out with him. If the physician does not have the time, he should, at the very least, delegate someone else (e.g., a skilled nurse or rehabilitation counselor) who does have the time to talk with the patient about his specific problems. Here again the doctor is functioning as the captain rather than as the whole team.

The physician (as in the two cases cited above) recognizes that the reactions of the patient to surgery—in one case taking the form of panic, and in the other taking the form of a severe clinical depression—may be just the first stages of a process which will continue over a long period of time: the grieving over the loss of a valued part of the body, the loss of one's former body image, or the loss of a "function." The grief, fear, anger, and anxiety that patients feel about the surgery which produces these losses may be expressed through actions rather than being verbalized. It is these peculiar actions which are labeled by others "the emergency."

As with the cases described, handling such an emergency might involve (1) joint counseling between the patient and the spouse; (2) arranging visits by other patients who have completed the "dreaded" surgery successfully; and (3) sufficiently frequent visits with the physician to allow the patient to become gradually informed about his condition, the procedures to be done, and the medical and surgical management involved. The doctor may also describe some of the reactions that other patients have had to the surgery (initially and later). He can assume that the family is having some difficulty coping with the situation, especially if the patient is having an extreme reaction to the illness or procedure. The doctor can encourage rapid rehabilitation after the illness by meeting with the family and the patient, opening communication channels, and arranging for the patient to resume many normal activities as soon as possible.

THE SUICIDAL PATIENT

As mentioned in Chapter 11, it is often difficult to distinguish between those patients who are seriously considering and planning to kill themselves from those whose motivation is primarily a "cry for help." Patients with serious suicide intent have a specific plan, imagine themselves dead, have a narrowed focus of vision in which other courses of action seem impossible, and often behave in a way in which their suicidal behavior is not detected, except inadvertently. On the other hand, with people who threaten suicide but are less inclined to the actual deed, a plan, if present, is vague or clearly not designed for implementation. This person does not imagine himself dead. He may have unsuccessfully tried a number of other measures to get support and attention, and the "call for help" is often fairly explicit.

One assumes that the vast majority of individuals who attempt and threaten suicide are ambivalent about the idea, and that if someone (e.g., a physician) can understand and respond to their anguish they may be willing to consider other options. Suicide attempts and threats are generally thought to be "two-person events." The intent of the suicidal person is to punish or in some way deal with the emotional entanglements of a relationship. Many persons who plan and/or threaten suicide have had a recent disappointment or loss in a major "love" relationship: They were jilted by a boyfriend, had a quarrel with a parent, etc.

Clearly a therapeutic strategy involves: (1) assessing the lethality of the suicide attempt or threat; (2) establishing rapport with the patient to see "where they are coming from" and what kind of intervention might re-establish some kind of equilibrium; (3) assessing the level of depression or affect disturbance (do they need medication?); and (4) linking the patient with experiences and people who are experienced in supporting and helping him recover. Patients are sometimes treated harshly by their medical caretakers following a suicide attempt on the theory that "scaring the patient" will avert further attempts and make the patient realize the folly of his action. By and large, this is an ineffective and hostile way of dealing with the problem. The need for a detailed interview to sort out whether the suicide attempt is motivated by the desire for revenge ("they'll be sorry when I'm gone") or involves a feeling of total despair and hopelessness when the patient feels he has lost something or someone who can never be replaced is illustrated by the following examples.

Example
An adolescent girl takes 25 aspirin tablets in a suicide attempt. The attempt may be "phoney": The patient has no intention of killing herself but is expressing a desire to punish her family who have not been paying a great deal of attention to her; she is also expressing her sufferings over being jilted by her boyfriend. During the interview the girl expresses open hostility toward her mother. At no time does she seem really depressed; instead, she shows anger, sarcasm, and skepticism about whether anyone wants to help her. She finally calms down somewhat when she starts seeing a kind and reasonably mature student nurse who talks with the patient daily about plans after high school, what she has to look forward to, how parents are never entirely understanding, etc. The girl and her family are referred for family counseling, and no further suicide attempts are made.

Example
An adolescent girl refers herself to a doctor when she realizes she is repeatedly thinking about killing herself by taking large amounts of her mother's medication. She too has been jilted by a boyfriend recently, but for this patient the rejection reminds her strongly of the time her father "abandoned her" 5 years ago when he deserted the family. The new rejection seems to her the confirmation of her fear that she is indeed totally unlovable and will always remain so. Treatment includes referral to a mental health counselor for long-term therapy, possibly working with the family, arranging for the patient to join an adolescent group at the local mental health center, and getting her involved in "candy striper" work at a local hospital with pediatric patients, proving to her that she can be very important to other people. If her suicidal thoughts do not rapidly diminish despite frequent visits to the physician and the counselor, antidepressant medication would be in order.

These two situations of a "suicidal patient" are superficially similar. The motivations of the patients and the extent of their depression and impulsiveness, however, are very different. Treating them in the same way would have been ineffective and perilous. In both cases emergency management involved meeting the patient's unique needs, maintaining self-esteem, providing sufficient therapeutic contact to form a beginning alliance with the patient, and mobilizing those parts of the patient's support system which could help the patient be less dependent on any one person for her source of self-esteem and satisfaction.

Unfortunately, suicidal assessment is rarely so straightforward and simple. A number of suicide attempts are precipitated by the use of drugs or alcohol, and attempts appear to increase when similar attempts are publicized in newspapers or on television. Successful suicide attempts among males increase with age and are considerably higher among individuals divorced or living alone than among those who are married. Among teenagers and young adults, being part of a racial minority, having a weapon, and using alcohol vastly increase the odds of both suicide and homicide attempts.

Assessing the motivation of a person who presents to an emergency room of a general hospital because of suicide threats or suicidal intent raises still another set of issues. Studies by Bassuk et al. (1) note that in studies of patients in crisis admitted because of suicidal intent the vast majority were chronic schizophrenic patients who had learned previously that the route to readmission to a hospital was to profess suicidal thoughts. The authors concluded that admission was probably reinforcement of a pattern of flight and antithetical to the development of coping skills in those individuals with schizophrenia, personality disorders, or addictive problems. Clearly, it is crucial to take a detailed history of previous admissions, illnesses, and coping patterns to determine under what circumstances admission for suicidal intent is helpful and when it may be harmful and regressive.

There is a final caveat about suicidal patients: The vast majority of people who kill themselves have talked about suicide on at least one occasion with their physician over the past year. Being available to listen, inquiring about suicidal ideas with the patient, making a no-suicide contract, and assessing whether the "latest threat" is serious or "crying wolf" are a heavy but necessary burden for the physician who must manage suicidal patients on a regular basis.

VIOLENT PATIENTS

Patients can become violent from a large variety of causes. Sorting out the probable cause of their behavior is often the critical determinant in making an appropriate management and treatment plan, although there are often common management strategies. Common sources of violence include the following: (1) acute intoxications (alcohol, PCP, amphetamines, rarely minor tranquilizers such as diazepam); (2) a confused patient with mild delirium or dementia aggravated by environmental change or stress (a new patient in a nursing home); (3) individuals with explosive personalities where the violence is triggered by environmental or interpersonal conflicts; (4) paranoid personalities whose violence is triggered by an environmental stress which sets off reactions of jealousy or rage; (5) persons with schizophrenia whose paranoid delusions are aggravated by environmental stress or change.

Management of the Violent Patient

Management of the violent patient often poses serious problems in an outpatient setting, where the threat to the physician's health, that of the staff, and that of other patients is real. Experts in violence (2) have suggested a "hierarchy of restraint" when dealing with the violent patient, starting with talking and progressing to physical restraint and then to "chemical" restraints.

Talking Restraints

With all violent patients, it is important that the person talking with them do so with confidence and clarity as well as respect. Paranoid patients, especially, require considerable physical distance; they respond with more anxiety when "crowded" or approached too closely or quickly. Clarification of your role, setting limits, listening actively with empathy, and seeking to identify the problems are critical. Talking with the patient in a quiet setting, with few distractions is also helpful:

"Mr. Smith, my name is Doctor Hammond. This is the emergency room of Harborview Hospital. I'd like to talk with you in the room down the hall. I wonder if you could tell me what's going on. The policeman said that you had been beaten up in a fight and couldn't tell him where you lived."

The purpose of this kind of intervention is to clarify who and where you are, what you intend to do with the patient, and why you are talking. The strategy is to involve the patient in verbal interaction and to establish a relationship and some basis for assessing the patient's problem.

Physical Restraint

If a patient is terrorizing the waiting room or the emergency room, it is crucial that he be brought under control as rapidly and humanely as possible. Often telling the patient in a calm but firm voice to stop his behavior and calm down produces such an effect. With paranoid men, women often pose less of a threat and are more effective than a man (including a physician). If this verbal intervention is not successful, calling for security to escort the patient either to a room outside the main waiting area or outside the facility is the next step. Obviously, a prior plan must be established to make this kind of intervention efficient or effective. There is much debate about whether the presence of uniformed policemen provokes violent behavior or is the necessary "show of force" to stop the patient's behavior. In some well-staffed settings, the use of sufficient security or emergency room male staff members to physically stop the patient's inappropriate behavior and assist in his taking medication to regain control is seen as the treatment of choice.

If a patient needs physical restraint, a plan must obviously be present ahead of time: Who "gives the orders"? Who orders the restraints? How many restraints are to be used? Are they to be cloth or leather?

The patient in restraints should be in a quiet area with a nonthreatening person taking a history or "talking down" the patient. If the patient is out of control, does not respond to isolation and verbal interventions, and the type of medication to give him seems in doubt, then physical restraints are the treatment of choice. Explaining what you are going to do and why is important:

> "Mr. Jones, you seem to be out of control, and we're worried that you might hurt yourself or someone else. We're going to have to put you in restraints to keep you from hurting anybody. We'll loosen them every half hour or so, and I or my assistant, Miss Rutherford, will be back every 15 minutes to talk with you to see how you are. Once you're calmer, we'll take the restraints off, one by one."

Chemical Restraint

For patients in whom a diagnosis has been established, specific medication can be administered to help alleviate symptoms: major tranquilizers for the schizophrenic patient in relapse, minor tranquilizers for the patient with DTs, sedatives for the person with an explosive personality disorder, etc. Unfortunately, a large number of patients present to the emergency room for whom it is difficult to establish a clear diagnosis, and for some of these medications are contraindicated.

Patients for whom PCP intoxication is suspected may be given sedatives but not major tranquilizers, which may aggravate their condition. Patients "coming down from a bad trip" (from hallucinogen intoxication) should be "talked down" by someone with sufficient time and skill to do this. (The process often takes 8 to 12 hours and requires frequent reality orientation, clarification of who and where the person is, etc.) The most effective person to do this is often a "street person" with sufficient drug experience himself to identify the specific affective or confusional state through which the patient is presently passing. Patients intoxicated with opiates may improve with the administration of opiate antagonists. Care should be taken that such patients are observed for a sufficient period of time: Narcotics often persist in the body considerably longer than their antagonists and have persistent respiratory and central nervous system depressant effects. Wherever possible, when a chemical restraint is needed it should be administered by mouth rather than by injection. When an appropriate "show of force" and firmness is displayed by those in charge, reluctant patients often swallow liquid medications; this is desirable as it avoids an unpleasant struggle between the physician and the patient who is resisting the syringe. Even for rapid tranquilization, Dubin (2) recommends oral medications, which he has found clinically to be as effective as parenteral agents. Specific protocols for effective management of violent patients are outlined by Dubin and Lurie (2a).

HOMICIDAL PATIENTS

The homicidal or potentially homicidal patient who occasionally presents to an emergency room or a physician's office is a major diagnostic dilemma in terms of both medical and legal management. Motivation and causes of homicidal behavior include: (1) greed and malice; (2) psychoses in which there is a paranoid misinterpretation of another person's actions, including a delusional notion that one is being attacked and so must "kill or be killed"; (3) temporal lobe epilepsy; and (4) the temporary loss of control in an explosive (or sometimes "ordinary") personality. Even if the homicidal attempt is initially identified by a law enforcement agent, the physician has the obligation, because of his training and diagnostic abilities, to try to sort out the reasons for the homicidal attempt.

In most states civil commitment procedures require that a person making threats or attempts to harm someone else be committed for at least 72 hours so that a psychiatric evaluation can be performed. In less dramatic cases, the physician himself may have to decide whether someone is of danger to someone else. (Currently, if a physician has a patient in treatment who threatens to kill another person, the physician is under a legal obligation to warn that other person. He is legally liable if he does not.)

Some of the factors identified by Miller (3) as predisposing an individual to violence include the following: The person (1) was beaten as a child; (2) had a high incidence of head injuries as a child; (3) had behavioral problems as a child; (4) has a history of emotional deprivation; (5) has parents who were likely to have been alcoholic; and (6) had a tendency to carry knives as a child.

Immediate precipitants of attempted murder include: (1) the recent loss of a parent or lover; (2) something in the situation being construed as a "threat to manhood";

(3) the victim representing for the murderer some specific aspect of himself which he finds weak or unacceptable, and which he would like to destroy; (4) the murderer seeing the victim as "not human"; (5) the murderer having or imagining that he has group support or sanction for the murder.

As a large number of murders in America involve the use of guns, the availability of the murder weapon, combined with the sudden impulse to commit the act and often aided by alcohol- or drug-induced lowering of social inhibition for violence, may conspire to permit the actual murder attempt to occur.

Data compiled by the U.S. Commission On Violence suggest that the victim is often known to the murderer, the murderer is likely to be young (late teens or early twenties), and the murderer is usually male, although the incidence of female murderers is increasing.

THE CHILD ABUSER/THE ABUSED CHILD

Having experienced child abuse himself often predisposes an individual to become a child abuser and/or a person of violence. Chronic child abusers (in contrast with a person who has a single episode of loss of control) often show some of the following characteristics: (1) the abuser was often an abused child himself; (2) he is isolated, with few friends and family to provide support; (3) he is untrusting and has a history of being unable to accept help from others, and therefore avoids contact with social and health care agencies or providers; (4) he has high standards and a high level of expectation for both himself and his children; and (5) he has a poor self-image and looks to the child for psychological support. These factors, combined with a precipitating crisis (e.g., a child who will not stop crying or the recent loss of a job or a lover) may be enough to trigger a battering situation.

Once an abusive situation is identified, the next steps are quite variable. If the child is extremely young, he is often removed from the home because of the extreme danger to physical life posed by any additional battering. If the child is older, intensive counseling with the parents and the child separately, and then together as a family (with someone there to act as an advocate for the child), is often recommended. If the abuse is severe and repeated, and the parent(s) resist treatment, the agency evaluating or working with the situation (often children's protective services) may recommend that the child be placed outside the home for an extensive period and sometimes permanently. Procedures and practices vary enormously, however, from state to state and even from community to community.

It is crucial (and required by law) that every physician report any case of *suspected* child abuse, as little other advocacy exists for the abused child. Only minor inroads have been made on this problem, which is considered by some to be the leading cause of death in children. There is a final sobering thought on the subject: Whereas 5% of child abusers are psychotic and 20% abuse their children because of a momentary loss of impulse control, the remaining 75% of parents show chronic and deliberate abuse of their children (4–6).

REFERENCES

1. Bassuk, E., and Gerson, S. (1980): Chronic crisis patients: a discrete clinical group. *Am. J. Psychiatry*, 137:1513–1517.
2. Dubin, W. (Jefferson Hospital, Philadelphia), and Petrich, J. (University of Washington School of Medicine, Seattle): Personal communication.
2a. Dubin, W. and Lurie, H. J. (producers and script) (1982): *The Diagnosis and Treatment of the Violent Patient* (videotape). University of Washington, Seattle.
3. Miller, D. (1973): The violent individual. *Audiodigest Psychiatry*, 2:19.
4. Rothenberg, M. (1974): The war of the eggs: child abuse revisited. Address for the Department of Psychiatry and Behavioral Sciences, University of Washington School of Medicine, Seattle.
5. Helfer, R. E. and Kempe, C. H. (1968): *The Battered Child*. University of Chicago Press, Chicago.
6. Kempe, C. H., and Helfer, R. E. (1972): *Helping the Battered Child and His Family*, Lippincott, Philadelphia.

14

Psychiatric Complications of Medical Drugs

Because many drugs commonly prescribed by primary physicians have psychiatric symptomatology as some of their side effects, it seems useful to list them here. This listing is by no means comprehensive, and neither the rationales for using the drugs nor the reasons for their side effects are included. There are excellent and comprehensive publications describing these psychiatric symptoms in some detail. A bibliography of some of these publications is included at the end of the chapter.

Psychiatric Side Effects of Ordinary Drugs

Drug	Side effects
Barbiturates	Excitement, hyperactivity, visual hallucinations, depression, delirium-tremens-like syndrome, confusion, disorientation, ataxia, impaired memory.
Bromides	Disorientation, memory impairment, mental confusion, hallucinations, gross confusional states, headaches, tremors.
Anticonvulsants	Tactile, visual and auditory hallucinations, delirium, agitation, depression, paranoia, confusion, aggression. These usually occur with high doses or high plasma concentrations.

Anticholinergics and atropine compounds (belladonna alkaloids, Cogentin®, scopolamine)	Confusion, memory loss, disorientation, depersonalization, delirium, auditory and visual hallucinations, fear, paranoia. These side effects occur more frequently in the elderly and children, and with high doses. Mistakenly using eye drops for nose drops may produce sudden delirium, incoherent speech, and high fever.
Major tranquilizers	Akathisia (motor restlessness—patient looks agitated), extrapyramidal syndrome (oculogyric crises), orthostatic hypotension, tardive dyskinesia.
Minor tranquilizers	Rage, excitement, hallucinations, depression, suicidal thoughts. These symptoms can occur with ordinary doses, whereas depression and hallucinations usually occur on withdrawal.
Tricyclic antidepressants	Anticholinergic psychosis: increased depression, depersonalization, hypomania, marked sedation, agitation with some patients, hallucinatory confusional state (particularly with the elderly), mental confusion.
Antihistamines	Anxiety, hallucinations, delirium, especially with overdosage.
Cimetidine	Visual and auditory hallucinations, paranoia, bizarre speech, confusion, delirium, disorientation, depression. These are more frequent with high dosages, especially with the elderly or with renal dysfunction.
Antiparkinsonian drugs	Confusional states, excitement, hallucinations.
Levodopa	Delirium, depression, agitation, hypomania, nightmares, night terrors, visual and auditory hallucinations, paranoia. These are seen more frequently in the elderly, with increased risk after prolonged use.
Phenacetin	Depression of mood, energy, and mental functioning.
Disulfuram	Delirium, depression, paranoia, auditory hallucinations. Not related to alcohol reactions.
Indomethacin	Depression, confusion, hallucinations, anxiety, hostility, paranoia, depersonalization—especially in the elderly.

Methyldopa	Depression, hallucinations, paranoia, amnesia.
Salicylates	Headache, weakness, paresthesias and tremors, hallucinations.
Sulfonamides	Headache, malaise, dizziness, paresthesias, tinnitus. In children there may also be sleep disturbance, nightmares, confusion, disorientation, illusions, hallucinations.
Penicillin	Mental confusion, hallucinations, hallucinatory confusional state with anxiety and motor agitation (from depot penicillin).
Isoniazid	Depression, agitation, auditory and visual hallucinations, paranoia.
Guanethidine	Depression (mild), ejaculatory delay.
Digitalis glycosides	Nightmares, euphoria, confusion, delusions, amnesia, belligerence, visual hallucinations, paranoia. Usually with excessive dose or high plasma concentration, especially in the elderly.
Rauwolfia alkaloids/reserpine	Depression—occurs commonly with doses higher than 0.5 mg daily and may continue for months after drug is stopped.
Corticosteroids	Mania, depression, confusion, paranoia, visual and auditory hallucinations, catatonia, euphoria. Symptoms are more common with high doses or a rapid increase in dose, with depression often occurring when the drug is withdrawn. Occasionally psychotic symptoms are present which mimic schizophrenia or affective psychosis.
Oral contraceptives	Depression, especially with drugs with high progesterone and low estrogen; decrease in libido, especially with continuous rather than sequential pills.
Pentazocine	Nightmares, hallucinations, disorientation, panic paranoia, depersonalization, depression.
Phenylephrine	Depression, visual and tactile hallucinations, paranoia, usually from overuse of nasal sprays.
Propranolol	Depression, confusion, nightmares, visual and auditory hallucinations, paranoia. Sometimes reported with usual dosages or after dosage increase.

BIBLIOGRAPHY

Greenblatt, D. J. and Shader, R. I. (1974): *Benzodiazepines in Clinical Practice*. Raven Press, New York.
Hollister, L. E. (1973): *Clinical Use of Psychotherapeutic Drugs*. Charles C. Thomas, Springfield, IL.
Kaplan, H. S. (1975): The effects of drugs on sexuality. In: *The New Sex Therapy*, pp. 86–103. Brunner/Mazel, New York.
Pare, C. M. B. (1973): Psychiatric complications of everyday drugs. *Practitioner*, 210:120–126.
Shader, R. I., editor (1972): *Psychiatric Complications of Medical Drugs*. Raven Press, New York.
Shader, R. I., editor (1975): *Manual of Psychiatric Therapeutics*. Little, Brown, Boston.

15

Systems Strategy: Crisis Intervention in Office Practice

Since the beginning of community psychiatry 15 to 20 years ago, when many of the principles of public health began to be applied to mental health, increasing attention has been focused on the reactions of individuals, families, and communities to acute stress situations. Increasing evidence suggests that during an intense crisis an individual's vulnerability to emotional disorder increases significantly; how the crisis is resolved determines very much the degree of subsequent emotional morbidity. While trying to grapple with and resolve the physical, psychological, and social aspects of a crisis, an individual is particularly subject to influence by key persons in his social network. This fact is the theoretical basis for crisis intervention strategies developed by health and mental health personnel (1).

A final but central notion to the concept of a crisis is that it is a breakdown of an individual's or family's normal homeostatic pattern. The implication of this, of course, is that the physician or other helper who assesses a crisis must look not only at the specific events which appear to have initiated the stress but also at the more subtle breakdown and changes in the functioning of the person's world. A death in the family may have to be assessed not only from the point of view of personal loss but also from the standpoint of the change in financial security, the need to change living arrangements, the decrease in social contacts in general, and the change in social status. Feelings related to these secondary changes are extremely important.

Some of the components of acute crisis intervention in any setting include: (1) identifying what the crisis is; (2) working in the "here and now" to develop specific ways to stop the crisis; (3) mobilizing appropriate supportive figures and institutions within the community to help the patient; and (4) having sufficient time, personnel, and follow-up capacity to carry the person or his family through the crisis—through item (2), above—to a level of functioning equal to that existing prior to the crisis.

Any crisis has precipitating causes, and identifying these causes and the methods by which these factors can be modified to prevent further crisis is as important as successful treatment of the acute crisis. The physician therefore must be prepared to call on his staff and colleagues and on persons who are part of the patient's own milieu to effect a long-term solution to the problem.

Example

> A young mother comes to a physician's office saying that she is so nervous she is falling apart and must have some tranquilizers or she will go crazy. Inquiry reveals that her husband, who used to work days, has just begun working the night shift. There are two children in diapers and three children under 5 for whom the mother is caring without assistance. During a recent financial crisis, the checking account was overdrawn, so this month's pay check must be used to pay back the bank. The woman feels that the marriage is deteriorating, and that her husband does not love her anymore. She has come to the doctor today because she just realized that she gets so angry at the youngest child she sometimes really feels like murdering him.

The crisis appears to be the culmination of many factors leading to the acute symptoms of being overwhelmed, panicky, unable to make decisions, and filled with intense rage. Steps the doctor might take include the following:

1. Diagnose that this is indeed a crisis.
2. Ask an office nurse, a public health nurse, or a social worker to go to the home and assess what is really happening there.
3. Suggest to the husband that he come in to talk over the possibility of changing his working hours so that he could give his wife some physical help during the periods of the day when she is feeling most harassed. Here, the physician might have to convince the husband that the house and child care chores are really too much for one person to handle without occasional breaks. The physician may also have to be supportive during the husband's initial difficulty in retaining his self-esteem and sense of masculinity while he changes diapers, feeds the baby, etc.
4. (This step could be an addition to or a substitution for step 3.) Inquire about any relatives who might be called on to help or investigate the possibility of getting someone else (e.g., a homemaker) to come in to help with the children when they are particularly demanding or difficult.
5. Make arrangements for the physician, nurse, receptionist, or someone else from the office to see the patient often enough to allow her to ventilate her feelings to someone other than her husband. This "objective outsider" could also help the patient move toward doing some constructive problem-solving.
6. Make a referral to a community financial planning resource which could work out an appropriate budget for reducing the family debts and thus ease some of the acute financial worries. Frequently banks are of great assistance in advising an individual or family about consolidating debts and paying them off in a rational way.

7. Make specific, concrete recommendations for the husband and wife to spend some time together outside the home. Suggest that a relative or neighbor come in and baby-sit so that the couple can get away at least for a hamburger or a movie now and then.
8. Consider prescribing medications such as a minor tranquilizer or a tricyclic antidepressant.
9. Know the resources of the community well enough to suggest an appropriate nursery school for one of the children. As nursery schools frequently refuse to take a child who is not toilet-trained, the physician may have to make a personal plea to the nursery school director to accept the child. A cooperative play group would also be a good strategy for both the children and the mother (as the mother would have contact with other mothers with similar problems). Likewise, cooperative baby-sitting arrangements among mothers are becoming more and more common, where "payment" is made on the basis of baby-sitting time, rather than money.
10. Refer the couple, if necessary, for some additional specialized help in solving a specific problem. For example, a parent-effectiveness training group might help the woman and her husband learn how to handle the children, a life planning or assertiveness course might help the woman meet her own needs outside the family, etc.

A primary physician is also likely to see many acute crises taking the form of acute depression related to a separation in the family, death, impending divorce, loss of a job, breakdown of a hoped-for marriage or promotion, impending retirement, etc. Crises often occur around specific developmental changes in a person's life, particularly during adolescence, at the time of the birth of the first child, when first separated from home, and pre- or post-retirement.

The crisis may present in many forms: a student deciding to drop out of school, a leading citizen getting a first driving-while-intoxicated citation, a suicide attempt, an episode of marital infidelity and subsequent guilt, etc. The important thing for the physician to remember is that he alone need not have all the responsibility for solving the crisis. As mentioned in Chapter 1, his office staff can learn to provide supportive contact and initiate constructive problem-solving if both he and they are aware of community resources which might be called on to help solve the crisis. The doctor can use his professional clout to call in the rest of the family and diplomatically persuade them to relate to the patient in a different way. Giving the anxious and distraught patient mentioned above a pill and sending her on her way "hoping for the best" may make the physician feel that he did something but will not help in the long run or prevent her return.

To be equipped as a mini-crisis intervention center, the primary physician's office should have the following.

1. A list of all the community resources designed to assist with the kinds of trouble patients or their families may present. Hopefully, the physician or his staff

has a friendly enough relationship with these resources that they can be called on for information and consultation, and will accept referrals when necessary.

2. A staff whose members work well together and have enough rapport with each other and the physician that they can quickly and easily adopt helpful roles in addition to their prescribed roles of receptionist, office nurse, etc. (Chapter 1).

3. Dual competence in some office tasks so that when a crisis does come up, one person can take time to deal with it while the office continues to function smoothly. Other patients are not short-changed in this situation as the intervenor's regular duties are automatically assumed by other staff members. The crisis may not have to be dealt with exhaustively the same day it occurs or comes to the physician's attention, but it is necessary that someone have sufficient time to investigate the components of the crisis so as to map out all the ingredients of its solution. This approach is quite similar to problem-oriented charting, where a variety of problems are listed along with specific strategies for addressing each one, including those which have no apparent or immediate solution.

In addition to these items, the following should also be present.

4. The physician should feel comfortable in setting limited goals for patients and having limited expectations of treatment. Doctors become so accustomed to "curing" that they may have difficulty recognizing that at times simply improving a chronically bad situation may be all that is either feasible or desirable.

5. The physician and his team must understand that families and patients generally have a great deal of innate strength. Once an acute problem is solved, it may be legitimate and desirable for the physician to withdraw rather than be constantly available in an advice-giving capacity. At the same time, the doctor must have the ability to sense when his continued support is needed (even on a casual basis) to prevent a chronically difficult situation from erupting into an acute crisis. Simply knowing that "someone is available" should the need arise often provides enough psychological comfort to keep an explosive person or situation under control.

6. The physician and his team must be able to consult with other agencies undertaking crisis intervention, e.g., the hospital emergency room, police, schools. Sometimes a "crisis" exists simply because an agency or institution becomes alarmed: The crisis may be as much in the feelings of helplessness of a school counselor or a harassed policeman as in the situation itself. Here the doctor can help the institution or individual use the same problem-solving approach: Clarify the problem and examine various solutions. For example, those schools which suspend pupils for smoking cigarettes may profit by the physician's abilities to arbitrate between school, pupil, and family and calm down both "the system" and the "culprits" involved.

REFERENCE

1. Caplan, G. (1981): Mastery of stress: psychosocial aspects. *Am. J. Psychiatry*, 138:413–420.

16

Adult Psychotic Illnesses

Patients are defined as psychotic when their mental functioning is sufficiently impaired to interfere grossly with their capacity to meet the ordinary demands of life. The primary physician encounters few psychotic patients in his practice, but he should have some awareness of the different types of psychotic illness, what strategies are most likely to be effective for interrupting the course of the illness in its early stages, how to alleviate residual problems when the patient has returned from the hospital, and how to use various treatment modalities.

Psychotic illnesses (Table 16-1) fall roughly into the following categories: (1) psychoses associated with organic brain syndromes (e.g., delirium and dementia, with global cognitive impairment); (2) schizophrenic disorders; (3) psychoses related to mood disturbances (major depressive disorder with psychotic features, manic-depressive disorder with psychotic features) (Chapter 11); and (4) illnesses with a mixture of affective and schizophrenic features (schizoaffective disorders).

MENTAL STATUS EXAMINATION

The mental status examination is a standardized procedure of structured questions and observations which assist the clinician in making a judgment about the functioning of a patient. A mental status examination is particularly useful for determining whether the patient has a condition which contains psychotic features or one which includes elements of organic brain disease. A mental status examination is an ancillary measure to confirm "hunches" elicited by a detailed history which either the patient or his relatives provide. Because some parts of the mental status examination include questions which are rarely included in social conversation, it is important to preface these questions with an explanatory remark. For example:

> I'm going to ask you an odd question which will help me understand your thinking. First I'm going to ask you to interpret proverbs or sayings, and I'd like you to tell me what they mean. The first one is, "Don't cry over spilt milk."

If the patient is obviously oriented to who he is, the place at which the examination is being conducted, and the date, it may be all right to omit that part of the mental status examination. At the same time, routinely including most parts is often important, as a person may appear normal even if he has severe memory or thinking problems. The following are the major dimensions of a mental status examination (1). Any item may be noted to be present (mild to severe) or absent.

Appearance

The more bizarre the appearance of the patient or the more unobservant of social amenities he is, the more likely it is that a psychotic process is part of the clinical picture. (The economic status of the patient, of course, must be considered; that is, poverty may result in ragged clothing; and a well-dressed individual may be severely disturbed.) A person neglectful of his appearance and body may be psychotic, forgetful (e.g., senile), or depressed.

Body condition: unkempt, dirty.
Clothing: disheveled, dirty, bizarre.
Unusual physical features: mutilations, scars, deformities, odd personal features.

Behavior

The patient's behavior often provides clues about his state of mind. Posture, facial expression, speech patterns, body movements, assessment of feelings, and an assessment of the relationship with the physician all provide behavioral clues which help determine the level of functioning and the presence or absence of psychotic thinking. All of the items to be assessed under "behavior" rely largely on the examiner's perceptions, not on the patient's self-report. Specific items to be evaluated include the following.

1. Posture.
   a. Slumped in a chair or otherwise drooping posture—suggesting depression.
   b. Rigid or tense—suggesting anxiety.
   c. Atypical or bizarre posture—suggesting a psychotic disorder.
2. Facial expression.
   a. Anxious/fearful—suggesting anxiety.
   b. Depressed—suggesting depression.
   c. Angry/bizarre/inappropriate—suggesting a psychotic state.
3. Speech.
   a. Tempo increased—suggesting mania, drug intoxication.
   b. Tempo decreased—suggesting depression, hypothyroidism, drug intoxication, occasionally mental retardation, occasionally expressive aphasias.
   c. Volume increased—suggesting mania, drug intoxication.
   d. Volume decreased—suggesting depression.
   e. Atypical—e.g., slurred, suggesting intoxication; bizarre use of language, suggesting schizophrenia.

TABLE 16-1. *Psychotic illnesses: symptoms and treatment*

Psychosis	Major symptoms	Drugs of choice	Treatment plan
Organic brain syndrome (organic psychoses)	General: disorder of memory, judgment, affect, orientation, intellectual functioning.	Tranquilizers only for agitation. Usually all medications are to be avoided.	Structured environment, clear directions, consistent therapeutic plan; reality orientation and remotivation.
Chronic brain syndrome, irreversible (dementia)	Symptoms as above. With vascular insufficiency, may show fluctuating levels of functioning. Memory loss or inappropriate affect may be first symptom.	Same as above.	Same as above.
Chronic brain syndrome, acute, reversible (delirium)	Same as above but often related to external or metabolic intoxication. May present with clouded sensorium, confusion, and trouble paying attention.	Same as above.	Diagnostic assessment to find and treat intoxication; sometimes EEG monitoring and psychological testing.
Schizophrenias	General: bizarre delusions or somatic or grandiose delusions or persecutory delusions, auditory hallucinations, loosening of associations and illogical thinking. Deterioration from a previous level of functioning. Continuous duration of at least 6 months.		
Brief reactive psychosis	Panic, agitation, hallucinations, loose associations, some delusional thinking; sometimes the sense of falling apart. May be triggered by environmental stress.	Major tranquilizers, although often needed only acutely for initial symptom removal.	For acute illness, rapid mobilization of support, acute hospitalization, work with family, follow-up.
Disorganized (hebephrenic) psychosis	Giggling, grimacing, flattened affect, regressed behavior. No systemized delusions or hallucinations.	Major tranquilizers.	Structured environment; may need day care or adult foster placement.
Catatonia	Mutism, stereotyped behaviors, automatic obedience, and major symptoms (above).	Major tranquilizers.	Structured environment; mental hospital; day care or adult foster care.

Paranoia	Grandiose thinking, paranoid ideas, delusions and hallucinations often persecutory, and major symptoms (above).	Major tranquilizers.	Supportive but not overly friendly. Needs life planning; can often work and socialize.
Undifferentiated psychosis	Grossly disorganized behavior, delusions, hallucinations, flat or inappropriate affect, tangential thinking, and major symptoms (above).	Major tranquilizers (may need combination which controls agitation and overactivity plus thinking disorder).	Structured environment, socialization groups, and very persistent medical follow-up.
Major depressive episode with psychosis	Depressed mood, slowed thinking, sleep and eating disturbances, somatic delusions, anxiety or agitation. Symptoms of major depressive episode (anhedonia, sleep disturbance, appetite disturbance, psychomotor agitation or retardation, plus delusions or hallucinations with content about guilt, inadequacy, disease, death, etc., or mood incongruent delusions or hallucinations (e.g., persecutory delusions).	Tricyclic antidepressants; may have to combine with major tranquilizers or use ECT, especially if suicidal and unresponsive to tricyclic antidepressants.	Very close follow-up, mobilization of family and other support; group or individual treatment. If suicidal: hospitalization, suicide precautions, support by family and therapeutic team.
Depression of old age	Depressed mood, sleep and eating disturbances, severe anxiety, agitation, somatic delusions, paranoid ideas.	ECT, especially if suicidal and unresponsive to tricyclic antidepressants; sometimes with addition of major tranquilizers.	Hospitalization, support by family and therapeutic team, suicide precautions.
Manic-depressive psychoses	Recurrent or simultaneous manic or depressive episodes; often strong family history. In mania: elation, pressured speech, hyperactivity, grandiosity, sexual preoccupation. In depression: akin to psychotic depressive reaction with a lot of hostility showing through.	Lithium carbonate (on a maintenance basis). Major tranquilizers or tricyclics, acutely.	May need highly structured environment including hospital. Watch for suicide attempts when patient switching from depressed to manic phase.

NB: A recent book, *Clinical Use of Psychotherapeutic Drugs* (by Leo E. Hollister; Charles C Thomas, Springfield, IL, 1973), has an excellent and detailed description of antipsychotic, antimanic, antidepressant, and antianxiety drugs, as well as the use of drugs with children with major psychological disturbances.

4. Body movement.
   a. Increased—suggesting mania, anxiety.
   b. Decreased—suggesting depression, sedation, some schizophrenic disorders.
   c. Atypical—bizarre use of body, suggesting a movement disorder (e.g., a tic) or some kinds of schizophrenia.
   d. Restless—suggesting anxiety, drug side effects (e.g., akathisias secondary to major tranquilizers).
5. Feelings (affect and mood).
   a. Mood inappropriate to thought content (e.g., patient smiles when talking about mother's death)—suggesting schizophrenia.
   b. Mood lability: mood swings during interview—suggesting organic brain disorder, bipolar affective disorder, cyclothymic disorder.
   c. Predominant mood: depressed, anxious, elated, absent or blunted, hostile.
6. Relationship to interviewer.
   a. Domineering.
   b. Overly submissive and compliant.
   c. Provocative (e.g., seductive/hostile).
   d. Suspicious (does the patient include you in a paranoid delusion?).
   e. Uncooperative.

Perceptions

With certain organic states (e.g., intoxication and delirium) as well as with schizophrenic disorders, there are often abnormalities of perception, especially hallucinations. Auditory hallucinations are most frequently associated with schizophrenic disorders, whereas intoxication or delirium is more frequently associated with visual or unusual hallucinations (e.g., hallucinations of delirium tremens, which include visual and tactile hallucinations of bugs crawling on the skin). In toxic states, as well as with sleep deprivation and severe states of anxiety, illusions (misperceptions of reality—a tree mistaken for a person) are sometimes present. Asking about all of these phenomena as well as noticing their possible presence during the interview is necessary (e.g., does the patient turn suddenly, as if in response to voices).

1. Perception.
   a. Illusions present.
   b. Auditory hallucinations (present or previously reported).
   c. Visual hallucinations (present or previously reported).
   d. Other types of hallucinations.

Thinking

Assessment of both the process and the content of thinking is an essential part of the mental status examination. In some psychotic disorders (e.g., schizophrenia), the content of the thinking (e.g., paranoid delusions of persecution) as well as the form of the thinking (e.g., loose associations, nonlogical sequences of thought) may be disordered. Certain aspects of thinking, especially recent memory, attention span, judgment, and ability to calculate, are frequently impaired with either acute or chronic organic brain disease. The ability to think abstractly may be impaired with schizophrenia, organic brain disease, mental retardation, and limited formal education. Orientation is impaired in acute disorders such as dementia and acute psychotic states (e.g., reactive psychoses, schizophreniform disorder). Because social niceties may be maintained even if a person has extremely poor memory, it is usually important to formally inquire about each of these areas to make sure one is not inadvertently missing a deficit of thinking. Specific "topics" to be inquired about include the following:

1. Orientation.
   a. Disoriented to person. (What is your name?)
   b. Disoriented to place. (What is this place?)
   c. Disoriented to time. (What day is this?)
   d. Orientation is lost in delirium, acute schizophrenia (at times), or severe chronic organic brain conditions (senile dementia).
2. Intellectual functioning.
   a. Impaired level of consciousness (lost in delirium).
   b. Impaired attention span: Noted by observation throughout the interview but also by asking the patient to remember digits forward and backward (e.g., repeating five digits forward and four backward). May be impaired in dementia, delirium, and states of severe anxiety.
   c. Impaired abstract thinking: Tested by asking patient to interpret proverbs: "Don't cry over spilt milk." "Two heads are better than one." "The grass is greener on the other side of the fence." "People who live in glass houses shouldn't throw stones." The ability to abstract may be impaired in dementias, delirium, schizophrenia (proverbs are often very personalized), or where the intellectual or educational level is limited.
   d. Impaired calculation ability: Tested by asking patient to do simple addition, multiplication, and subtraction (e.g., "serial sevens": subtract 7 from 100 and keep subtracting). May be impaired in dementias and with massive anxiety.
   e. Impaired intelligence: Evaluated by estimating the patient's current level of intellectual functioning and seeing if this corresponds to the intellectual abilities of the patient, as estimated by his verbal facility, school attainment, income, and job status. In toxic states, dementias, and some chronic schizophrenic states, the patient appears to have significantly deteriorated from his previous level of functioning. Fund of normal information may be tested by asking the names of five large cities, identification of famous people, etc.
   f. Impaired insight: Patient has little understanding of his psychological problem, blames others, or distorts or denies the situation. May be seen in a wide

variety of conditions, ranging from antisocial individuals to schizophrenia to chronic dementias. May be explored by asking person what is wrong with him, why he is in a hospital or nursing home, etc.

g. Impaired judgment: Patient has impaired ability to manage activities of daily living or to make reasonable life decisions. May be tested by asking patient common sense questions: "What would you do if you found a stamped, addressed letter?" "What would you do if you noticed a house on fire?" "What would you do if you were lost in a store?" May be impaired in schizophrenia, dementia, or sometimes severe anxiety states. Also may be impaired with significant mental retardation.

h. Impaired memory: Impaired immediate memory (within 10 seconds).

i. Impaired recent memory (several minutes to several months): Cannot remember three objects after 5 minutes, cannot remember what he had for breakfast, the current President, his current address or phone number.

j. Impaired remote memory: Cannot remember significant events from the past, including place and date of birth, date of marriage, kinds of employment and places of employment, names of his children. (Immediate and recent memory are expecially susceptible to impairment with organic brain disease, both acute and chronic, as well as depression. Remote memory is rarely lost, except in severe dementias or chronic schizophrenias.)

TYPES OF PSYCHOSES

Psychoses with Organic Brain Disease

A psychosis secondary to an organic brain disorder may be due to a variety of etiological factors, ranging from head injuries, encephalitis, and brain tumors to acute and chronic intoxications (lead, alcohol, bromides, etc.). Although specific labeling of these disorders may be left to specialists, it is important for the primary physician who suspects an organic impairment to assess orientation, memory, intellectual functioning, and judgment, as these areas are the most likely to be impaired in organic brain disease.

The major categories to be looked for are: (1) *Delirium:* Consciousness is clouded; attention is reduced; there is disorientation and memory impairment; there may be speech incoherence and perceptual disturbance (e.g., hallucinations). The clinical course is rapid in onset and related to a specific organic factor (a blow on the head, a poison, a specific viral agent). Deliriums are usually brief, self-limited, and reversible. (2) *Dementia* is the other major organic brain disease diagnostic category. Here there is a loss of intellectual abilities sufficient to interfere with social or occupational functioning. Findings include: (a) impaired memory (especially recent memory); (b) possible impaired abstract thinking and judgment; (c) possible organic language disorder, motor disorder, or failure to recognize or identify familiar objects; and (d) a personality change. The state of consciousness is not clouded. There is a history of a specific (presumed) organic etiological agent. In some elderly people, a major depressive illness often mimics dementia. At times, an acute intoxication (e.g., alcohol, cannabis) may resemble either a delirious state or a dementia.

Management of Organic Psychosis

Thorough Work-Up

Because a wide variety of medical, degenerative, and neurological illnesses may produce a clinical picture corresponding to an organic psychosis, it is imperative that a detailed work-up be done to rule out illnesses such as subdural hematomas. Only after such a work-up can one conclude, for example, that the clinical picture is consistent with senile or presenile dementia (i.e., an irreversible picture arising in late life, the former arbitrarily occurring after age 65), for neither of which is there currently an effective treatment.

Mimicking both organic and nonorganic psychoses are states such as endocrine abnormalities, e.g., thyrotoxicosis. Chronic subdural hematomas and brain tumors simulate degenerative processes. Drug intoxications produce disorientation and hallucinations similar to schizophrenia; and infectious diseases (e.g., syphilis) may also be mistaken for other kinds of nonorganic and organic psychoses.

As part of a work-up, it is useful for a primary physician to consider using a checklist to look at the differential diagnostic possibilities for the patient with an organic psychosis. Is it likely to be degenerative, demyelinating, malignant, vascular, endocrine, traumatic, infectious, allergic, or an intoxication? Appropriate tests (and conclusions) are determined after the preliminary evaluation using such a checklist (2).

With a number of elderly patients who have a mild underlying organic brain syndrome, a sudden physical crisis ranging from the flu or a cold to constipation may trigger a full-blown organic psychotic picture, with delirium, confusion, paranoia, and delusional thinking. With elderly patients, therefore, it is particularly critical to search for any current decompensation in physical status which may have triggered a toxic acute organic syndrome. Similarly, over-the-counter sleeping medications or other sedatives in such a patient with borderline intellectual functioning may produce symptoms of a toxic organic psychosis (toxic delirium). This is especially true for medications containing scopolamine, which is often poorly tolerated in the elderly. The differential diagnostic possibilities in this age group, therefore, should start with a careful scrutiny of the more mundane aspects of the elderly person's life and physical functioning.

A Structured Environment

When managing a patient with severe organic brain syndrome of psychotic proportions, it is crucial that a highly structured, predictable, and stable environment be established to help the patient function at his maximal level. Specific routines and procedures, involving both personnel working with such a patient and the patient himself, should be worked out with the cooperation of the entire staff; such routines should be posted and, where appropriate, given to the patient. In order to make a patient's environment as predictable and stable as possible, it may be wise to designate only a few specific staff persons to work with the individual. Visits with friends and relatives should be designed to be as nonthreatening as possible for the patient and should be carefully explained to the patient ahead of time.

An intense reality orientation program should be established for patients who are disoriented (Chapter 9). Every attempt should be made to involve a patient as much as possible in meaningful activity and to maintain and expand his areas of intellectual functioning. As soon as feasible, the patient should be encouraged to spend time specializing on a regular basis with at least one other patient, and a concerted effort should be made to increase the patient's areas of social functioning. One way to start this is by making sure the patient eats his meals with someone else and is not sitting in front of the television set all day long. Those patients who have specific neurological deficits, of course, should have specific remedial therapy under the supervision of an occupational therapist.

Psychological Testing

Psychological testing is considered in more detail later (Chapter 19). However, it is worth mentioning here that psychological testing for the degree of organic impairment should be done at the start of treatment and sequentially as treatment proceeds. This allows an assessment of progress and aids in delineating those areas of continued impairment.

Medications

Medications are usually contraindicated for an organic brain syndrome, whether acute (reversible) or chronic (irreversible), because of the confusing effects the medications have on the clinical picture. (If the patient is less alert, is it because of the medication or his disease process?) If the patient is extremely agitated, some sort of tranquilizer may be indicated acutely; however, the dosage should be maintained at the lowest possible level so that the patient can maintain optimal contact with his environment and the people within it, rather than being "snowed" into indifference. The patient may need sleeping medication, but this should also be carefully monitored.

Disorientation at Night

Certain individuals with an organic brain syndrome become quite disoriented and delusional at night, even though they are relatively well oriented during the day. It may be very important that night lights, frequent checks by the night nurse or aide, and possibly nighttime sedation be considered for such patients, as this experience of disorientation is obviously terrifying for the individual involved.

Electroencephalographic Monitoring

For those acute and chronic brain syndromes that are secondary to intoxication (metabolic or environmental), a clinical picture of delirium is usually present; in these cases the patient has greater difficulty attending, as he experiences a reduction in his level of consciousness and cognitive functioning. Electroencephalographic (EEG) slowing closely correlates with this kind of clinical picture, and so the patient's progress can often be followed by monitoring the EEG (3).

The Schizophrenias

Most schizophrenic illnesses begin during adolescence or young adulthood and often occur at times of stress: when the patient is separating from home or family or when some of the conflicts of normal maturation occur (e.g., the need to make vocational choices or to demonstrate sexual competence and assertiveness).

The *paranoid schizophrenias* tend to begin somewhat later than other types. Chronic cases of *disorganized (hebephrenic) schizophrenia* (outbursts of giggling or grimacing, regressed and disheveled appearance, occasional incontinence) and *catatonic schizophrenia* (mutism, stereotyped behaviors, automatic obedience, and maintenance of a particular bodily posture for long periods of time) are seen less frequently with the advent of more effective treatment measures.

We now know that rapid and vigorous intervention often prevents such illnesses from reaching the level of chronic, regressed, and deteriorated behavior formerly associated with the picture of the person with a schizophrenic illness. Drug therapy, intensive supportive follow-up of the patient and his family, adult day treatment services, and prolonged availability to manage or handle the patient through his job, personal, or financial crises are very important and help greatly to reduce the likelihood of additional episodes.

It is sometimes quite difficult for the clinician to distinguish between a true schizophrenic illness—wherein thinking becomes progressively delusional and the patient seems to be deteriorating and withdrawing into his own fantasies, projections, and morbid or bizarre preoccupations—and a severe version of an "identity crisis" that occurs with many adolescents (Chapter 7). The diagnosis of schizophrenia is not made based just on "crazy" behavior; schizophrenia is a severe disorder of thinking and behavior. (A detailed description of the criteria and the illness may be found in Chapter 7.)

During an identity crisis, on the other hand, an adolescent patient may seem crazy and fragmented because of panic and agitation about his life situation, his repudiation of former values, and his putting into action many of his fantasies and wishes in order to be free of family and responsibility. Distinguishing between an identity crisis and a schizophrenic illness involves looking at the degree to which a person is able to function socially and intellectually, how aware he is of the process he is experiencing, and how fragmented his thinking is. By the very nature of the processes involved, the person with an identity crisis has a heightened awareness of what he is experiencing, whereas the person with psychotic decompensation may be experiencing increasing withdrawal into his own peculiar and private world of highly personalized and frequently jumbled thoughts, perceptions, and feelings. The distinction is illustrated by the contrast between the sadness, cynicism, and disenchantment of the protagonist in J. D. Salinger's *The Catcher in the Rye* and the nightmarish, panicky thoughts, feelings, and delusions plaguing the schizophrenic protagonist of Hannah Green's *I Never Promised You a Rose Garden*.

People having an identity crisis often respond to supportive counseling by an outsider who has sufficient time to sit down and listen to the conflicts manifested by the contradictory behavior and thinking. The appearance of schizophrenia in an adolescent or adult is much more ominous. The patient with a schizophrenic breakdown may come to the physician's attention because of gradually deteriorating school performance, withdrawal, bizarre ideas or thoughts, or sometimes a suicide attempt. Any of these may be accompanied by delusions or hallucinations and irrelevant, disorganized, or tangential thinking.

If a first episode of psychosis is apparently triggered by environmental stress and has an acute onset (rather than a gradual deterioration of functioning), it is a brief reactive psychosis, even if it resembles schizophrenia in its symptoms. If it lasts more than 2 weeks, however, it is called a *schizophreniform disorder*, and if it lasts more than 6 months it is called a *schizophrenic disorder*. This new scheme is an attempt to label more accurately brief psychotic episodes which do not, in fact, become a schizophrenic disorder and do not imply a poor prognosis or a chronic course.

When a diagnosis of schizophrenia is made (Table 16-1), some of the following steps can be taken:

Use of Medications

Medications in schizophrenic illnesses are useful for reducing psychotic thinking, including autistic preoccupations, hallucinations, and loose associations. Medications are also useful for reducing the degree of agitation or panic experienced by the patient, and they allow the patient to sleep. Sleep loss alone tends to aggravate psychotic symptoms and even produces hallucinations if the loss is sufficiently prolonged. Unfortunately, there are so many antipsychotic medications at the present time it is often difficult for the primary physician to know which or what to use. Excellent advice suggested by May (7) is that the physician become familiar with one drug from each of the five major tranquilizer categories, each of which would have specific indications for its use, and each of which would have individual and specific side effects. Although the distinctions and separations between the drugs are rarely clear-cut, the various categories (Table 16-2) include the following distinguishing characteristics:

Halogenated Phenothiazines

A drug such as chlorpromazine is useful in acutely disturbed, hallucinating schizophrenic patients. Advantages include the drug's rapid action, its availability in a variety of forms (oral and injectable), and its variety of dosages: 25 to 1,000 mg/day in the usual patients, or up to several thousand milligrams per day in severely

TABLE 16-2. *Antipsychotic drugs: pharmacological profile of factors that may influence drug selection in medically ill patients*

Drug	Sedation[a]	Extra-pyramidal side effects	Anti-cholinergic activity	Postural hypo-tension	Slowed cardiac conduction	Representative brands
Phenothiazines						
Chlorpromazine	3	2	2	3	—	Thorazine
Thioridazine	3	1	3	3	3	Mellaril
Mesoridazine	3	1	3	3	3	Serentil
Prochlorperazine	2	2	2	2	—	Compazine
Perphenazine	2	2	2	2	—	Trilafon
Trifluoperazine	2	2	2	2	—	Stelazine
Fluphenazine	1	3	2	2	—	Prolixin
Thioxanthene						
Thiothixene	2	2	2	2	—	Navane
Butyrophenones						
Haloperidol	1	3	1	1	—	Haldol
Droperidol	1	3	1	1	—	Inapsine
Dibenzoxazepines						
Loxapine	2	2	2	2	—	Loxitane
Indolics						
Molindone	2	2	2	2	—	Moban

From ref. 6.
[a]Rating: when compared to other drugs of the same class: 1 = least, 2 = intermediate, 3 = most.

agitated homicidal or manic patients. Disadvantages include its side effects of drowsiness and sedation, as well as orthostatic hypotension and parkinsonian-like effects found with large dosages.

Phenothiazines with a Piperazine Side Chain

A compound such as trifluoperazine might be especially suited to a chronic patient whose primary symptoms are a thinking disorder but without agitation or panic, or with an apathetic, retarded, or withdrawn catatonic patient. These compounds are given at lower dosages, are extremely potent, and are often useful in long-term treatment because of their gradual buildup of medication levels within the body (hence a missed dose or two does not immediately jeopardize the patient's clinical status). Disadvantages include the strong likelihood of extrapyramidal and other parkinsonian-like side effects in the course of treatment, sometimes with an alarming clinical picture such as an oculogyric crisis. Other disadvantages include their "lag time" of 1 to 3 weeks for maximal effect.

Mercaptophenothiazines

The mercaptophenothiazines, including thioridazine, are excellent for producing an immediate response. Thioridazine is often useful in agitated, acutely disturbed, hallucinating patients. Advantages include the rarity of parkinsonian-like and antiemetic side effects. Disadvantages include the danger of chorioretinitis with dosages over 900 mg/day, somewhat slowed cardiac conduction time, and the danger of orthostatic hypotension.

Butyrophenones

Compounds such as haloperidol are useful for both chronically ill and more acutely disturbed patients. They may be given by a variety of routes (oral, injectable). Like the piperazine side chain compounds, their major disadvantage is their marked propensity to produce parkinsonian-like symptoms.

Long-Acting Injectable Tranquilizers

At the present time, long-acting injectable tranquilizers include drugs such as fluphenazine decanoate. These medications are often particularly useful with patients who have been discharged from a psychiatric service and are adamant about not needing any medication. Adverse effects include extrapyramidal symptoms, as well as (like other high-potency antipsychotic medications), the possibility with chronic usage of the development of tardive dyskinesia: "purposeless, repetitive, and involuntary movements of the mouth, tongue, and face which may occur during or following the cessation of treatment with long-term neuroleptic medication" (4).

Caveat

Some useful concepts to consider when administering antipsychotic medication include: (1) use only one drug at a time as the side effects are additive; (2) use an effective enough dosage to control symptoms but try to discontinue or reduce the medication from time to time in view of the possibility of tardive dyskinesia; (3) explain clearly and often the rationale for the medication, preferably in a friendly and nonauthoritarian way. By the very nature of their illness, patients with schizophrenia are especially sensitive and irritated by efforts to control them and often resist such efforts assiduously.

Mobilizing a Support System

In addition to medication, prompt mobilization of the patient's support system is vital. This support system may include the classmates, advisors, and teachers of a college student, as well as the infirmary staff if the patient is temporarily hospitalized; the family, if they are coping with the situation rationally enough to be supportive; the spouse, girlfriend, or boyfriend; co-workers and understanding employers; and certainly the physician and his office staff. A "support system" refers to the network of relationships and activities which allows the patient to feel cared about—those persons with whom he can interact socially and emotionally during the crisis he is facing. The support system for an individual experiencing a schizophrenic illness can establish a structure that will reintegrate the patient with reality and help him continue in his normal activities (e.g., classes, job). Members of a support system can also be alert to possible suicidal preoccupation and monitor the level of the patient's dysfunction. The combination of medication and an active support system is extremely helpful in getting a person with schizophrenia over the initial acute episode.

After this stage of the illness, the task becomes somewhat more difficult, as many patients with less-acute schizophrenic illnesses resist continuing their medication and accepting further treatment. For younger patients, an adolescent or young people's therapy group is a good answer if expert psychiatric consultation is available and the effects of the group on the patient can be closely monitored. Such a group may be part of the school system (if the school has some sophistication about mental illness and is willing to try to maintain such patients in school), or it may be connected with a mental health clinic. Alternatively, groups may be established by a physician and his staff in the office. The group is a good forum for discussing issues bothering the patient: conflicts about growing up, anxieties about separating from the original family, sexuality, coping with social and work pressures, etc.

After an acute episode, prevention of relapse and rehospitalization depends, at least initially, on whether the patient is willing to continue medication and also whether he has accepted a trusted figure in his life—one who not only listens empathically but who can also work with him on long-term life planning. The physician or someone he designates can certainly be that person. If the doctor does not have the time to do this himself, he must formally hand the patient over to someone who does have the time: a minister trained in counseling, someone on his office staff, or a counselor in the community with psychiatric consultation and backup available. Accepting the patient's word that "everything is fine now" is perilous even if it seems expedient to do so at the moment, as the relapse rate for schizophrenics can be very high. Lehman states that with drug maintenance and follow-up therapy about 10 to 15% of patients in remission relapse within a year, compared to 35 to 40% who relapse without follow-up treatment (5).

In conclusion, the more the schizophrenic patient continues to have in the way of support, family, personal satisfactions (e.g., art, photography, music, friends, hobbies, a regular job), the better is his chance of recovery. For this reason, keeping the patient in the community, if possible, is the optimal goal. Sending him—even if he seems "crazy"—off to a hospital many miles from home will cut him off, perhaps permanently, from his sources of "nourishment." If referral to a mental hospital seems necessary, the stay should only be long enough to allow for medication adjustment and some degree of personality reconstitution. Treatment should then be transferred to community resources as soon as possible.

Psychotic Depressions

Patients with severe depressive illnesses are discussed in Chapter 11.

THE EX-MENTAL PATIENT

Many physicians come in contact with patients who have been in a mental hospital but have now returned to the community. The stereotypical view of such patients is that they are still more or less "crazy," resist treatment, and are "hopeless cases." Many persons who have been hospitalized on and off for years do exhibit one or more of these behaviors. On the other hand, many ex-mental patients are only mildly "eccentric" and many others would blend into society if their previous history were not known. Many ex-mental patients are capable of productive lives; their lack of a job may be related as much to their social naïveté and candor about their previous illness as to current disability.

The primary physician who is faced with a person who has just come out of a mental hospital has a very important role in helping the patient reintegrate into the community. The first order of business is to make sure that the individual continues his medication, particularly if the history is one of chronic schizophrenic or manic-depressive illness. If possible, the patient should be urged to join a program(s) that involves him in social activity and encourages problem-solving in relation to joining the community: how to get and hold a job, how to tell people that he has been in a mental hospital, what alternatives are available if he feels he is "coming unglued," how to relate to his family, and support for continuing to take medication. If such programs do not exist in the community, and if lack of local mental health resources results in a high proportion of rehospitalization of these patients, the physician can be the moving force behind establishing a day treatment program for such patients, sometimes under the auspices of a church, or a social service agency. Monitoring of medication and continued support remain essential roles of the physician, however.

Many community mental health centers provide comprehensive adult day treatment services for the individual who has had a psychotic illness in the past (particularly a schizophrenic illness) and who continues to need supportive services (including medication, recreation, socializing, support and problem-solving for tasks of daily living, and reintegration into the community). Such a program is often extremely helpful in spotting early relapse, supporting continued medication management, and building a supportive network for the more-regressed, chronic patient for whom the major therapeutic task is to maintain the patient outside the hospital.

The physician must also provide personal support to both the patient and his family so that they feel they have someone to turn to when a family problem is having a destructive effect on the patient or the family members. For many families, a psychotic episode is akin to venereal disease: Everyone is acutely conscious that "it exists," but everyone assiduously avoids discussing it. It can be very destructive for a patient to return from a mental hospital and find that he is treated in a peculiar way and his family has withdrawn from him. It is unclear to him how he can re-enter the family system, gain acceptance, and talk frankly about some of the things which concern him. In the case of some patients who have had chronic psychotic illnesses, medication, family counseling, etc. may not always help the family or prevent recurrence. Nonetheless, many persons who have had psychotic illnesses have made a recovery sufficient to be able to hold jobs, raise a family, and remain creative. The crucial thing is for the physician and his team not to fall prey to believing in the stereotype of the ex-psychotic patient—pathetic, hopeless, and not really worth much time and effort.

REFERENCES

1. Johnson, C. W., Snibbe, J. R., and Evans, L. A. (1975): *Basic Psychopathology: A Programmed Text*. Halsted (Wiley), New York.
2. Brosin, H. W. (1967): Acute and chronic brain syndromes. In: *Comprehensive Textbook of Psychiatry*, 1st ed., edited by A. M. Freedman and H. I. Kaplan, p. 708. Williams & Wilkins, Baltimore.
3. Engel, G. L., and Romano, J. (1944): Delirium. II. Reversibility of the EEG, with experimental procedures. *Arch. Neurol. Psychiatry*, 51:378.
4. Ravins, P., Tune, L., and McHugh, P. (1981): Tardive dyskinesia. *Johns Hopkins Med. J.*, 148:206–211.
5. Lehmann, H. E. (1967): In: *Comprehensive Textbook of Psychiatry*, 1st ed., edited by A. M. Freedman and H. I. Kaplan, p. 646. Williams & Wilkins, Baltimore.
6. Sack, R. L., and Shore, J. H. (1981): Psychopharmacology in medical practice—the benefits and the risks. *West. J. Med.*, 134:223–234.
7. May, P. R. A. (1976): Integrating treatment with patient needs. In: *Alternative Treatment for Schizophrenia*. Audiodigest Psychiatry, Vol. 5, Glendale, California.

17

Posttraumatic Stress Disorder in Vietnam Veterans

The symptoms of posttraumatic stress disorders have been recognized for a number of years, largely from observations of individuals who have survived natural catastrophes. The emergence of large numbers of Vietnam veterans with this disorder, however, has made its recognition in primary care settings of major importance. It is estimated that 60% of Vietnam veterans who actually saw combat are currently suffering from posttraumatic stress disorder (1). This translates into one-half to three-quarters of a million Americans. The suicide rate among this group is estimated to be 33% higher than that of the general population (controlled for age, sex, and race). Forty percent of the veterans were divorced within 6 months of returning from Southeast Asia, and the number hospitalized for alcoholism has doubled during the past 7 years.

In testimony before Congress in 1980, Dr. John P. Wilson, project director for the "Forgotten Warrior" of the Disabled American Veterans, identified the characteristics of Vietnam veterans suffering from posttraumatic stress disorder. The following is adapted from Wilson's testimony: (2)

1. *Emotional responses:* Emotional numbing, depression, anger, and rage; anxiety, with specific fears related to the combat experience; emotional constrictional sleep disturbance and recurring combat nightmares; hyperalertness and irritability; avoidance of activities that remind the person of war activities; suicidal feelings and thoughts; survivor guilt; flashbacks to traumatic events and intrusive traumatic thoughts; severe identity problems and crises.

2. *Cognition:* Fantasies of retaliation and destruction; cynicism and mistrust of government; alienation; value confusion, with both humanistic and self-indulgent contradictory values; negative self-image and low self-esteem; memory impairment

during times of stress; excessive sensitivity to issues of fairness, equality, justice, etc.

3. *Interpersonal relationships:* Problems with intimacy; problems with authority figures; emotional distance from children and concern about his anger alienating family members; inability to talk about war experiences; a tendency to explode into sudden fits of rage and anger, especially when under the influence of drugs.

Wilson also identified phases through which many veterans pass when experiencing their posttraumatic stress disorder:

1. *Emergency phase:* A panic state, in which the individual feels exhausted, vulnerable, and helpless.

2. *Denial:* The person is emotionally numb, feels constricted and confused, has a distortion of the meaning of past and present events, and fantasizes a great deal to deal with his current feelings.

3. *Flashback phase:* Recurring nightmares, intrusive thoughts, and flashbacks about combat experiences occur. The person may be preoccupied about the war and have a compulsion to talk or think about war experiences. There are many fears about losing control or merging with a victim. They experience survivor guilt and have startle reactions, hyperalertness, and vigilance. They re-enact traumatic events and use "survivor tactics."

4. *Reflective-transition phase:* The individual develops a larger perspective. Symptoms of earlier phases subside, and more appropriate coping mechanisms emerge. The individual has less rage, anger, and cynicism, and begins to think about the future and positive ways of relating and working.

5. *Integration phase:* The individual has successfully integrated his combat experiences into a coherent sense of self and a coherent identity.

The process of integrating the stressful events from combat takes time and usually requires a specific therapeutic atmosphere in which the veteran feels that the therapist can understand his combat experiences and is not "out to exploit him." Because of these constraints, the most effective therapy usually has occurred under the auspices of Vietnam Outreach, which is a branch of Disabled American Veterans. A trained counselor who himself has had combat experience in Vietnam may be a prerequisite component to attain credibility with the suspicious or cynical veteran (although nonveterans are occasionally successful).

The critical role of the primary physician is to identify the person experiencing the disorder. Often such a person, because of his explosiveness and anger, is viewed as having an antisocial personality disorder or as being psychotic. A detailed interview will reveal, however, that there is no disorder of thinking; nor does the person have a basic disregard for the feelings and rights of others, and no premorbid history of antisocial behavior. The symptoms appear to be primarily related to the stressful events themselves. If one has a blood relationship with this person previously, can show genuine interest, and can establish real rapport, then referral or even some sorting out of treatment priorities with the person may be possible. The development of peer support and understanding, however (a lack of which appears to be a major precipitant of the stress disorder in the first place), can best be accomplished by referring the individual to a group therapy situation where true combat peers can be found.

REFERENCES

1. *Forgotten Warriors: America's Vietnam Era Veterans*. Disabled American Veterans, 807 Maine Ave., S.W., Washington, D.C. 20024, January 1980.
2. Wilson, J. P. (1980): Toward an understanding of post-traumatic stress disorders among Vietnam veterans. Testimony before U.S. Senate Subcommittee on Veteran Affairs, May 21, 1980, Washington, D.C. (Dr. Wilson's address: Dept. of Psychology, Cleveland State University, Cleveland, OH 44115.)
3. Disabled American Veterans, 807 Maine Ave., S.W., Washington, D.C. 20024. Additional information is included in: Williams, T., editor (1980): *Post-Traumatic Stress Disorders of the Vietnam Veteran*. Disabled American Veterans, Washington, D.C.
4. Figley, C. R. (1978): *Stress Disorders Among Vietnam Veterans*. New York, Brunner-Mazel.
5. Horowitz, M. J. (1976): *Stress Response Syndromes*. Philadelphia, Blackiston.

18

The Alcoholic Patient

Alcoholism is America's number one drug problem. Many primary physicians know this and yet are reluctant to look for clues to alcohol problems among their patients or, even if unmistakable evidence is present, to do much about it. The reasons for this are complex but include the following: the fact that many physicians drink a lot (a facetious definition of an alcoholic is a patient who drinks more than his doctor); the fact that for doctors, as for other individuals, drinking is often associated with "good times"; the fact that there is cultural ambivalence about alcohol ("a real man can drink his buddies under the table, but drunks are disgusting"); and the fear of an angry or embarrassing response from a patient who is furious about being questioned on the subject.

The statistics are alarming. There are more than 10 million individuals with alcoholic problems in the United States and 40 million others directly affected by the 10 million (the families).* For this reason, it is important that each primary physician have some knowledge of how to identify individuals with drinking problems, have some notion about how to treat them or refer them, and have strategies to try to motivate patients with alcohol problems to look at themselves and begin to change their drinking behavior.

DIAGNOSIS OF ALCOHOLISM

Definitions of alcoholism vary extensively. Rigid criteria have been established by the National Council of Alcoholism (1) and include physiological dependence, tolerance to alcohol, alcohol-associated physical illness, laboratory tests that reveal high alcohol levels, and psychological dependence. Such criteria, however, veer toward physiological and "traditional, stereotyped" definitions of alcoholism rather

---

*Alcoholism is implicated in a major way in the four leading causes of death (accidents, homicide, suicide, and alcoholic cirrhosis) of American males aged 25 to 44.

than defining it as a disease, the effects of which cause severe marital and family problems, job difficulties or absenteeism, and depression. As Valliant (2) observes: "Diagnosis is the first step in treatment, but it is most difficult, and more than half the alcoholics seen by physicians go undiagnosed. This lack of recognition exists because different social groups regard alcohol abuse so differently, because individual use patterns differ so widely, because the alcoholic's denial is so convincing, because many physicians recognize only stereotypes of alcoholic drinkers, and because alcoholics are adept at concealing overt signs of intoxication."

Considering the possibility of alcohol as a contributing or central factor in the life or physical difficulties under investigation, asking about alcohol usage is crucial. Diagnostic questions include the following (2):

1. Has the patient tried to stop drinking to prove he can, changed brands, or otherwise tried to limit his drinking?

2. Has the patient begun to sneak drinks or become more irritable when people comment on his drinking?

3. Does the patient ever regret what he has said or done while he was drinking?

4. Has the patient ever experienced blackouts (memory lapses while intoxicated)? Do his hands shake the morning after? Does he drink in the morning to steady himself?

If the answer to one or more of these questions is yes, alcoholism is a probable diagnosis.

Many alcoholics have alcohol-related problems without being physically dependent on alcohol—the "incubation period" of the disease (alcoholism) being very long (in contrast with drug abuse, which has a short incubation period). The natural history of alcoholism often involves periods of being abstinent, as well as other periods where control over drinking is lost.

Cohen (3) observed the following: "One characteristic of the alcohol-dependent person is a general inability to consistently drink moderately. Some are so lacking in control that one drink may mean drinking until unconscious. For others, the dyscontrol is incomplete. They drink without impairing themselves or others for shorter or longer periods of time. Then, at some point, due to some noxious mood, perhaps, their control is lost... common characteristics of many chronic alcoholics are their enormous ability to deny the seriousness of their alcoholism, and a well-developed capacity to rationalize and minimize the consequences of their drinking behaviors. These factors not only bring them into treatment late, but justify their early withdrawal by dropping out and pronouncing themselves cured."

Beliefs specifically held by alcoholic individuals have been identified and can help make the diagnosis (as such ideas are not held by social drinkers or recovered alcoholics) (5). These may be described as follows (4):

1. A preoccupation with drinking is characteristic of the alcoholic (in contrast to the social) drinker.

2. The alcoholic does not recognize what is happening or that he is out of control because it would be too frightening for him.

3. The alcoholic believes that his actions result from his personality and so he becomes filled with self-loathing.

Factors which correlate on a long-term basis with the development of alcoholism are now becoming clear (5). Childhood emotional problems, family instability, a "bad childhood," low IQ, and "oral dependent traits" did not correlate with the development of alcoholism, whereas the following factors did:

Culture: Being from a culture which forbids children to drink but encourages young adults to get drunk. In one inner-city study, 25% of those of Irish descent developed alcoholism, whereas only 4% of those of Italian descent did. (There is also a high incidence among Scandinavians and Native Americans.)

Heredity: Twenty-four percent of those with an alcoholic parent developed alcoholism, whereas only 7% of those without an alcoholic parent developed the disorder.

Premorbid delinquency: Thirty-eight percent of delinquents developed alcoholism, although during adolescence most alcoholics were not delinquent.

TREATMENT OF ALCOHOLISM

Treatment for the patient with alcoholism (2) must obviously be differentiated between acute treatment for the individual with alcohol intoxication and withdrawal, and longer-term treatment for the overall condition. Intoxication expressed by slurred speech, nystagmus, motor incoordination, and a fluctuating mental state can usually be treated by bed rest or, if there is extreme excitement, with 5 mg haloperidol, i.m. Physiological withdrawal syndrome (delerium tremens, DTs) on the other hand, begins 6 to 24 hours after heavy drinking has stopped and shows the following signs: sweating, tachycardia, confusion, agitation, hyperventilation, and elevated systolic blood pressure. Treatment usually involves large doses of chlordiazepoxide, usually 100 mg orally when the patient presents, and another 100 mg in 1 hour if the patient continues in severe distress. Chlordiazepoxide should then be given, 25 to 100 mg p.r.n. at 4- to 6-hour intervals, with the total dose not exceeding 400 to 600 mg in 24 hours. The first 24-hour dose is cut in half the second day, and again in half the third day. Medication is discontinued altogether on the third or fourth day. If more than 400 mg chlordiazepoxide is required during the first 24 hours, Valliant recommends that 50 mg oral chlorpromazine be added for each additional 100-mg dose of chlordiazepoxide, and that this medication, like chlordiazepoxide, be cut in half the second day (2).

Apart from this acute treatment, the longer-term treatment of the patient with alcoholism involves both a *change in ideas and beliefs* as well as a *change in behavior*. A change in beliefs involves the following (4):

1. Willingness to accept the diagnosis.

2. An admission that others are not to blame and an acceptance that much of the alcoholic's pain comes from drinking, as well as the recognition that problems will worsen if the drinking continues.

3. An awareness that help is available through counseling, Alcoholics Anonymous (AA), etc. and that, with help, the patient can stop drinking.

Bean observed that patients relapse when one or more of such "sober" beliefs revert to "drinking" beliefs: "I can drink and control it when I'm feeling great/I want to drink when I'm feeling awful/I am in despair and think it will never get any better" (4).

Overall, factors contributing to the recovery from alcoholism include the following (5):

1. Finding a substitute (usually a gratifying behavior) that can replace the alcohol.
2. Behavior modification, including disulfiram (Antabuse®), compulsory supervision, or physical ailments (e.g., ulcer symptoms) immediately aggravated by alcohol.
3. Finding close relationships that have not been injured by the patient's prior drinking.
4. Finding a new source of hope and self-esteem. (For 40% of abstaining men in a study sample, this source was Alcoholics Anonymous.)

The Role of the Primary Physician

Treatment of the alcoholic patient in an outpatient primary care setting is fraught with frustration: broken appointments, pseudoagreements, resumption of drinking when "everything seemed to be going so well," etc. There are no magical answers to questions on ways to motivate the alcoholic patient, but there are some common experiences to consider: (1) Many alcoholics, like other patients, are lonely, depressed, or feel inadequate, and they believe that drinking makes them feel better (even if the drinking is causing the depression, destroying their relationships, and thereby producing the loneliness, etc.). Providing something else besides alcohol that can make such a patient feel better (e.g., a supportive relationship with a physician) is often a useful approach. (2) Problem drinkers often involve other people in their lives by getting them to assist and help perpetuate the drinking. Identifying such patterns and dealing with the other people involved may assist in clarifying the issue and interrupt the drinking pattern. (3) Because alcohol is seen to have an adaptive function in an individual's life, lectures about the dangers of drinking or how one is "ruining his liver" usually are useless in producing change. This is not to deny that an occasional patient will make the rational decision to stop drinking when the doctor honestly and nonjudgmentally discusses with him the effects of the drinking on his health, family, social, and economic status. More often, the physician or counselor must try to identify the one "sensitive" area through which he can reach the patient. This area may be the patient's intellectual functioning, the integrity of his body, a child whom he loves, or a marriage on which he is dependent. Motivation for help may come by the patient deciding to make the great sacrifice—giving up alcohol—if a "greater reward" is clearly evident. (4) During and immediately after the period of detoxification or other stressful event related to alcohol (e.g., an arrest for driving while intoxicated), the patient may be most amenable to change (although if the patient is a chronic heavy drinker it may take several months of abstinence before the patient's judgment and nervous system are not influenced by a withdrawal state).

To help with both behavioral and belief changes when treating the alcoholic individual, a contract between the treating physician and the patient should be negotiated. A grandiose scheme—"sobriety for 5 years"—is rarely helpful or feasible, even if the patient agrees. Instead, specific, short-term goals which the patient can manage have much more likelihood of success. Such goals might be staying sober for a month, no arrests for drunken driving for 6 months, or even coming to the doctor's office every week to talk. Most patients with drinking problems are agreeable to the notion of change but hate to give up drinking in order to accomplish it. For this reason, even if total abstinence seems like a desirable goal to the physician, limited abstinence or even some social drinking (with the likelihood of a predictable "slip") may be the only kind of drinking contract to which the patient will initially agree. Asking the problem drinker (to whom alcohol has been a periodic solace) for total sobriety is like asking the professional athlete to give up athletics: The sacrifice may be seen as devastating.

If abstinence is the immediate goal of a contract, using disulfiram may help meet this goal. The usual way to administer the drug is a maximum of 500 mg/day as a single dose for 1 to 2 weeks, followed by a daily maintenance dose of 125 to 250 mg/day. Patients should be warned of the effects of drinking while taking disulfiram. They should also carry a card or wear a bracelet stating they are taking the medication in case they experience a reaction to it; the card or bracelet also warns that if they are unconscious they should not be given an alcohol-containing medication. The reaction which follows drinking while the person is on disulfiram may include flushing, throbbing in the head and neck, headache, respiratory difficulty, nausea and vomiting, sweating, chest pain, hypertension, and syncope. A reaction to disulfiram alone may include drowsiness, impotence, headache, and occasionally psychotic thinking.

Negotiating with the patient about disulfiram often helps clarify whether the patient is indeed motivated to stop drinking, as many patients who have been unsuccessful in stopping their drinking themselves still refuse to consider disulfiram, calling it "a crutch"; alternately, they may intend to use the medication for a short period to help them through an immediate crisis but then resume drinking. The medication may also be seen as a way to placate boss and family, with the patient having mixed feelings about long-term use. Exploring these ideas about what disulfiram means to the particular patient is obviously crucial if the drug is to be used successfully.

Individual Therapy

Depending on the individual's needs, problems, and personality, the treatment of choice may be individual, group, family, or aversion therapy. In the author's experience, patients who do particularly well in individual therapy are those who are shy (and thus would be extremely hesitant to reveal their problems in a group setting) or those who appear to drink in response to a particular psychological stress of which they are not fully aware (when they have been rejected by someone, when they feel lonely, when they start to become aware of unacceptable sexual or aggressive impulses).

When the drinking is precipitated by some internal conflict or need, talking about this need or conflict with a professional person may help the patient resolve the conflict (and cure the drinking problem) or at least recognize the danger signals. People with drinking problems often have extremely low self-esteem initially; drinking contributes to this by adding feelings of guilt and self-reproach. For such persons, individual treatment is preferable to a more confrontive situation; in the latter situation, group or family members may attack the patient, causing him either to collapse in an orgy of self-recrimination or try to respond to the attacks. In neither situation can he critically examine why he "needs" to drink.

Some alcoholics periodically show up intoxicated for treatment. Many professionals feel that the treatment is pointless at such times and that a new appointment should be made for a time when the patient is likely to be sober. There is considerable debate about whether a person with a very severe drinking problem can benefit from individual psychotherapy until he is "dry" for at least a month or two. Although this period of drying out would certainly be helpful, patients with other psychological or addictive disorders (e.g., drug addicts) are not rejected simply because they recently used a habitual way of dealing with stress and anxiety. It is the author's opinion that persons with drinking problems should not be rejected for this reason either.

Many primary physicians or psychiatrists who see large numbers of alcoholic patients feel that working with the entire system in which the alcoholic is involved is essential for effective treatment. The primary component of this system is likely to be the patient's family. The therapist should help the spouse or the family recognize which of their actions or attitudes aggravates the drinking. For example, a discussion in terms of one of the "scripts" mentioned above may help a wife recognize how her habit of alternatively punishing and forgiving her husband may perpetuate his problem. Many communities have resources where family members can get support and help for themselves if the strain of living with an alcoholic becomes too severe, and where they can learn to deal intelligently with the drinking member of the family (e.g., Al-teen).

Employer Confrontation

Employer confrontation is a technique used by many large companies for their personnel with drinking problems. The company tries to clarify and document the ways in which alcohol is impairing or interfering with the employee's ability to function on the job. Armed with these data and offers of moral support and perhaps time off from work for therapy sessions, the company sets a limit on the employee's behavior: Either his performance improves or he will be dismissed. This strategy is effective with both lower-level employees and management-level personnel. The physician, with the patient's permission, can help the employer set up such a program for the employee, or the physician may consult with the employer on a long-term basis. In general, this technique has been found to be extremely effective in "rehabilitating" an alcoholic who is still employed and who wishes to keep his job.

Hospital and Residential Treatment

Many alcoholics who have been drinking heavily for a long period find it impossible to stop drinking if they remain in their usual milieu. In such cases, admitting the patient to the hospital is helpful, as it removes him from surroundings which may have been permitting or encouraging the drinking. There are other indications for the admission of an alcohol-dependent patient to a general hospital, suggested by the Committee on Alcoholism and Drug Dependence of the American Medical Association (6).

1. A patient diagnosed as alcoholic by a physician or hospital should be admitted if he has: (a) an infectious disease; (b) hyperthermia; (c) a history of convulsions or a poorly controlled seizure disorder and has been drinking; (d) is hemorrhaging or unconscious; (e) wants to be withdrawn from alcohol for the first time or after a relapse from sobriety; (f) has a disulfiram-alcohol reaction.

2. A person should be admitted with the tentative diagnosis of alcoholism if he: (a) has been drinking and is unconscious; (b) is agitated and tremulous, suggesting acute withdrawal; (c) has convulsions, hallucinations, or DTs, suggesting a complicated withdrawal state; (d) is suffering from a disease related to alcoholism (cirrhosis, neuropathy, pancreatitis) and wishes to be withdrawn from alcohol; (e) has a disease or posttraumatic injury usually not requiring hospitalization but also has a history of prolonged drinking or of heavy alcohol consumption immediately prior to the illness.

3. An alcohol-dependent patient should be admitted to the psychiatric unit or a psychiatric consultation should be obtained if he: (a) is overtly psychotic; (b) is so severely depressed that he is probably suicidal; or (c) represents a serious management problem because of extreme confusion or behavioral problems.

After the acute, "drying-out" phase of alcohol treatment, which is primarily medical, the patient may enter a residential program. Such programs usually last 3 to 6 weeks and include individual and group therapy, starting the patient on disulfiram, and introducing him to Alcoholics Anonymous. The group therapy may include confrontation experiences where the patient is challenged by other patients about the true nature of his behavior and problems. Other residential treatment programs feature aversion therapy; such techniques usually involve the patient taking an emetic at the same time he is consuming his favorite alcoholic beverage, which in turn leads to vomiting and the association of such vomiting with drinking.

Group Therapy

There are many group techniques available for alcoholics at the present time, and it is often difficult to choose among them. Groups differ in their organizational structures (T-groups, Alcoholics Anonymous, etc.). They can be supportive, religious, highly confrontive, extremely nondirective, or extremely directive (as in a court-established group for drunk drivers). Groups often differ from each other even if they bear the same label. For example, Alcoholics Anonymous groups may differ widely depending on the socioeconomic status and educational level of their members, the style of the leader, the type of agency originally referring most of the members, etc.

The way in which a referral is made has a great deal to do with whether a patient will accept a group, and the way a person is welcomed into the group is equally important. Thus persons sent to alcoholism groups by a court usually continue to maintain that "I don't have a problem" or "The only problem I have is that I got caught." This resistance to treatment can sometimes be dealt with effectively if the leader and other group members are willing to be empathic and understanding but at the same time confrontive. When a patient is referred to an alcoholism group by a physician he trusts, he is much more likely to accept the group. His adjustment and willingness to accept treatment in the group will be helped if the physician explains carefully beforehand what is likely to happen in the group and what the process is. It is also useful for the physician to give the patient the name of a specific person he will meet in the group (usually the leader) and to call the agency sponsoring the group to explain the patient's problems.

One distinct psychological advantage that self-help groups such as Alcoholics Anonymous have over other groups is their emphasis on the experience of the members in having overcome their problems. Rather than talking about their problems with a therapist who can "understand" but has never experienced the problem, alcoholic patients may receive special support and inspiration from other members of a group who have "licked" the problem themselves. In addition, such groups often focus more on what the members are accomplishing day by day in their struggle for sobriety, rather than on the problems remaining; this tack is often experienced as much more supportive than the usual therapy groups, where there is more emphasis on looking at and dealing with continuing problems.

Problems in Implementing Treatment with Alcoholic Patients

The physician may find implementation of an appropriate treatment plan more difficult in the case of those patients who are of the same social class or milieu as the physician. Without realizing it, a physician can sometimes be manipulated into treating this patient as "special" and exempt from the usual kinds of inquiry and confrontation. Obviously, this dilemma is even more painful when one physician must confront another about a drinking problem (e.g., a chief of staff in a hospital and a junior colleague). The inclination to "be a nice guy" and "give him one more chance" is very strong, but giving in means that the problem drinking will probably continue.

Most physicians find alcoholics extremely ungratifying and frustrating patients. They often miss appointments; they sometimes lie about whether they have been drinking; and they may try to con the doctor out of tranquilizers. The moral revulsion about people with drinking problems who cannot "hold their liquor" and embarrass and upset their families remains strong in many people, including physicians; when the patient has gone on a bender for the umpteenth time, this underlying moral position is likely to prompt the physician to toss the patient out. It is important for the doctor to recognize that, in many ways, patients with alcohol problems resemble other patients with chronic illnesses and complaints, be they physical or emotional. One does not ordinarily "fire" the hostile diabetic or the nagging hypochondriacal patient. Instead, one tries to understand the meaning of the symptom, to set appropriate limits, and to work gradually to alter the chronic maladaptive behavior pattern. This takes much time and patience, as does treating an alcoholic. It is almost inevitable that the alcoholic will have ups and downs, will resume drinking and then indulge in maudlin fits of remorse. The physician should realize that the (perhaps few) good working sessions with a patient may indeed be very helpful over the long run, even if the drinking behavior recurs from time to time.

REFERENCES

1. Criteria Committee, National Council on Alcoholism (1972): Criteria for the diagnosis of alcoholism. *Ann. Intern. Med.*, 77:249.
2. Valliant, G. E. (1978): Alcohol and drug dependence. In: *Harvard Guide to Modern Psychiatry*, edited by A. M. Nicholi Jr., pp. 567–577. Belknap/Harvard, Cambridge, MA.
3. Cohen, S. (1976): *Drug Abuse and Alcohol Newsletter*, Vol. 8.
4. Bean, M. H. (1980): Remarks made at a Cambridge Hospital symposium on alcoholism. To be distributed as part of *New Directions in Alcoholism Treatment*, Human Services Development. 1616 Soldiers Field Road, Boston, MA.
5. Valliant, G. E. (1980): Remarks made at a Cambridge Hospital symposium on alcoholism. To be distributed as part of *New Directions in Alcoholism Treatment*, Human Services Development, Boston, MA.
6. Committee on Alcoholism and Drug Dependence (1969): *JAMA*, 210:105.

19

Psychological Testing

Psychological tests may be viewed as "behavioral bioassays," tests administered under controlled and standardized conditions to patients; the yield is objective, psychological data relevant to diagnosis and treatment. No test, however, is a substitute for a careful clinical evaluation. The reliability, validity, and interpretation of psychological tests, like tests of body chemistry, depend on the skills and expertise of the person administering the test, except in those cases where interpretation is done by computer.

Psychological testing should be used as any other confidential information is to be used: with a great deal of discretion and with all the care and regard with which one handles any confidential medical information. Unfortunately, the results of testing are sometimes released without careful assessment as to how they will be used. Labels of "schizophrenic" or "sociopathic" may accompany people around for years (reappearing whenever the patient applies for a job, tries to get into college, or tries to get a civil service rating). These labels may be inaccurate; they are frequently irrelevant to current functioning; and the employer may be scared off by the "diagnostic label." Test scores should therefore be released with extreme caution and never without a clinical description of the patient's current functioning.

In general, psychological tests can be enormously helpful to the physician for both diagnostic assessment and to help define the focus of treatment. With judicious use, they may provide valuable data useful for improved patient care. This chapter describes some of the tests that are commonly used to assess various aspects of psychological functioning.

TESTS OF INTELLIGENCE: THE WECHSLER TESTS

It should be noted that an intelligence test is an indirect means of assessing an individual's present level of performance. The score is most useful when considering an individual's scholastic skills and accomplishments.

Wechsler Adult Intelligence Scale

The Wechsler Adult Intelligence Scale (WAIS) is one of three tests derived from the Wechsler-Bellevue Intelligence Scale. The WAIS consists of 11 subtests: six verbal tests and five performance tests. Verbal subtests include arithmetic, vocabulary, comprehension, general information, similarities, and digit span. Performance subtests are digit symbol, picture completion, block design, picture arrangement, and objective assembly. For several of these subtests, scoring is done on the basis of speed and accuracy of performance. The 11 subtests further break down into three groups: verbal comprehension, perceptual organization, and memory.

Normative data for WAIS scores have been obtained for various age groups between 16 and 64. A person's test performance indicates his ability in relation to his age group and not the entire population. Scores are highly reliable and correlate with educational and occupational achievements.

Wechsler Intelligence Scale for Children

The Wechsler Intelligence Scale for Children (WISC) is designed to be administered to children aged 7 to 15 and consists of 12 subtests: six verbal scale and six performance scale. The scales are similar to those in the WAIS. The twelfth scale of the WISC, mazes, does not appear on the WAIS.

Wechsler Preschool and Primary Scale of Intelligence

The Wechsler Preschool and Primary Scale of Intelligence (WPPSI) is the third scale developed from the Wechsler-Bellevue Intelligence Scale. This test was designed for children aged 4 to 6.5. The scale consists of 11 subtests, although only 10 are used to determine intelligence quotient (IQ). Eight of the 11 subtests are downward extensions of those found on the WISC; the remaining three subtests are memory or visual-motor tests because children in this age group have not yet acquired writing skills. Like the WAIS and the WISC, the WPPSI is a fairly accurate measure of intelligence for a specific age group.

TESTS FOR ORGANIC IMPAIRMENT

Performance on tests for organic impairment indicate an individual's level of visual-motor coordination. Scores which suggest impairment may be related to such conditions as brain damage, psychotic disorders, and other pathological states. Highly irregular performance scores may also be due to organic disorders or educational and environmental deprivation; certain emotional disturbances also affect test performance.

Bender-Gestalt Test

The Bender-Gestalt Test is the common name for the Bender Visual Motor Gestalt Test. As the name implies, this is a test of both visual perception and motor performance. Nine simple designs, each on a separate card, are given to the individual, one at a time. The person is asked to either copy the figure or study the design and then draw it from memory; this test is usually given as a copying test.

Scoring is done on the basis of drawing errors. Performance scores do not depend on drawing ability; rather, they reflect maturation and organic condition. The greater the number of drawing errors, the greater is the amount of impairment. Because this test can be quickly scored, it may be useful as a rapid screening device.

The Bender-Gestalt is a nonverbal performance test and is therefore most useful in children under 10 years of age. It is often effective in identifying the likelihood of a perceptual-motor problem or minimal brain dysfunction in children. Scores are subject to fluctuation and therefore must be interpreted cautiously.

Benton Visual Retention Test

The Benton Visual Retention Test is similar to the Bender-Gestalt Test in that it is a series of 10 geometric designs on individual cards. Subjects reproduce the drawings from memory after studying the card for a fixed amount of time. This is a test of visual and motor performance as well as of recall and spatial perception.

Scoring is done on the basis of total errors and number of drawings reproduced correctly. The higher the number of errors and the lower the number of figures reproduced, the greater is the impairment.

Like the Bender-Gestalt Test, the Benton Visual Retention Test is useful for determining brain injury in children. Unlike the Bender-Gestalt test, this test is also useful for adults, emotionally disturbed children, and schizophrenic patients.

PERSONALITY TESTS

Many tests for personality assessment exist, and their major value to the primary physician is to assess the degree of mood disturbance or personality disorganization. If the patient has a physical complaint, the test can often indicate whether it is based on an emotional or an organic problem.

California Psychological Inventory

The California Psychological Inventory (CPI) is a self-report inventory consisting of 480 true or false items. Approximately half of the items were drawn from the Minnesota Multiphasic Personality Inventory (MMPI) described below. The 480 items break down into 18 scales: Three scales are validity scales, and 15 are personality scales of such factors as dominance, self-control, socialization, self-acceptance, responsibility, and some achievement-related items.

The CPI has undergone extensive research and development and is empirically related to personality traits. The CPI was developed for use in normal populations aged 13 and over. Prediction of delinquency and school performance is possible with the CPI. Cross-cultural studies on some scales show promising results for determining traits within different cultures.

Minnesota Multiphasic Personality Inventory

The Minnesota Multiphasic Personality Inventory (MMPI) is the most widely used self-report personality inventory. The MMPI consists of 550 affirmative statements to which a response of true or false is given. Item content varies widely and includes health, psychosomatic symptoms, attitudes on sexual, religious, political, and social matters; questions on education, family, occupation, and marriage; neurotic and psychotic behavior manifestations; and phobias. The primary use of the MMPI is in differential diagnosis for adults 16 and over.

Scores on the MMPI are provided for 10 clinical scales: hypochondriasis, depression, hysteria, psychopathic deviate, masculinity-femininity, paranoia, psychasthenia, schizophrenia, hypomania, and social introversion. The MMPI is designed to assess traits characteristic of disabling psychological abnormality and is appropriately used in a clinical setting rather than as a screening procedure for occupational or educational purposes. In general, the greater the number of deviant scores, the greater the likelihood that the individual is severely disturbed.

Scoring can be done either by hand or computer. Computerized scoring and interpretive services are available through the Mayo Clinic, The Psychological Corporation, or the Roche Psychiatric Service Institute.

PROJECTIVE TESTS

In contrast to tests already described in this chapter, projective techniques are relatively unstructured tests. Test instructions are general; the subject is free to respond in any manner his personality dictates. There are therefore no right or wrong answers, and reliability and validity are difficult to assess.

Projective tests are designed to measure all aspects of personality: conscious, unconscious, and latent. Test interpretations reflect the subject's overall personality, not selective traits. The subject is supposedly unaware of which psychological aspects are being scored; intellectual, interpersonal, emotional, and behavioral characteristics form the global personality picture.

Rorschach Test

The Rorschach Test consists of 10 bilaterally symmetrical inkblots, one to a card. Five of the cards are shades of black and gray; three include pastel shades; two include splashes of red. Cards are shown one at a time, and the person is asked to describe what he sees. Scoring is a composite of location (area of inkblot to which subject refers), determinants (includes reference to form, color, and movement), and content (such things as human, animal, or inanimate objects).

The Rorschach is used in children as young as 3 years and is valid through adulthood. Responses tend to depend, to some extent, on age, intelligence, and education. Interpretation is difficult because responses vary widely in content and number; and in the absence of norms and validation, interpretation reflects characteristics of the examiner as well as the subject.

Thematic Apperception Test

The Thematic Apperception Test (TAT) is somewhat more structured than the Rorschach. Nineteen cards make up the TAT; 18 cards are vague black-and-white pictures and one card is blank. Subjects are asked to make up a story for each picture including events leading up to the situation, what the characters think and feel, as well as the outcome of the story. The blank card requires the subject to create first a picture and then a story using no cues.

The TAT is used, like the Rorschach, to assess personality. The subject's present emotional and physical environment will influence responses. Like the Rorschach, reliability and validity of the technique are not completely established.

MEASURES OF ANXIETY AND DEPRESSION

Many patients seek medical attention for illnesses having no organic base. Underlying many of their physical complaints are symptoms of anxiety and/or depression. These symptoms are, however, often masked or expressed in subtle ways. This section includes tests to assist the physician in quantitatively measuring clinically significant symptoms of anxiety and/or depression.

Taylor Manifest Anxiety Scale

The Taylor Manifest Anxiety Scale (TMAS) is a self-report inventory. Patients are asked to respond to 50 questions as "true" or "false"; all 50 questions must be answered. Like the CPI, much of TMAS is an adaption of the MMPI. This test is usually given to adults, although a scale for children has been developed. A short form, 20 items, has also been developed for the adult scale.

There has been some controversy as to whether the TMAS actually measures manifest anxiety. It may assess a more general area of emotional responding. Responses may reflect the patient's awareness of, and willingness to express, his emotional feelings. The scale was designed to measure an individual's general drive level; anxiety is considered to be another term for drive level.

State-Trait Anxiety Inventory

The State-Trait Anxiety Inventory (STAI) consists of two 20-item scales: one to measure state (situational) anxiety and one to measure trait (general) anxiety. These two scales may be used together or separately. If used together, the state anxiety scale should be administered first.

Responses to the state anxiety scale reflect how the individual feels at the moment he answers the questionnaire. To each item, a response of "not at all," "somewhat," "moderately so," or "very much so" is given. The trait anxiety scale is a measure of how the person generally feels and responses to each item are "almost never," "sometimes," "often," or "almost always." Numerical ratings for each scale are identical; each item is scored on a unit scale from one to four. For both scales, higher scores indicate higher anxiety levels.

Hamilton Anxiety Scale

The Hamilton Anxiety Scale is a multiple-item rating scale which is completed by the physician or psychologist and used for patients diagnosed as having neurotic anxiety. Although it is used to determine anxiety in other conditions (e.g., depression, phobias, and schizophrenia), it is not intended for these uses.

Scoring is on a five-point scale, ranging from zero (symptom not present) to four (sympton very severe). The very severe rating is seldom seen in outpatients. Symptoms included on the scale are: anxious mood, tension, fears, insomnia, depressed mood, or intellectual, somatic (muscular), somatic (sensory), cardiovascular, gastrointestinal, genitourinary, and autonomic problems. The last item is a measure of behavior during the interview. Each of these symptoms is of equal value for scoring purposes.

Hamilton Depression Scale

The Hamilton Depression Scale is a 21-item rating scale which is completed by a physician or psychologist on the basis of a clinical interview. It is intended for the evaluation of patients already diagnosed as depressed. Items on the scale cover a wide range of symptomatology, including depressed mood, guilt feelings, anxiety, and sleep and appetite disturbances.

Beck Depression Inventory

The Beck Depression Inventory (BDI) is a self-rated scale which measures the behavioral and subjective manifestations of depression. The original 21-item scale can be completed in about 10 minutes; a modified 13-item short form is also available. There is apparently no loss of reliability and validity with the short form.

Symptomatology covered by the BDI includes sadness, guilt, anorexia, work difficulty, and self-image. Symptom severity is rated on a four-point scale. The BDI correlates well with other tests of depression and does discriminate between anxiety and depression.

Hopkins Symptom Checklist

The Hopkins Symptom Checklist (HSCL) is a 58-item self-report inventory used for outpatients. Scoring is done on the basis of five symptom clusters: somatization, obsessive-compulsive behavior, interpersonal sensitivity, depression, and anxiety. Scores on this rating scale reflect not only the existence of a symptom but also the extent of the symptom.

Over the last 15 years, the HSCL has undergone extensive evaluation and development, and appears to be a valid and reliable means of assessing anxiety and its correlates.

When given to outpatients, the HSCL-58 can be employed as a screening procedure to determine the current status of the patient. Interpretation of these scales will also alert the physician to those patients who require professional help.

NOTE

Comprehensive and critical reviews of most published tests are provided in the series of *Mental Measurements Yearbooks* (edited by O. K. Buros, Gryphon Press, Highland Park, N.J.).

20

Behavioral Approaches in Office Practice

The term "behavioral therapy" means different things to different people. It may mean giving candy to a child who has successfully completed his potty training, or it may mean giving an emetic to an alcoholic with his favorite beverage, thereby setting up an association of drinking with nausea and unpleasant aftereffects. This chapter describes very briefly some techniques of behavior modification and behavioral therapy which might be applicable to office practice and suitable for dealing rapidly—and hopefully, effectively—with certain kinds of symptoms, eliminating or at least alleviating them.

The assumption behind most behavioral approaches is that behavior is learned and can therefore be unlearned. The behavior which can be learned includes not only things a person does but feelings he has about himself, his body, other individuals, etc. Behaviorists often try to focus on specific areas of doing or feeling which the patient would like to change; this is somewhat in contrast to more traditional approaches to psychotherapy. In the latter the focus is on the relationship between the therapist and the patient, and how the relationship can be used to produce understanding, insight, and emotional comfort, and, over time, produce changes in behavior and feeling. The measure and criteria for behavioral change are usually spelled out ahead of time, so that both patient and therapist can know how closely they are approaching "the cure," which usually means removal of the specific symptom for which the patient entered treatment (rather than, as in traditional psychotherapy, the production of "growth," greater awareness, increased productivity, a greater sense of self-fulfillment, etc.). Behavioral as well as more traditional approaches have an important role in the primary physician's armamentarium.

RELAXATION THERAPY

Relaxation therapy allows a patient to learn gradually how to systematically relax the various parts of his body. Mastery of the technique results in some relief from tension-induced states (e.g., tension headaches, "cramps" in various body parts, feelings connected with neckache and backache).

There are a number of techniques, but most involve the patient becoming more aware of his own tensions and then learning to decrease them. For example, the patient may receive written instructions for systematic relaxation. He either lies supine or sits in a comfortable position, legs crossed and eyes closed, concentrating on his breathing, counting the breaths, and willing progressive relaxation of his toes, his feet, etc. Alternately, the patient may tense a particular muscle to its maximal amount, hold the tension for several seconds, and then relax. The patient practices these exercises at home until he has mastered their elements sufficiently to gain relief from his particular tensions. Descriptions of this technique are found in many books on yoga and in human awareness books (1).

Some of the relaxation techniques recommended to patients at the University of Washington (Department of Psychiatry and Behavioral Sciences) are included below. The therapist records the protocol on a tape cassette and gives it to the patient to play and practice at home. Obviously, this method could be used by primary physicians with their patients (2).

Relaxation of Arms (Time: 4 to 5 Minutes)

Settle back as comfortably as you can. Let yourself relax to the best of your ability.... Now, as you relax like that, clench your right fist... just clench your fist tighter and tighter, and study the tension as you do so.... Keep it clenched and feel the tension in your right fist, hand, forearm.... Now relax.... Let the fingers of your right hand become loose and observe the contrast in your feelings.... Now let yourself go and try to become more relaxed all over.... Once more, clench your right fist really tight... hold it and notice the tension again.... Now let go, relax; your fingers straighten out, and you notice the difference once more.... Now repeat that with your left fist. Clench your left fist while the rest of your body relaxes; clench that fist and feel the tension... and now relax.... Again, enjoy the contrast.... Repeat that once more, clench the left fist, tight and tense.... Now do the opposite of tension—relax and feel the difference.... Continue relaxing like that for awhile.... Clench both fists tighter and tighter, both fists tense, forearms tense, study the sensations... and relax; straighten out your fingers and feel that relaxation.... Continue relaxing your hands and forearms more and more.... Now bend your elbows and tense your biceps, tense them harder and study the tension feelings.... All right, straighten out your arms, let them relax and feel that difference again. Let the relaxation develop.... Once more, tense your biceps; hold the tension and observe it carefully.... Straighten the arms and relax; relax to the best of your ability.... Each time, pay close attention to your feelings when you tense up and when you relax.... Now straighten your arms, straighten them so that you feel most tension in the triceps muscles along the back of your arms.... Stretch your arms and feel that tension.... And now relax.... Get your arms back into a comfortable position.... Let the relaxation proceed on its own.... The arms should feel comfortably heavy as you allow them to relax.... Straighten the arms once more so that you feel the tension in the triceps muscles; straighten them.... Feel that tension... and relax.... Now let's concentrate on pure relaxation in the arms without any tension.... Get the arms comfortable and let them relax further and further.... Continue relaxing your arms even further.... Even when your arms seem fully relaxed, try to go even further; try to achieve deeper and deeper levels of relaxation.

Relaxation of Facial Area With Neck, Shoulders, and Upper Back (Time: 4 to 5 Minutes)

Relax your entire body to the best of your ability.... Feel that comfortable heaviness.... Let all your muscles go loose and heavy.... Just settle back quietly and comfortably.... Wrinkle up your forehead now; wrinkle it tighter.... And now stop wrinkling your forehead; relax and smooth it out.... Picture the entire forehead and scalp becoming smoother as the relaxation increases.... Now frown and crease your brows and study the tension.... Let go of the tension again.... Smooth out the forehead once more.... Now, close your eyes tighter and tighter- ...feel the tension... and relax your eyes.... Keep your eyes closed, gently, comfortably, and notice the relaxation.... Now clench your jaws.... Relax your jaws now.... Let your lips part slightly.... Appreciate the relaxation.... Now press your tongue hard against the roof of your mouth.... Look for the tension.... Let your tongue return to a comfortable and relaxed position.... Now purse your lips, press your lips together tighter and tighter.... Relax the lips.... Note the contrast between tension and relaxation.... Feel the relaxation all over your face, all over your forehead and scalp, eyes, jaws, lips, tongue, and your neck muscles.... Press your head back as far as it can go and feel the tension in the neck; roll it to the right and feel the tension shift; now roll it left.... Straighten your head and bring it forward, press your chin against your chest.... Let your head return to a comfortable position, and study the relaxation.... Let the relaxation develop.... Shrug your shoulders, right up.... Hold the tension.... Drop your shoulders once more and relax.... Let the relaxation spread deep into the shoulders, right into your back muscles; relax your neck and throat and your jaws and other facial areas as the pure relaxation takes over and grows deeper... deeper... ever deeper.

Relaxation of Chest, Stomach, and Lower Back (Time: 4 to 5 Minutes)

Relax your entire body to the best of your ability.... Feel the comfortable heaviness that accompanies relaxation.... Breathe easily and freely in and out.... Notice how the relaxation increases as you exhale... as you breathe out just feel that relaxation.... Now breathe right in and fill your lungs; inhale deeply and hold your breath.... Study the tension.... Now exhale, let the walls of your chest grow loose and push the air out automatically.... Continue relaxing and breathe freely and gently.... Feel the relaxation and enjoy it.... With the rest of your body as relaxed as possible, fill your lungs again.... Breathe in deeply and hold it again. That's fine, breathe out and appreciate the relief.... Just breathe normally.... Continue relaxing your chest and let the relaxation spread to your back, shoulders, neck, and arms.... Merely let go... and enjoy the relaxation. Now let's pay attention to your abdominal muscles, your stomach area. Tighten your stomach muscles, make your abdomen hard.... Notice the tension... and relax.... Let the muscles loosen and notice the contrast.... Once more, press and tighten your stomach muscles.... Hold the tension and study it.... And relax.... Notice the general well-being that comes with relaxing your stomach.... Now draw your stomach in, pull the muscles right in and feel the tension this way.... Now relax again.... Let your stomach out.... Continue breathing normally and easily and feel the gentle massaging acting all over your chest and stomach.... Now pull your stomach in again and hold the tension.... Now push out and tense like that; hold that tension... once more pull in and feel the tension... now relax your stomach fully.... Let the tension dissolve as the relaxation grows deeper. Each time you breathe out, notice the rhythmic relaxation both in your lungs and your stomach.... Notice how your chest and your stomach relax more and more.... Try to let go of all contractions anywhere in your body.... Now direct your attention to your lower back.... Arch up your back, make your lower back quite hollow, and feel the tension along your spine... and settle down comfortably again relaxing the lower back.... Just arch your back up and feel the tension as you do so.... Try to keep the rest of the body as relaxed as possible.... Try to localize the tension throughout your lower back area.... Relax once more, relaxing further and further.... Relax your lower back, relax your upper back, spread the relaxation to your stomach, chest, shoulders, arms, and facial area.... Relaxing the parts further and further and ever deeper.

Relaxation of Hips, Thighs, and Calves Followed by Complete Body Relaxation (Time: 4 to 5 Minutes)

Let go of all tension and relax.... Now flex your buttocks and thighs.... flex your thighs by pressing down your heels as hard as you can.... Relax and note the difference.... Straighten your knees and flex your thigh muscles again.... Hold the tension.... Relax your hips and thighs.... Allow the relaxation to proceed on its own.... Press your feet and toes downward, away from your face, so that your calf muscles become tense.... Study that tension.... Relax your feet and calves.... This time, bend your feet toward your face so that you feel tension along your shins.... Bring your toes right up.... Relax again.... Keep relaxing for a while.... Now let yourself relax further all over.... Relax your feet, ankles, calves, and shins, knees, thighs, buttocks, and hips.... Feel the heaviness of your lower body as you relax still further.... Now spread the relaxation to your stomach, waist, lower back.... Let go more and more deeply.... Make sure that no tension has crept into your throat; relax your neck and your jaws and all your facial muscles.

Now you can become twice as relaxed as you are by taking in a really deep breath and slowly exhaling.... With your eyes closed you become less aware of objects and movements around you.... To prevent any surface tension from developing, breathe in deeply and feel yourself becoming heavier.... Take in a long, deep breath and let it out very slowly.... Feel how heavy and relaxed you have become.

As you relax you should feel unwilling to move a single muscle in your body.... Think about the effort that would be required to raise your right arm.... As you think about raising your right arm, see if you can notice any tension that might have crept into your shoulder and your arm. . . . Now decide to lift the arm but to continue relaxing. . . . Observe the disappearance of the tension.

Just keep on relaxing. . . . When you wish to get up, count backward from four to one. . . . You should then feel fine and refreshed, wide awake, and calm.

RECIPROCAL INHIBITION

Reciprocal inhibition, a technique developed and perfected by Wolpe (3), Lazarus, and other behaviorists, is particularly useful for treating phobias or other specific situations which evoke anxiety in the individual. The technique involves either the use of a relaxation strategy (e.g., the one listed above) or the evocation of some pleasurable or anxiety-reducing activity (e.g., being held or eating). Prior to the "actual therapy session," the patient and his therapist (who might be a primary physician) construct a hierarchical list of those items that produce the patient's anxiety, with the least anxiety-provoking items listed first and the last item being something about which the patient is most uncomfortable. The patient then begins his relaxation routine and tries to remain relaxed while the therapist enlarges on each item, beginning with those least likely to produce anxiety. A number of sessions are required before the patient will be able to retain his relaxed state when his most agitating fantasies are evoked.

Example of hierarchy
Imagine a toy airplane.
Imagine a picture of a real airplane.
Imagine driving to an airport.
Imagine being at the airport with a real airplane.
Imagine standing next to the real airplane.
Imagine getting into the airplane.
Imagine sitting down in a seat on the airplane.
Imagine the take-off of the airplane. It is a perfect take-off and the weather is perfect.
Imagine the take-off of the airplane. It is nighttime and you cannot see very well.
Imagine taking off in a rainstorm. It is a perfect take-off.
Imagine taking off and riding in a big storm, with thunder, lightning, a lot of turbulence and bumpiness.
Imagine landing on a clear day, a perfect landing.
Imagine landing in a rainstorm with a lot of wind and bumpiness.

Thus while the physician is talking about increasingly disturbing aspects of riding in an airplane, the patient with the airplane fears is simultaneously doing something to relax (e.g., focusing on breathing and relaxing body parts, eating). Reciprocal inhibition techniques have sometimes been coupled with hypnosis. These methods seem particularly useful in the treatment of circumscribed functional disorders (e.g., specific phobias) which the patient is motivated to change (i.e., where the symptom does not appear to be an attention-getting device).

BEHAVIOR MODIFICATION

The supposition behind behavior modification (and much behavioral therapy in general) is that behavior is determined by its consequences (4). Dysfunctional behavior was, at one time, learned and then reinforced by subsequent events. For instance, a child with frequent temper tantrums presumably first "stumbled" on this behavior, but the tantrums became reinforced by the kind of attention he received (either positive or negative). The child then learned that attention could be gained by producing a tantrum, and each incident reinforced the behavior. There are three principal strategies used to modify such behavior:

1. *Positive reinforcement:* Positive rewards are given for specific behavior which is new, acceptable, or particularly desirable (especially if it replaces undesirable behavior). This specific (desirable) behavior should be very clear to the person observing, counting, and rewarding the behavior.

2. *Extinction phenomena:* Behavior which is undesirable is simply ignored, with the notion that it is a demand for attention and will gradually disappear if attention is not forthcoming.

3. *Negative reinforcement:* Punishments, spankings, deprivations, etc. are meted out in response to bad behavior. This is sometimes extremely effective. Its major difficulty is that even though negative behavior may disappear in response to this strategy a great deal of innovative socially adaptive and positive behavior may disappear as well, as fear may become generalized to appropriate as well as inappropriate behavior.

Examples

Positive reinforcement: For every half-hour that a child can sit still in a classroom, he receives one point, one M & M candy, or one penny that he can use to purchase various pleasures. This strategy is particularly useful with a disruptive child, one whose major goal seems to be to upset everyone in the classroom. These tangible rewards can gradually be replaced by social rewards (e.g., praise or giving the child a position of leadership). It is crucial, however, to identify specific items which would indeed be rewarding for this particular child and to zero in on specific aspects of the child's behavior that one wants to encourage.

Negative reinforcement: The child swears in class. Every time he swears at a classmate or a teacher, he is promptly removed from the classroom and sent to the principal's office and, on occasion, given a stern lecture by either the principal or the teacher. If the principal is stern enough, it is conceivable that the swearing behavior will disappear, but it is equally likely that the child will develop a strong aversion to schoolteachers and learning, and later drop out of school.

Positive reinforcement: A child is withdrawn at home. The withdrawn behavior is partially reinforced by the sarcasm used by the parents every time he becomes very assertive or talkative. The first step in a behavior modification program might be to count the amount of time the child is socially interacting and ta
king. Increased talking and social interaction are rewarded with praise, attention, and smiles. The parents, on their part, should keep track (perhaps with the child's help) of the number of sarcastic remarks and frowns they themselves use; they can reward themselves with a "night on the town" when they have decreased their sarcasm level to an acceptable point.

As one can see from the last example, the principles of behavior modification work equally well with adults. The essential first step is to carefully analyze and count the behavior one wants changed. Having this baseline data, one can properly assess whether the behavior is getting better, is unchanged, or is getting worse. For example, patients who are obese may start by counting the number of mouthfuls they chew in a day (using a mechanical counter such as the kind used by toll takers). After establishing the baseline data, the number of mouthfuls can be systematically reduced, possibly by using some kind of reward system (e.g., self-rewards with money, entertainment) in exchange for fewer mouthfuls and the accompanying weight loss (5,6).

DESENSITIZATION AND HYPERSENSITIZATION

Desensitization and hypersensitization, a technique somewhat similar to reciprocal inhibition, is based on the premise that if a person is exposed to gradually increasing amounts of a stimulus he dislikes, it will become increasingly more neutral for him. As is mentioned in Chapter 23, desensitization to discussions of sexual material is extremely useful (for both patient and physician) as a preparation to the treatment of patients with sexual dysfunctions.

The same is true in the more prosaic situations: The process of studying anatomy with cadavers in medical school is one in which the feelings of the medical student gradually change from horror and/or nausea to relative indifference to nudity and death. The goal, of course, is to develop an interest in the structures of the human body without the feelings of revulsion. Curiously enough, medical schools often do such an excellent job of desensitizing, the student often turns into the doctor who sees his patients as "simply the sum of their anatomy and physiological functioning."

Frequent, carefully controlled and structured exposure to subject matters one dislikes, coupled with the reassurance and support of a mentor, can be an effective way of applying desensitization principles in office practice. For example, the physician who has many adolescent patients who use profanity finds that his receptionist cannot get used to this new speech pattern and reacts with distaste and evident irritation. A plan of attack would be to record the words she most dislikes and ask her to listen to the tape a number of times during the day as well as to say the words to herself several times a day. Within a rather short time, the words will cease to have the same impact.

Another style of desensitization is a "flooding" procedure, whereby a person is bombarded with the stimuli he finds uncomfortable under the assumption that "the first 5 minutes are the hardest." Unfortunately, this sink or swim approach may "turn off" the person altogether, so that he goes out of his way to avoid any further contact with the stimuli. One of the explanations for "traumatic neuroses" (where, for example, a person refuses to ride in or drive an automobile after a car wreck and becomes anxious at even the thought) is that the individual has become so overwhelmed by unmanageable anxiety that he continues to link the original stimulus with the present anxiety.

RESENSITIZATION

The term resensitization is a bit awkward, but the concept and its application are becoming increasingly valid to many behavioral scientists. We are coming to realize that many people have been led, through childhood experiences, to pretend, in effect, that some parts of their bodies do not exist, and they have therefore become insensitive to certain kinds of pleasurable experiences of the senses (e.g., touch, sight, or smell). This kind of "partially aware existence" deprives an individual of a great deal of potential pleasure. A resensitization exercise instructs a patient to start experiencing parts of his body, experimenting with different smells, tastes, etc.

Obviously this kind of technique is usually more applicable to "human growth and potential" programs than to specific treatment of any clinical malady. Nonetheless, an "uptight" or rigid individual whose only interests are perfectionism on the job and autocracy at home enjoys very little of life and living. A resensitization "prescription"—if the doctor can persuade the patient to carry it out—may help to relax and revivify this person, and allow him to discover aspects of himself of which he has been unaware for a considerable time. Perls described ways in which persons can "rediscover themselves" by almost deliberate instruction in "how to do it." (7) Some books give specific instructions that a patient might be able to practice by himself (1) or with friends or family (8,9).

ASSERTIVENESS TRAINING

Assertiveness training (6) involves making a "contract" with an individual who is to develop and try new behavior he feels is desirable but has been reluctant to try without support (e.g., being directly and forcefully assertive with peers, parents, colleagues, family, etc.). The patient can be helped to try some of these new behaviors by first practicing the behavior in a "game."

Example
A person who has trouble asserting his rights at work and saying "no" might begin practicing his new firmness skills with people with whom he is not intimately involved or who do not particularly matter to him. For example, he might order various items he does not want from the nearest mail order store and then return them, stating that they were unacceptable, that he did not want them or they did not fit, etc. Obviously, if this were carried to extremes, difficulties might develop with the store; but practicing to say "no" in a nonthreatening situation may be the first step toward being able to say "no" to the boss.

Assertiveness training for children who allow themselves to be scapegoated and bullied might involve teaching them what they might say in typical confrontations and teaching them how to fight. At the same time, the physician, and by extension teachers and parents, should support and encourage legitimate areas of pride and self-confidence for this child whose self-esteem, if he is bullied, must be very low. This assertiveness training really involves teaching and practicing roles, and learning through doing; it is quite different from the usual psychotherapeutic premises, which suggest that attitudes and feelings must change before behavior changes.

BIOFEEDBACK

There is currently considerable interest in the way biofeedback and medication may be useful in changing autonomic functioning (e.g., in hypertension, management of vascular headaches). Through the use of electroencephalographic or body temperature monitoring systems, patients can become aware of what they must do (either through relaxation, self-hypnosis, or simply by changing their feelings) to alter their blood pressure, heart rate, etc. Many studies of this sort are under way and are leading to the development of guidelines or teaching methods which could be used by the primary physician to treat certain patients. Courses on the use of biofeedback techniques are currently available in many medical schools and some psychiatric institutions such as the Wenning Foundation, Topeka, Kansas, which has been a pioneer in the development of biofeedback as a treatment technique. A popular description of biofeedback is found in the work of Karlin and Andrews (10).

SOCIAL SKILLS TRAINING USING BEHAVIORAL PARADIGMS

A behavioral program which reinforces thinking and problem-solving sequences, rather than isolated behaviors, has been developed by Trupin et al. (11) (Chapter 7). The sequence—called SIGEP, for Stop, Identify (the problem), Generate (alternatives), Evaluate (choose the best one), and Plan (how to implement)—is a scheme which can be extremely helpful with both impulsive children and impulsive or disorganized adults, especially those recovering from a serious mental illness. Some physicians, after instructing a patient in the particular components of the SIGEP program, then work with the patient on specific problems in the session, using the scheme. They then also assign "homework" so the person can develop further skills in this method outside the physician's office. Often such a program is self-reinforcing because of improved behavior in school or at home; with disorganized individuals, however, reinforcement for continuing with the method and not reverting to planning by impulse may have to be done by the physician in an explicit and deliberate way.

MAKING A BEHAVIORAL CONTRACT

The concept of behavioral contracts is mentioned in several other chapters (Chapters 4, 11, and 18): making a contract with a patient who has a drinking problem about what his goals are, making a behavioral contract with a depressed patient for specific increased functioning every day, etc. However, it may be useful to explore the behavioral contract in general here.

Behavioral contracts are particularly useful (1) with patients who have had previous psychotherapeutic encounters; (2) when an individual appears to agree with a doctor's treatment suggestions but his behavior shows that he is resisting treatment; and (3) as a way to assess motivation when there is doubt about the extent of the patient's commitment. With the present concern about patient care assessment and appraisal, and the increased desirability of being able to set specific objectives for patient treatment (both medical and psychological), the contract has emerged as an extremely useful tool. Establishing a behavioral contract allows the physician and the patient to collaborate on establishing specific goals to be reached through the treatment program and at the same time allows them to evaluate whether they have reached the goals.

A valid goal in the case of an angry patient might be becoming aware of and writing down every time he feels angry, and then working out with the doctor other ways of dealing with the anger besides "exploding." In the case of an alcoholic, doctor and patient might agree on a treatment goal of being dry for a month, with the patient's part of the contract relating to abstinence, and the doctor's part being the agreement to supply the disulfiram and to see the patient every week. The resulting contract effects behavioral change or else (if the patient refuses the disulfiram clause) forces the patient to examine the depth of his motivation. It is a way of assessing commitment while avoiding direct confrontation by challenging the patient with a statement like, "I don't believe that you really want to give up drinking right now."

Establishing behavioral contracts that contain specific rewards for fulfilling the contract and specific penalties for "goofing up" is becoming an increasingly popular way of dealing with certain kinds of troublesome school behavior. For instance, it might be agreed with a child that he will have to spend 15 minutes in the "time-out room" every time he disrupts the class, but after he has 3 or 4 days of non-disruptive behavior the teacher will take him out for a hamburger. If the contract is in writing and signed by both student and teacher, it seems more binding on both, and it may be a strong incentive for the child to try to change his behavior. Contracts between parents and children, where parents agree to certain concessions in writing in return for certain behavioral changes on the part of their children (also in writing) may force both parents and children to become more responsible in their demands on each other and avoid the sudden "power plays" and angry outbursts which sometimes occur in families. For example, "You can have the car Saturday night if you come home on time every school night this week. Shall we put it in writing?"

Some behavioral contracts are drawn up between "educational agencies" and the adults who want to change their own behavior and involve appropriate penalties for violations. For example, a health-care group might charge $200 for a program designed to help people give up smoking, but it will return $150 of the fee if after 3 months the person has succeeded in staying off cigarettes. The contract is specific and, because money is involved, may induce a high motivation to change behavior.

Resolutions appear to have more meaning to many people when they are written. If a formal contract exists between patient and physician, it is easier to avoid misunderstanding, to review the treatment objectives, and to reassess their respective roles in the treatment; ultimately, the contract can help decide if there has been any improvement.

REFERENCES

1. Lewis, H. R., and Streitfeld, J. S. (1972): *Growth Games.* Bantam, New York.
2. Modified from Kohlenberg, R., and Carr, J.: Relaxation exercises. Used in course work within the Department of Psychology and the Department of Psychiatry and Behavioral Sciences, University of Washington, Seattle.
3. Wolpe, J. (1969): *The Practice of Behavior Therapy.* Pergamon Press, New York (see particularly Chapters VII and VIII).
4. Patterson, G. E., and Gullion, M. E. (1971): *Living With Children.* Research Press, Champaign, IL.
5. Levitz, L., and Stunkard, A. J. (1974): A therapeutic coalition for obesity: behavior modification and patient self-help. *Am. J. Psychiatry*, 131:423.
6. Liberman, R. P. (1972): *A Guide To Behavioral Analysis and Therapy*, p. 137. Pergamon Press, New York.
7. Perls, F. (1972): *In and Out Of the Garbage Pail.* Bantam, New York.
8. Gunther, B. (1971): *What To Do Until The Messiah Comes.* Collier, New York.
9. Gunther, B. (1973): *Sense Relaxation.* Pocket Books, New York.
10. Karlin, M., and Andrews, L. M. (1973): *Biofeedback.* Warner Paperback Library, New York.
11. Trupin, E., Gilchrist, L., Maiuro, R., and Faye, G. (1979): Social skills training for learning disabled children. In: *Behavioral Programs for the Developmentally Disabled*, edited by L. A. Hamerlynck. Brunner–Mazel, New York.

21

Life Planning

The vicissitudes of national elections, the women's movement, and such books as *Future Shock* (1) have not only indicated the major ways in which societal attitudes can change but also demonstrate the enormous number of personal moral and value changes which occur during many people's lives. All of us have noticed a trend toward couples living together and even having children with no intention of getting married. "Illegitimate" pregnancy is no longer a disgrace in many circles. Some people are making career changes every few years, with a year off every now and then as a looking-around period.

As more is known about adult development (Chapter 8), it is clear that upheaval and rethinking of priorities and reassessing one's life is sometimes the norm rather than the exception. The institution of marriage seems more fragile with each passing year. Even within stable marriages, wives are assuming head-of-household status for longer periods, and the number of single-parent households increases with each passing year. The primary physician can no longer be secure in giving the advice to troubled individuals that his predecessors might have given. Sometimes a well-reasoned opinion of 5 years ago is no longer relevant.

Everybody's life changes, of course, but nowadays changes occur much more rapidly. The assumptions about ourselves and the world in which many of us grew up no longer apply, although, of course, we as individuals may not be aware of this new inapplicability. For instance, 25 years ago many Americans had unquestioningly assumed that the President of the United States was relatively infallible, that the family was the "basic unit" of America, that "nice people do not get divorced," and that free, mixed discussions of sexuality and readily accessible films depicting explicit sexual activity were taboo except for "stag parties." Yet much of this has changed. Added to this is the enormous physical mobility characteristic of American life at the present time. Forty million Americans move every year, and many others have significant life changes that produce stress, temporary social isolation, and difficult adjustment to new situations.

Beginning in the 1970s, when interest in studying adults throughout their life cycles began to increase, it became clearer that change is necessary and inevitable but that people were often unable to organize their thinking in a sufficiently focused way to determine the direction and types of changes that were needed or even desirable in their lives. Added to this was the belief (now decreasing, with the increasing public awareness of these issues) that if someone questioned the patterns of his life or wanted to go in a different direction he was perhaps "sick" and needed to become a "patient" in order to come to terms with various conflicting feelings and wishes.

With the rising interest in adult development, however, new methods and techniques taken from psychology, education, and personal growth technology became available. A person or group, following a series of structured exercises, could not only become more aware of options, value changes, and the changes in his priorities on a "gut level" throughout his life, but he or they could also develop specific plans for putting such revelations into action. These techniques are loosely called "life planning." Clinical observation has suggested that such life planning can help individuals: (1) anticipate and plan for inevitable life changes (e.g., retirement); (2) assess where one is in one's life; and (3) be the basis of "non-illness" interventions to help individuals (including physicians and their families) enrich the quality of their lives, their time, and their relationships.

The purpose of life planning is just what it says: to allow a person to become much more aware of where he is at this moment, where he wants to be in the future, and how he can get there. In other words, rather than accepting whatever happens to him as "fate" or inevitable, life planning allows the person to have a hand in designing his own future. Objectives are established, "personal myths" are examined (and irrelevant parts discarded), and goals that once were valid are re-examined in the light of present needs and interests. Past influences in present choices are sometimes examined, and focused decision-making on how to increase the use of one's creative abilities is begun.

Although many life planning centers began in response to the needs of women re-entering the job market or redefining themselves as more than "just wives", the methods of life planning have been used with increasing frequency by both men and women. One center in Seattle, the Individual Development Center* (I.D. Center) has developed a curriculum in which the following issues are addressed over a period of 6 weeks in six 2-hour group sessions: (1) influences that have shaped one's past life and self-image, including school experiences, influences of family and other interpersonal influences, career, fantasies, previous employment; (2) a systematic analysis of work the participant has done, as well as a documentation of work skills, specialized knowledge, and natural abilities; (3) an analysis of the current life situation (including activities which increase or decrease anxiety, self-

---

*Individual Development Center, Ms. Alene Moris, Director, 1020 East John Street, Seattle, WA 98112.

esteem, pleasure, and energy) and an analysis of current values; (4) an analysis of current time expenditures, expenditure of discretionary income, investment in health, current friendship patterns; and (5) a compilation of long- and short-term goals, what implementing them would mean in terms of the participant and his family, and how it would have an impact on their current economic situation, self-concept, and life style. Participants are expected to complete homework assignments and to analyze in writing various facets of their lives which can then serve as the basis for group discussion.

Life planning methods and exercises have, in this author's experience, been very useful with professional groups, as well as with individual patients whose clinical complaints center around career dissatisfaction and mid-life reassessment, rather than symptoms of pathology. A sample of specific life planning exercises, taken from a variety of sources and clinically applicable to both individuals and groups, are included here:

1. *Values clarification:* Whether an individual is facing a mid-life crisis, a pre-retirement crisis, a reassessment mobilized by the children leaving home, or whether someone merely wishes to re-examine the direction in which he is going, he needs to try to clarify basic values. This has specific relevance when contemplating a move or a career change: the older person saving for retirement to a small golfing community in Arizona may find after his move that he really misses New England, his old friends, and his support system far more than he enjoys the golfing opportunities. He is now "stuck" and wishes that he could have foreseen his reactions. A recent publication, (2) originally designed to help students clarify their values, includes a number of exercises helpful for clarifying such values. The following exercise (adapted from that book) is particularly helpful in this regard. The instructor (physician/leader) asks the person to draw up a list of 20 things he likes to do. After the 20 things are listed (in no preferential order) the person is asked to code the list, using the following symbols:

$—beside each item which costs more than $10 each time it is done.
A—beside those items he prefers to do alone.
P—beside those items he prefers to do with other people.
LP—beside those items he enjoys equally alone or with other people.
PL—beside those items which require planning.
N5—beside those items which he would not have done 5 years ago.
R—for those items involving risk (by self-definition).
I—for those items involving intimacy (by self-definition).
S—for those items which can be done only one season of the year.
U—for those items he thinks other people would consider unconventional.
CH—for those items he hopes his children will have on a similar list at his age.
F—for those items he thinks will not appear on his list 5 years from now.

Finally, to the far left, he is asked to list the five most important things currently, number 1 first, etc. To the right side, he should mark with a "B" the three things he anticipates will become the three things in the future which will have the most importance (e.g., 10 years from now). At the conclusion of this exercise, the person is asked to make a statement in writing summarizing his data and observations about himself.

2. *Analysis of present situation:* It is often difficult to describe how one "feels" about his present situation. Many times it seems preferable not to face the realities and to avoid thinking about the situation directly, carrying on in as routine a way as possible, hoping that somehow, someway, things will get better by themselves. Sometimes, upon analysis, time itself is seen as one's best ally; more often, however, procrastination is a self-defeating tactic which exacts a high price in psychic energy and physical vitality.

Sometimes when one faces a difficult decision, the problem obscures the whole life picture. It is necessary to stand back and "see the forest." It is necessary that a patient (or any person assessing his life situation) consider the total situation and not just problem areas. The following exercises (modified from those developed at the ID Center) allow one to list the dimensions of the present situation which are both positive and negative (individuals list items under each heading):

  a. *Anxiety increasers:* Tasks or circumstances which tend to heighten tension or which cause the person to feel insecure or worried.
  b. *Anxiety reducers:* Tasks or circumstances which tend to relieve tension, or which help meet needs for security and belonging.
  c. *Exhausters:* Tasks or aspects of life which tend to tire the person out of proportion to the real energy expended.
  d. *Energizers:* Anything in the person's life which actually seems to release or create new energy; a task which leaves him more invigorated than when he started.

At the completion of such exercises, a person is then asked to make a statement: "Upon examination of this analysis, I realize that _____. If I am to continue much as I am doing now (making no conscious decisions), the likely consequences would be _____."

3. *New goals:* Developing specific goals, both short- and long-term, can provide a focus for helping decide where one wants to go and provide a means to get there. Balanced goals—between career, personal goals, and in terms of relationships—should be included. General goals (e.g., "security" or "happiness") are much too vague to fulfill. Restating a security goal as "getting a job with a bigger salary" comes closer to articulating it in specific terms.

To emphasize the need for balanced goals, three rather artificial categories may be set up: relationships, individual goals, work/job goals. In reality, these goals impinge on and blend with one another. Goals should first be brainstormed; later on, one can choose specific ones on which to work.

4. *Longitudinal life assessment:* A graphic way (literally) to describe and chart one's life so far is to make a "life line" across a sheet of paper, with the beginning of the paper (on the left) representing birth. The line can then be drawn to the point where the person is now in terms of years, rising like a fever chart for "high points"

and sinking near the bottom of the page for bad times or low points. Each high and low point should be labeled. The chart serves as an excellent focus for discussion, graphically condensing a great deal of material.

5. *Life roles:* A person is asked to list 10 roles which are considered to be the most important in his life (e.g., husband, father, teacher, friend of X, and so on). The person is asked to check the four roles which are the most important or give the most satisfaction. He is then asked if the amount of time spent in any of these roles would change if he had only 1 year to live, and if there were any roles he would eliminate altogether. After writing these down, the person is asked to discuss the conclusions with someone else.

6. *Identity questions:* A person is asked to list 30 words or phrases which describe who he is. He is then asked to list, in order, the five which are the most important.

7. *Projective questions:* A series of structured questions that are likely to provoke anxiety and which have a very personal quality are given to a person one by one to complete in written form. The most effective use of these questions is to have some time for discussion after each question or two.
   a. What would "heaven on earth" be for you?
   b. If you were marooned on a beautiful island with abundant food and water but could bring only half a dozen individuals with you, who would they be? What activities would you do with these individuals?
   c. If you had 6 months to live, how would you like to spend the time?
   d. If you were to die today, what would you like inscribed on your tombstone? What would you like people to remember about you after your death? If that is not how they see you now, is there any way to change things so they could see you the way you would like to be seen?
   e. If you suddenly won (on a quiz show) one million dollars, what would you do with it?
   f. If you were 20 years old again, what would you do differently? What would happen if some of those things you think you would do differently were incorporated into your life now?
   g. Are there any individuals in your life whose influence has had a bad effect on you? What would you like to say to each individual if you had the chance?

These exercises and others from the sources cited can be compiled by an individual physician to fit the needs of his particular patient population or any individual patient. They can be useful in helping guide a patient toward an examination of current and alternative life styles and values. As the directions imply, however, they should not be asked in a casual way. Sufficient time must be taken for thinking about the questions, answering them in writing, and discussing them. Ultimately, the questions are designed to look at such issues as:

1. Can I simplify my life but keep it productive and interesting?
2. How important is money to me in my overall scheme of things?
3. How much time do I have to do the things I really want to do, and how can I make more time for these things?

4. How much anxiety does my current style of living generate and is it worth it?

If change is contemplated, these types of exercises also force the individual to focus on:

1. How much would I have to give up?
2. Where would I live and how?
3. Could I give up existing commitments; if so, which ones?
4. Would the change turn into another rat race, and how could I prevent this from happening?

The purpose of life planning is to allow the individual, with the help of his physician or counselor, to achieve the greatest possible intelligent and responsible control over the decisions in his life, and to free him from a reliance on "fate", chance, and luck.

REFERENCES

1. Tofler, A. (1970): *Future Shock*. Bantam, New York.
2. Simon, E. B., Howe, L. W., and Kirchenbaum, H. (1972): *Values Clarification*, p. 31. Hart, New York (modified).
3. Lurie, H. J. (1977): Life Planning: an educational approach to change. *Am. J. Psychiatry*, 134.8:878–882.

22

Marital and Family Counseling

Many couples and families come to a family physician with problems about how their relationships are functioning. Sometimes the problems are major, and it becomes evident immediately that interactional problems are so severe a referral to a professional therapist is crucial. However, marital or family problems sometimes emerge in oblique ways, and it is often unclear whether the situation would respond to brief educational intervention or to supportive counseling provided by a primary physician, or if it requires a referral. A referral may be appropriate either because of the length of time a successful intervention might take, or because the situation needs the skills and experience of a trained professional versed in the intricacies of untangling conflict-ridden relationships. This chapter looks at a variety of issues relevant to couples and families: assessment, the dimensions and strategies of supportive counseling, and the cases appropriate for referral.

DIAGNOSTIC ISSUES

Developmental Issues

Stress both within and between individuals may arise throughout the life cycle, and often at reasonably predictable intervals (Chapters 8, 11, and 23). It is often when such a developmental stress occurs that family members may call on a physician or counselor, sometimes with somatic complaints and sometimes with an explicit complaint about what is happening in the relationship.

Example
   A young mother, barely able to cope with two preschoolers and who receives very little support emotionally from her spouse, becomes pregnant. She is irritable and angry, and wants an abortion. Her husband is puzzled and opposed to the abortion. He believes the "problem" is his wife. She believes the "problem" is the marriage and that her husband expects too much from her. She comes to the physician because of fatigue and depression.

Maturational Issues

Many individuals, when young, courting, or newly coupled, romantically imbue their partner with superlative attributes; they often find qualities and strengths in their partners which they themselves are lacking. Sometimes these attributes and strengths are valid, of course, but often with time it becomes clear that these are projections, or that people want other qualities and behaviors than the ones with which they were originally enamored.

Example
A woman with doubts about her own values of child-rearing may be particularly taken with the strong religious and moral principles of the man she dates and subsequently marries. It is when they are raising children, however, that she becomes distressed and irritated by the husband's convictions which now strike her as "rigid and harsh." She herself since the marriage may have gradually developed her own values about child-rearing which she views as humanistic, kind, and supportive, but which her husband views as "coddling" and "wishy-washy." Thus as the relationship has evolved, the husband may see the evolution of his wife's values and beliefs as a betrayal of the original beliefs of the wife (which were actually only a mirror of his own beliefs). She in turn may believe that she has "married her worst enemy" now that her own ideas have evolved and changed.

Cultural Issues

Most people acquire a notion of what is a right or a wrong way to do things; they get these attitudes from their families and from the culture in which that family existed. The family of origin and the culture define, for example, how men should behave in general, how fathers should act, how much cursing is tolerated, appropriate sexual expression, how intimacy is expressed, and what kinds of decisions are made and by whom. Individuals are often attracted by differences in these areas, which they perceive as personality differences but which may really be the reflection of the familial and cultural differences between the individuals.

Example
A reserved and laconic WASP male from a reserved and rather proper family may be attracted by the emotional expressiveness, loquacity, and warmth of the Italian-American girl he is dating and subsequently marries. Under stress and during marital conflicts, however, he becomes even more reserved and quiet, and she becomes loud and even more emotionally expressive. A misunderstanding may be significantly aggravated by the way in which each person reacts when in conflict or under stress, especially because each of the individuals has a strong, unquestioned conviction that his is the only "proper" way to react or to conduct himself.

Communication Issues

Communication among couples and in families is often unclear and even destructive, particularly when the couple or family is in conflict or under stress. People have different meanings for different words, and particularly points made by one person may be only half-understood by another in the relationship.

Over time, certain complementary but destructive communication patterns can grow up between individuals. Each person plays a decisive part in the destructive interaction, although one or another of the individuals may be blamed for the problem.

Satir (1) described a number of faulty communication situations in families. She spoke of the *blamer* who characteristically directs his internal anger at other family members, pointing an accusing finger at other people and holding them responsible for anything that has gone wrong. Blamers characteristically think only of themselves and ignore the feelings their accusations arouse in other persons.

The *placator*, on the other hand, is all too ready to assume responsibility for whatever unfortunate thing has happened. He embraces this responsibility and assumption of guilt, disregarding his own feelings of hurt. He serves to complement the behavior of the blamer by being a willing scapegoat for the blamer's wrath.

The *dictionary* is a person who is primarily concerned about "being right" and leaves the human element out of the equation. Such a person is constantly citing authorities, immutable laws of nature, etc. He omits or considers irrelevant his own feelings and the feelings of the individuals with whom he is dealing.

The *irrelevant* person is one who simply avoids being pinned down in a situation, usually by putting up such a smoke screen of distracting signals, talk, and behavior that those conversing with him are never sure whether a point in decision-making has been reached.

Each of these dysfunctional communication styles elicits in the partner and children of a family some sort of complementary behavior, often another dysfunctional communication. Sometimes, even a "straight" (nondysfunctional) statement or question elicits a dysfunctional response. For example, a husband politely inquiring about an irregularity he noticed in the checkbook may get a hostile, blaming response from the wife, about "It's all your fault that I have to write checks, anyway. You should do them all." A mother who asks her child in a neutral way why he is 15 minutes late after school may be greeted by behavior from the child which is hyperactive, evasive, and joking (irrelevant). The persons in these or similar situations may be trying to avoid accepting responsibility in a situation or being controlled by the other person.

Complementary patterns of poor communication may gradually develop in a marriage or family, becoming so much a part of the milieu that unless there is an outside observation individuals are never aware of the ways in which they characteristically respond to each other.

Personality Pathology Issues

Although everyone has longstanding traits through which he deals with conflict or uncertainty—and which are generally called personality traits—some individuals have traits that are sufficiently exaggerated or dysfunctional as to be called personality disorders. The labeling of such disorders may come from psychiatric nomenclature (e.g., "passive-aggressive" as a description of someone who repeatedly and habitually resists authority through negativistic, pseudocompliant means). Labeling may also be done using transactional analysis (2) nomenclature (e.g., the person playing a "Yes, but" game in response to suggestions he has asked for). In severely dysfunctional marriages, Martin (3) found that certain personalities tend to be attracted to each other. These include the following (3):

1. *The "love-sick" wife and the "cold-sick" husband:* In this relationship the "hysterical" wife, who has a poorly formed sense of her own identity, forms a parasitic relationship with her "obsessional" husband. In such situations, the wife typically complains that her husband does not love her but also deprecates and destroys every source of self-development and individuation. The husband, though competent, has emotional constriction or seething conflicts held in check by rigidity and constriction of emotional expression. Martin avers that such couples are "the most common and most difficult psychotherapeutic problem."

2. *An "in-search-of-a-mother" marriage:* In such a relationship, the husband is "hysterical," tending to be passive and dependent, with a dominant wife who has an obsessive-compulsive personality. The pattern of the marriage is such that the man characteristically marries young and appears to marry for love. His wife works and helps him in his career until they have children. Dismayed at her inability to take complete care of him, he then searches around for a younger woman to do the job.

3. *The "double-parasite" marriage:* In this marriage the passive-dependent wife and the passive-dependent husband are married to each other. They tended to be either indigent—with neither partner able to carry the responsibility for the marriage and with "alcoholism, drugs, anxiety, depression, and inability to work" characterizing the marriage—or else have inherited wealth but are "emotionally incapable of being good parents and hostilely project their inadequacies onto the mate." Each partner expects the other to take care of him and make the marriage work, and neither can grow or fulfill the other's needs.

4. *The paranoid marriage:* One or both partners in this marriage hold distortions or denials of reality. There may be agreement between the two about the same delusions which permits them to get along in the marriage (but terribly outside the marriage). There may be a situation in which one partner delusionally and constantly blames the other (thereby permitting that partner to function all right outside the marriage but terribly within it). In some paranoid marriages both partners share a distorted self-protecting view of the world, representing a type of marriage which Ford and Herrick called, "two against the world" (4).

"Transference And Projection" Issues

Marital relationships over time tend to elicit emotions which are often reminiscent of emotions from childhood, particularly toward frustrating or nurturing authority figures. As transactional analysis experts have observed, one spouse often interacts with the other as if he were a child (e.g., "You should do this"). The other spouse, in turn, may respond as a child ("I won't do it, you can't make me"), and the battle is on. Transferring such reactions and affective states unconsciously from one's own childhood into a current marriage or family situation is called transference and can be examined when such repeated patterns become apparent.

Another unconscious pattern is that of the parent who projects on the child an image of someone from the past (e.g., "You look just like your uncle who landed in jail, and you're going to turn out like him too"). Being treated repeatedly as if he is to behave in a certain way may induce in the "victim" of such "projective identification" a pattern of behavioral response which indeed corresponds closely to the projection. Such a pattern, though sometimes easy to identify, is usually difficult to treat.

DIAGNOSTIC PROCEDURES FOR MARITAL AND FAMILY ASSESSMENT

To complete an assessment of a marital or family conflict, it is crucial to "see the situation in action." Frequently statements a person makes about a relationship are a distortion (often inadvertent) of the real situation. For some individuals, it may be easier to talk about how mean and cruel the spouse is without mentioning (or perhaps even being aware) how provocative they themselves are, and how much the spouse is "set up" to act in the cruel way. Similarly, a placating person may blame himself for the problems in the family or marriage without noticing that accepting the blame, no matter how unjustified, is his characteristic pattern.

When people talk about relationships, they may not indicate the extent of their hatred, love, or loyalty, all of which are critical ingredients when assessing whether the marriage or family unit can be mobilized to save itself. The degree to which people act as mature or responsible individuals within a relationship may also be inapparent from conversation or history-taking alone. For example, an intelligent, articulate businessman who appears to have everything under control judging by his own descriptions may act like a dependent child or a ferocious bully when seen in the context of his family. The lack of independence and development as a separate, autonomous individual is evident only when the person is observed reacting with his spouse or family present not by himself.

To assess the interaction of individuals within a marriage or family, the couple or family is usually given a series of structured tasks. Different family therapists use different specific tasks. The following, a modification of the "Structured Family Interview" from the excellent family therapy text by Glick and Kessler (5), presents one viable assessment model:

1. The interviewer asks each family member, "What is the main problem in your family at present?" Each is given a chance to speak. Usually the questioning begins with one parent. (The answers to this question help assess whether the perception is that this is indeed a marital/family problem or an individual problem.)

2. The interviewer asks the family to plan something they can do together. (The interviewer may stay or leave the room while this is going on.) The couple, without the children, is then asked to plan something just the two of them would enjoy doing together. If there is a family problem with an "identified patient," the child and first one parent and then the other are also asked to plan something they would enjoy doing together.

3. The marital pair is asked how they happened to meet and how they decided to get married. (Although Glick and Kessler suggest that this be done with just the husband and wife present, other therapists find that this is enlightening for the children as well, and demystifies the myth of parental infallibility.) Taking such a history helps focus on the mutual illusions of courtship and early marriage, and may help point up why there are problems now, as some of the illusions are challenged, given up, or outgrown. The history often uncovers resentments and bitterness which may have soured the relationship and which may never have been discussed.

4. The parents are asked to arrive at a mutually satisfactory interpretation of a proverb or saying they have been given and then teach it to their children. Such a task not only illuminates how the couple relate to each other in terms of power, compromise, and negotiation, it also may illuminate bizarre or distorted communication patterns between the couple and with their children.

5. Family members are handed cards on which they are asked to write down the outstanding fault of the family member to their immediate left. The therapist also adds some comment cards. The cards are then collected; the therapist shuffles them and reads each one aloud. He asks the family to decide which family member the comment applies to. Another section of this question involves asking each family member to state what he considers his outstanding fault.

6. Family members are handed cards on which they are asked to write down the most admirable quality ("the thing you like/admire most") of the person to their left. The therapist also adds a few cards of his own, the cards are collected, and as the therapist reads each one, the family is again asked to decide which family member the comment applies to. Each individual in the family is asked to say what he considers his own outstanding quality.

7. If the identified patient is a child, each family member in turn is asked which of the two parents the identified patient most resembles.

When dealing with a couple alone, some therapists during the assessment phase ask each member of the couple, in turn, to tell the other one what he would like to change to make the relationship better. Sometimes this question is structured by asking the couple to hold hands while the question is being asked and answered. (What can be helpful about observing this is to note the level of comfort or discomfort each member experiences in stating a position, trying to establish verbal intimacy, and trying to establish even a small amount of physical intimacy.)

When dealing with either a couple or a family, it is important to try to assess the level of humor, good will, depression, or hostility family members convey toward each other when they are together. If there appears to be only contempt, irritation, and virtually no respect within the marriage or the family, or if family members adamantly insist on choosing and keeping an identified scapegoat within the family system, the likelihood of the family working productively in family therapy may be considerably reduced.

COUNSELING STRATEGIES AND INTERVENTIONS

As mentioned earlier in this chapter, families with severe interpersonal problems are usually beyond the competence and the time available within the primary physician's professional life to permit treatment to be carried on effectively. On the other hand, many marital or family situations respond favorably to support, reassurance, guidance, and suggestion. In such situations the couple or family has a reservoir of basic good will, trust, and respect; the problems are situationally or developmentally induced; and the personalities of the individuals involved are not so maladaptive or intractable as to make compromise, change, modeling, or trying new behaviors an impossibility. The following are some guidelines for working with a couple or family (provided the previous conditions have been met):

1. A specific number of sessions to work on specific issues is agreed on. Usually this contract is reached by the middle or end of the session.

2. The therapist makes an alliance with each family or couple member present. Such a conscious move is essential to ensure that the physician or therapist will be seen as a person who does not "take sides." It is especially important in marital work that an alliance be made with the most reluctant/skeptical family member, as that person's agreement to participate is usually crucial for the success of the treatment.

3. A detailed history should be taken from each parent about their own families of origin: What were the rules (explicit and implicit)? What role did the parent play within the family (e.g., "mother's helper," "the baby")? Other considerations include: Who made the important decision in each parent's family? How were males treated in contrast to females? How would the nondominant parent achieve power (e.g., manipulation, argument, secret "deals" with the children)? Answers to each of these questions provide important clues to the ways in which each parent/spouse currently views the "proper" procedure in the current marriage together with the expectation of how the other spouse should behave.

4. Because most people caught up in a marital or family conflict want the other person to "change right now," it is important in family counseling to "cool the conflict." This may be done by making a contract to meet for a number of weeks or sessions, during which time there is an agreement that no major unilateral marital/family decisions will be undertaken. This "breather" will permit issues to be examined and alternatives for change explored (none of which can easily be done at the height of the conflict). Strategies which may help cool down the situation while it is being examined include:

a. Getting a historical prospective about the major complaints about the marriage or family problems:

> "George always was an impatient guy, but he got a lot worse after he got his promotion two years ago and had to travel a lot more."
> "Billy was always a bit hyper and obnoxious, but after his Dad and I got divorced 2 years ago and his Dad moved away, he really started acting up."

b. Having each family member develop a small, written list of major areas he would like to see changed in the family. This written list may then serve as the basis for negotiation of areas or issues within the relationship or system.

> "I'll promise to start coming home on time if Alice will give me 15 minutes to recover my wits and read the paper before she starts complaining about what's wrong."
> "I'll do my chores without being told if Dad will let me stay out later on Friday nights so I can go to parties with my friends."

c. Having each member of the couple complete a "marital assessment test" (e.g., those in Lederer and Jackson's book) (6). Each partner (married, contemplating marriage, or struggling with a shaky marriage) separately completes a particular test. When the results are compared, they are useful in estimating the degree of compatibility and likelihood of a successful marriage. Insights the tests provide can serve as a basis for discussion and negotiation between a married couple, helping each person expand his horizons within the marriage and encouraging each to try new things his partner likes but which he may not like himself. Test A deals with historical background. For example, "In our community, my parents were (a) considered important; (b) included among people with some standing; (c) average socially; (d) below average socially; (e) considered to be outsiders." Test B deals with past life experiences, present life experiences, attitudes, perceptions of the mate, expectations for the marriage and its relation to future plans, etc. Completing such a written test often provides a specific focus which can serve as a point of negotiation in a way that spoken words cannot.

d. Using life planning exercises (Chapter 21). Some life planning exercises, by forcing individuals to clarify values, perceptions of self, and personal goals, may also serve as a point of negotiation and compromise.

e. Development of an explicit "marriage contract." Sager (7) described how each individual has both explicit and implicit expectations of the marriage, and that teasing out what these are often determines the basis for negotiation. Components include such issues as expectations of the marriage (e.g., "a mate who will be loyal, devoted, loving, and exclusive"); intrapsychic and biological determinants (e.g., on the "closeness-distance continuum," does anxiety increase with closeness or self-disclosure); and external foci of marital problems (e.g., communication, life style, families of origin) (7).

f. Prescribing or advising various decision-making procedures or tasks in the family or marriage and examining the results (e.g., having Dad "discipline" Johnny for not doing his homework, in contrast to the current situation of Mom yelling and criticizing Johnny, which he blithely ignores). Tasks may also be explicitly positive ("I want you children to insist that Mom and Dad go out to dinner once this week. Bob, you can help Dad decide on the place to go; Sue, you can help Mom stop worrying about whether you and Bob will have enough to eat or get into trouble when they're out.")

THE NEED FOR REFERRAL

Although support, structured interviewing, and negotiation among couples and families sometimes help, often the "real" issues are considerably more subtle and deep-seated; these require the intervention of an expert who can unravel the difficulties, which may be out of conscious awareness. It is also important to be aware that when a couple or family seeks counseling, their motivation for treatment may be different from what they say. For example, when they both say they want "help," they may mean two separate things: One partner may have already decided on divorce, and the help he wants is to have that process facilitated; he may want to "dump" his mate on the counselor or doctor. Similarly, the semidelinquent child who is brought by his parents may be brought not, as the parents initially state, so the family can negotiate and learn to live together, but so that the child may be sent away to a residential treatment center or boarding school.

Having a slightly skeptical approach to marital and family motivation, therefore, is crucial. Marital and family therapy, beyond the supportive, clarifying, and somewhat simple structural techniques described here, is time-consuming, complex, and relatively exhausting. An appropriate referral for a difficult family or couple (despite what the couple or family says they want) may ultimately save the primary physician's time, energy, and frustration.

REFERENCES

1. Satir, V. (1972): *Peoplemaking*. Science and Behavior Books, Palo Alto, CA.
2. Berne, E. (1964): *Games People Play*. Grove Press, New York.
3. Martin, P. (1976): *A Marital Therapy Manual*, pp. 5–30. Brunner/Mazel, New York.
4. Ford, F., and Herrick, J. (1974): Family rules/family life styles. *Am. J. Orthopsychiatry*, January.
5. Glick, I. D., and Kessler, D. R. (1980): *Marital and Family Therapy*, 2nd ed. Grune & Stratton, New York (modified).
6. Lederer, W., and Jackson, D. D. (1968): *Mirages of Marriage*, p. 381. Norton, New York (modified).
7. Sager, C. (1976): *Marriage Contracts and Couple Therapy*. Brunner/Mazel, New York.

23

Sexual Counseling Roles of the Physician

The area of sexual counseling has been seen as the physician's "territory" for a number of years—to the dismay of many physicians, who often feel inadequate for the task. This chapter focuses on several aspects of sexual counseling; roles played by the physician are those of teacher, facilitator, permission-giver, and, if adequately trained, sex therapist. Much of the material in this chapter is a compilation of ideas, techniques, and materials a primary physician might use in his office. The description of specific techniques of sexual therapy are intended more for information than as guidelines for how to conduct treatment. (In the author's opinion, techniques of sexual therapy should be learned with the help and supervision of an "expert" accustomed to employing them.) However, providing information, taking an adequate sexual history, and knowing about educational or therapy resources, whether books, movies, or special clinics, should be a part of the repertoire of each primary physician.

WHO WANTS HELP AND WHY?

Patients coming to a family physician often have sexual concerns and questions. Planned Parenthood, adapting ideas of Annon (1), conceptualized that the kinds of intervention required in treating sexual concerns of patients include the following, which they call the PLISSIT Model:

*P*ermission (for patients to ask questions about sexuality and receive reassurance).

*L*imited *I*nformation (to give patients information and facts about sexual behavior, including the wide range of individual sexual behavior).

*S*pecific *S*uggestion (which the physician may impart to the patients, regarding sexual communication to help with a dysfunction, recommendations to join a preorgasmic women's group, etc.).

*I*ntensive *T*herapy (where significant psychological and emotional problems are part of the sexual dysfunction and they require long-term treatment).

Implicit within the PLISSIT model is that the vast majority of sexual complaints require permission and limited information, and that a much smaller number call for specific information. An even smaller number need intensive therapy. The primary physician who is open, accepting, and comfortable with the subject of sexuality will be asked many questions by patients of different ages often in the course of nonacute care of physical problems, during the follow-up of chronic problems, or during normal health maintenance. A large number of questions reflect "development concerns" of the individual's particular life stage. Some of these include the following (2).

Prenatal Period

Especially during the first pregnancy, a woman may feel that she has become or is becoming sexually unattractive, particularly as her sexy figure is supplanted by a bulging abdomen and pendulous breasts. Coupled with the sense of being unattractive is the fear that sexual relations during the latter part of the pregnancy may injure the fetus, induce a miscarriage, or in some other way be harmful. This sense of doubt or guilt about sexual activity may create communication problems or produce sexual anxiety and unresponsiveness ("Let's hurry up and get this over with"), with sexual problems continuing later on. Giving advice while encouraging her questions and finding out her concerns often helps. The physician can alleviate guilt, clarify issues, and give permission for activity which will continue to be supportive to the couple and their relationship. Encouraging touching and coital positions which are less tiring to the female, informing couples of the continued need for foreplay, and spoken reassurance which are essential to many women during pregnancy can do much to maintain sexual and personal communication between the partners.

Neonatal Period

When a family physician sees a mother and child a few days after delivery, the mother wants reassurance not only about her child's general health but about her own and her baby's sexual health as well. Many mothers of first-born children have never observed a newborn child at close range. The presence of hormone-induced enlargement of nipples and labia in a female child, for instance, requires a reassuring "that's fine and healthy" statement from the physician. Similarly, a new mother, feeling pain from her episiotomy, will wonder "What's been torn up down there?" Positive statements should be made about resuming sexual activity, and advice should be given about exercises to restore muscle tone, normal body contour, and sexual responsiveness if the new mother has concerns in these areas.

Childhood

The interventions by primary physicians about the sexual concerns of children can have long-lasting therapeutic effects. It is the parents who are most concerned about the sexual expression of their young children. As they grow, the children themselves will have concerns about their bodies and their sexuality. During early childhood parents sometimes attribute to their children qualities associated with relatives: If a child masturbates or explores his body in a way that is normal for his age, it may still be seen as behavior of the kind that "got Uncle John into trouble." A positive explanation to the parents that their children's bodies are normal and healthy, and that their exploratory behavior is also normal and healthy, can help dispel some of this attribution.

Children, similarly, often wonder if their bodies are normal or if having sexual sensations or questions means that something is "wrong" (both physically and morally). If a primary physician has a comfortable relationship with a child, he can often make positive statements about a child's body during or at the conclusion of a physical examination. For example, "That's a fine penis." Talking comfortably with children, giving them books to read about their bodies and sexuality, and emphasizing the positive aspects of sexual development, self-exploration, and "good feelings" often help them regard their sexuality positively. This is preferable to the attitude that sex is something to be whispered about only with friends or to be ashamed of, denied, hidden, suppressed, or not felt.

Adolescent Concerns

Many adolescents have concerns about their looks, their popularity, their relationship with their parents, their future, and their sexuality. Because onset of puberty varies so greatly among children, they have a continual preoccupation about body size and genital adequacy. If adolescents trust their physician, they often inquire about body size: "I think my penis is too small" or "I think my breasts are too big." Being comfortable when discussing anatomy, pubertal changes, and sexual functioning can relieve much of the anxiety which adolescents experience when they feel that in some way they are "different."

Many girls are prepared for menstruation physically, but there is often little psychological reassurance about the possibility (and desirability) of remaining physically active during menstruation. Boys are rarely prepared for wet dreams and frequently go to great lengths to conceal "the evidence," feeling that something shameful or abnormal has occurred.

Masturbation is of even greater concern. There is an increasing body of evidence that individuals who become comfortable with their own sexuality as they grow up and who experience and experiment with sexuality at least to a limited degree adjust more comfortably to the explicit sexual roles expected of them as adults. For instance, girls who masturbate as teenagers are more apt to be orgasmic as adults, as they are more comfortable and familiar with their own sexuality and sexual response patterns. When asked about masturbation, the physician should answer, "It won't harm you; it's perfectly normal." If it seems appropriate, the physician can also mention its positive aspects, e.g., the relief of sexual tension and the promotion of an individual's awareness of his own body. The physician, however, should certainly be sensitive to the needs and beliefs of the teenager and not impose his own beliefs, which may be unwelcome or embarrassing.

A pelvic examination may be embarrassing for young girls and even for older adolescent patients. If the patient is treated with friendly respect—sometimes with even a bit of "distance"—the patient feels more at ease. When the physician calls the patient (whom he does not know socially) "honey" and talks about "you girls," the examination may have embarrassing sexual overtones and make the patient feel she is being demeaned and, in some undefined way, being "cheap."

A vast majority of teenagers want reassurance and factual information. Providing these routinely and without a lot of fanfare can be very helpful. Beginning with early physical examinations, the physician can make clear to both children and parents that he is available to answer any question pertaining to sexuality—privately with either the parents or the child. He may also point out to the parents that often children confide in the doctor only if they know that their questions will be held in strict confidence. Once he has parental permission, the primary physician may reassure teenagers that he will not pass on information to the parents. Both physician and teenager are then free to discuss such topics as male and female contraception, anatomy, sexual functioning, "crushes" (both heterosexual and homosexual), venereal disease detection and prevention, and sexual responsibility. (Incidentally, the family physician may play a role in reinforcing an adolescent's decision *not* to become involved sexually if he is uncomfortable or unready for such experiences.)

A physician can also help his adolescent patients by becoming informed about the ages of "normal" exploration of homosexuality. (The statistics may have changed since Kinsey; there is some suggestion that more college students are experimenting with both homosexual and heterosexual activity and seem interested in being "sexual" rather than identifying themselves as exclusively "one thing or the other.") A primary physician is wise to be "cool" about confessions of homosexual activity: Persons who subsequently became bisexual, homosexual, or heterosexual often report that their encounters with doctors around this topic have been disastrous. The physician tries to "cure" them at once, reassure them prematurely, or is so embarrassed by the topic that both patient and doctor retreat in confusion. (If the doctor feels especially uncomfortable about this topic, the patient could be referred to a competent counselor whom he knows and trusts and for whom the topic is less problematic.)

When doing sexual counseling with an adolescent patient or young adult, particularly shy ones who come either to seek birth control information or for premarital counseling, it is extremely important that the physician be comfortable with the language his patients use. "Screwing" and "fucking" may be more natural and comfortable to patients than "coitus" and "intercourse," though the physician may prefer the latter terms. If the adolescent detects embarrassment on the part of the physician when sexual concerns are raised, the patient may cease to admit having any sexual questions. If the physician can answer questions about rubbers and the clap, some patients may feel free to voice other concerns.

Adult Years

Recent studies of adult development (3) suggest that adults experience varying needs for personal and physical intimacy during adult life, and that couples negotiate different sexual patterns and roles as their relationship changes. A young couple in their early twenties may experience a difficult sexual and personal adjustment when negotiating sexual roles and prerogatives. For example, a man may feel that his role sexually is to initiate all sexual activity and to "teach his wife about sexuality." This rigid set of expectations, acquired from his own family and his social peer group, may directly conflict with his wife's expectations that she knows something about her own sexual needs and has the right to indicate such needs and desires. If the couple has trouble discussing these issues and expectations, it may become very important for the family physician to be able to serve as a negotiator for them, simply giving them some perspective about their differences and where their different expectations arose.

As their relationship continues, other stresses which are reflected in their sexual life may emerge. The desire for career achievement may make physical and personal intimacy seem of secondary importance. Children and their care may produce fatigue and a conflict about who gets the most attention and affection. A role conflict may appear when individuals are torn between being parent, spouse, lover, etc. Statements such as, "My husband's too tired to be interested in sex/My wife seems a lot more interested in the kids than in me/We try to have sex, but the baby keeps crying and it turns me off/We don't have any privacy anymore" call for an active problem-solving role for the primary physician to help couples develop their own solutions. The vast majority of such problems are not really sexual problems at all; they are problems of living which are beginning to jeopardize the intimacy of a relationship. Without appropriate intervention, such problems can lead to decreased sexual contact, feelings of estrangement, and development of more serious sexual problems.

The harrassed, depressed mother of young children who feels overwhelmed by the sexual demands of her spouse and the physical needs of her children may easily become nonorgasmic or simulate sexual enthusiasm so that she can "get it over with" and go to sleep. Similarly, the husband who feels that his wife spends all her time with and gives her attention to the children and is starting to treat him like one of them may become threatened and anxious, and develop partial impotence or premature ejaculation: He feels that the sexual experience is no longer a shared pleasure but something that his wife is "putting up with" for him. The primary physician who acts as a facilitator with the couple may be able to suggest ways in which the couple can work to maintain sexual intimacy (and thereby prevent more serious sexual difficulties from arising or the present ones from eroding the relationship).

Mid-life Transition

A variety of personal and sexual concerns emerge during the late thirties and early forties. They may be experienced as a chance to re-establish lost intimacy which was previously eroded by the demands of career, family, and community responsibilities, or they may be felt at the time an individual thinks about his current relationship and wonders, "Is this all there is? Is there something more that I'm missing?" Here the primary physician can offer suggestions for marital enrichment and for promoting open discussion about sexual fulfillment within the relationship. The physician can also dispel some of the myths associated with middle age (e.g., an inevitable decline in sexual interest and performance related to menopause).

Old Age

Because elderly persons are usually more reticent about presenting sexual problems and concerns than young people, it requires special sensitivity and tact to pick up these concerns. It is especially important that a primary physician be able to communicate information about sexual functioning. Elderly people often believe the cultural mythology that sexual expression is "finished" by the time one reaches old age. This clearly is not true, as sexual functioning can continue indefinitely. Older patients often need to be encouraged to remain sexually active, to exercise, to touch, and to be informed about the differences in sexual performance in elderly males (ability to have an erection, but desiring or reaching orgasm less frequently). Women outnumber men in this age group, and the primary physician should allay the guilt of older women who are distressed because they masturbate. It seems clear that physical touching, especially in this age group, is a comforting and restorative experience. Encouraging such touching, with or without erotic implications, may require the explicit sanction of a trusted physician.

TAKING A SEXUAL HISTORY

In addition to anticipating questions and concerns which normally arise during the life cycle, the primary physician must often ask detailed questions in order to gather sufficient data on which to base decisions about the intervention that would be most appropriate. Each individual grows up in a different family and has acquired different assumptions, myths, and values about how one should be, both as a person and as a sexual being, and what sorts of things are or are not proper in situations labeled "sexual." Sexual histories, therefore, in order to be complete must elicit not only detailed information about (1) specific symptoms of sexual dysfunction, but also about (2) areas of the relationship which are or are not satisfying, (3) how the partners communicate with each other (both sexually and nonsexually), and (4) where and how they learned their original attitudes toward physical and nonphysical communication. A person's values may either obviously or more subtly interfere with his sexual functioning. It is important, therefore, to inquire about attitudes on nudity, touching, and expressing emotion (or keeping feelings in), and whether the person views intercourse as a pleasure or a "duty." How does each partner view his own sexual role and that of his spouse? Where did he learn about these sexual roles?

Psychological factors, especially depression, anger, and conflict, may interfere with sexual functioning. Some clinics therefore ask the patient to list any specific "resentments" pertaining to sex (even if they seem trivial) which he bears toward the spouse. Patients are also asked to list five or more resentments about matters other than sex (4).

A person's feelings about himself as a sexual person also strongly influences sexual performance and satisfaction. The Group For the Advancement of Psychiatry (GAP) in its interviewing guide includes a questionnaire that measures "sexual appealingness (5)." Included in the questionnaire is a section entitled, "Feelings About Self as Masculine/Feminine." The section for the male asks such questions as: Do you feel masculine? Popular? Sexually adequate? Sexually inadequate? Do you have any feelings about being a "sissy?" Are you accepted by peers? What are your feelings about (a) body size (height, weight, etc.), (b) appearance (handsomeness, virility), (c) voice, (d) hair distribution, (e) genitalia (size, circumcision, undescended testicle), (f) virility, (g) potency, (h) ability to respond sexually?

Asking and getting detailed answers to questions such as these from both partners can provide significant information about how they view themselves as sexual beings. Additional questions should explore what each partner conceives is his sexual role vis-à-vis the other partner or the opposite sex in general. For instance, a woman may feel that her "role" is to be passive, allowing the male to make all the sexual advances and to be silent about those physical aspects of sexuality which she either enjoys or finds unpleasurable. This woman's sexual partner would be very unlikely to discover what pleased her. If the partner also has a strong taboo about talking about such things, he may never know if she enjoys their lovemaking. Conversely, a male may think that his role is to be the exclusive initiator of sexual activity; he is convinced that all women are "secretly longing to be raped" and want to submit to a macho male. This point of view may be quite repugnant to a woman who feels that sexual activity should be mutually agreed on, and that she does not want to be a "victim."

Information of this sort can be obtained by an empathic, thorough interview which maintains neutrality and is not a "cross examination." A detailed format for such an interview can be found in the work of Masters and Johnson (6) or the GAP report (5). Particularly relevant areas to cover include:

1. Description of the sexual problem.
2. Whether the problem has affected the partner's sexual functioning.
3. How the marital union has handled the problem.
4. The couple's concepts of effective male and female sexual function.
5. A precise enough definition of the problem to be sure that it is being labeled correctly. (For example, if a woman is considered "frigid" it may be extremely important to learn that she is orgasmic with masturbation—by definition, then, she is not innately "frigid." This redefinition by the therapist may have a strongly positive influence on the treatment.)

Additional data should be gathered about attitudes and their development: specific influences such as religious, familial, cultural, or traumatic; how the couple expresses affection; the couple's social and sexual adjustment before and after marriage; how each partner greeted the appearance of children; who makes decisions about when and how lovemaking occurs; communication patterns on sexual and nonsexual topics, etc. The analysis of these data should provide the physician with a clear picture of the extent and type of sexual dysfunction and some very good ideas about why this particular dysfunction came into being.

ALTERED STATES OF HEALTH AND SEXUALITY

Sexual functioning relies on vascular, neurological, and hormonal integrity as well as psychological factors (7). A disruption of these systems may affect sexual desire and/or performance.

The following is a list of diagnoses which commonly affect a person's sexual functioning. This list is not global nor does it imply that any of these conditions necessarily interferes with sexual response.

1. Systemic diseases—any chronic illness that results in general debility, pain, and/or depression which may decrease libido, affect arousal, or impair erection.
    a. Angina.
    b. Postmyocardial infarction.
    c. Hypertension.
    d. Infections.
    e. Malignancies.
2. Liver diseases—the damaged liver may fail to detoxify and excrete metabolic products and estrogen, resulting in decreased libido.
    a. Cirrhosis.
    b. Hepatitis.
    c. Mononucleosis.
    d. Azotemia.
3. Endocrine disorders—may affect either pituitary or gonadal functioning, with central nervous system depression, low androgen levels, general debility, and depression. Libido and erection may be impaired.
    a. Diabetes mellitus.
    b. Hypothyroidism.
    c. Hypopituitarism.
    d. Cushing's disease.
    e. Addison's disease.
    f. Hypogonadism.
4. Neurologic diseases—may affect the brain (rare) or interfere with peripheral nerve supply and/or spinal cord reflex center. If the brain is affected, libido and sexual behavior may be altered. Otherwise, the disease may affect erection, ejaculation, and/or orgasm.
    a. Multiple sclerosis.
    b. Spinal cord injuries or lesions.
    c. Amyotrophic lateral sclerosis.
    d. Disc disease.

e. Epilepsy.
5. Surgical conditions—may damage genitals or genital nerve supply or lower androgens, resulting in impaired libido, impotence, retarded ejaculation, or orgasmic difficulties.
   a. Obstetrical trauma.
   b. Oophorectomy plus adrenalectomy.
   c. Prostatectomy (radical perineal).
   d. Abdominal-perineal resection.
   e. Abdominal aortic surgery.
   f. Lumbar sympathectomy.
6. Local genital diseases—may damage genital organs and cause pain or irritation. This can result in dyspareunia, loss of libido, impotence, or orgasmic difficulties.
   a. Pelvic pathology, e.g., endometriosis.
   b. Vulvar and vaginal pathology.
   c. Conditions causing irritation, e.g., urethritis.
   d. Conditions causing pain on intercourse, e.g., priapism.
   e. Conditions affecting intromission, e.g., hypospadias.

Various drugs may alter libido or affect the sexual response cycle. If a patient is receiving a drug which may impair sexual functioning, he should be informed of this potential side effect. Even if no suitable drug alternative exists, the patient may be reassured of his own adequacy as a sexual partner. The categories of drugs which *may* affect sexual response include the following:

1. Antihypertensives.
2. Antianxiety agents (minor tranquilizers).
3. Antidepressants (tricyclics and monoamine oxidase inhibitors).
4. Antipsychotics (major tranquilizers).
5. Sedatives (alcohol, barbiturates, narcotics).
6. Antiandrogens.
7. Anticholinergics.
8. Antiadrenergics (e.g., rauwolfia alkaloids, ergot alkaloids, phentolamine).
9. Sex hormones (including those in birth control preparations).

Although the training of a sex therapist involves extensive training and supervision, it is important that the primary physician be aware of the specific ingredients of sex therapy techniques (as originally developed by Masters and Johnson).

CONTEMPORARY BEHAVIORAL TECHNIQUES APPLIED TO SEXUAL DYSFUNCTION

Masters and Johnson stress several steps in the sexual therapy process (6): a) gathering an extensive history from the partners individually and together, including a medical history and examination; b) having roundtable discussions between couple and therapist to combat misconceptions the patients may have about sexuality; and c) the therapy itself, where the focus is on changing the frame of reference of the couple and expanding their view of sexuality.

For many couples, "sex" means merely the act of intercourse. When sexual dysfunction occurs, this conception may be a contributing cause. Often the first step in a sexual therapy program involves teaching the partners to feel sensual pleasure that is not necessarily connected with intercourse—to focus on feeling and responding with pleasure to each other's touching and stroking. The partners learn to convey sensual feelings to each other and to communicate in ways which enhance pleasure. This is accomplished through exercises called sensate focus exercises. The couple practice touching and being touched, which teaches mutual trust and reshuffles "active" and "passive" roles and promotes the satisfaction of giving as well as receiving pleasure. The couple gradually becomes aware of the importance of other senses: the role of vision in lovemaking, the possible pleasure-enhancing effects of odors and their part in sexual arousal, or the heightening of sexual pleasure through sounds, e.g., music. Sensate focus or "pleasuring" is really the basis for all of the other more specific techniques involved in the treatment program.

Specific Problems

Premature Ejaculation

When treating a patient for premature ejaculation, after the couple has learned to feel and respond pleasurably to sensation in other parts of the body, the penis is stimulated manually by the female. When ejaculation is imminent, the "squeeze" is applied; with thumb on the frenulum and the first and second fingers on the dorsal surface of the penis (above and below the coronal ridge), pressure is applied for 3 to 4 seconds. The penis will lose 30 to 40% of its volume as a result of this maneuver, and ejaculation is averted. The manual stimulation of the penis is then repeated to the point of ejaculatory inevitability, the squeeze is again applied, etc. This exercise should be practiced until erection without ejaculation can be maintained for 15 to 20 minutes. The next stage requires the penis to be pushed or stuffed into the vagina with the female in the superior position. She remains motionless in order to accustom the male to intravaginal containment. Once the male feels comfortable with this step, some pelvic movements by the female may be begun, but when ejaculation again seems imminent, the penis should be withdrawn and the squeeze again applied. The couple should continue practicing the technique; sometimes it requires 6 to 12 months of practice after therapy sessions have ended.

Impotence

The treatment procedure for impotence first stresses clarifying to the couple that no man can will an erection, and that anxiety has an inhibiting effect and blocks the input of sensual pleasures which stimulate the erection. The focus initially is on re-establishing communication between the marital partners on nonsexual matters and trying to decrease the importance given to sexual performance. The couple concentrates on giving sensate pleasure to one another as an end in itself; the therapist should suggest that they not engage in intercourse during this phase of the treatment.

The sensate focus exercises should begin with stroking of arms, legs, back, etc. and then proceed to touching each other's pelvic areas under the direction of the partner, who indicates what pleases him most. The object is to establish communication and focus attention on giving pleasure to each other, rather than on being spectators of each other's performance.

The couple gradually begin to engage in manipulative play to erection, cease manipulation until the erection subsides, and then again return to play, ending in erection; in this way the man is assured that he can continue to achieve erection. As the male becomes more competent in his ability to retain an erection, the female may get astride him (sitting on his thighs, for instance) and actively stimulate the penis. If erection occurs, there may be intromission of the penis into her vagina in this position, accomplished slowly and undemandingly by the female. The next step involves the female thrusting backward and forward slowly, the object being that of penile containment rather than thrusting toward climax. Gradually the male takes over, thrusting slowly, concentrating on sensate pleasure and vaginal containment. Eventually the couple will interact sexually in a cooperative, nondemanding fashion to maintain the erection and to achieve maximal sexual pleasure.

Orgasmic Dysfunction in the Female

It is most important for the therapist to ascertain, during the history-taking, what things the male does (or fails to do) which please or displease the female sexually. This information can be obtained only by a careful exploration of the female's past sexual experiences and sexually tinged memories. Discussion sessions following sensate focus exercises should emphasize that orgasmic release and sexual excitement cannot be willed—orgasmic response in the female is a matter of accepting erotic stimuli and of communicating to her partner what aspects of sexual experience are pleasurable to her. The therapist should encourage the female to share her sexually stimulating experiences with the male.

After areas of sensitivity and pleasure have been discovered by the couple, genital play can be gradually initiated, the female sitting between the male's legs with her back against his chest. By squeezing his legs and directing his hands, the female guides the male's caresses. The male needs to be extremely responsive to the female's verbal and nonverbal directions, and he should be particularly careful not to approach the clitoris directly because of its great sensitivity. It is preferable to manipulate the general mons area, particularly the clitoral shaft, the inner thighs, and the labia (making sure that the clitoral area is lubricated by moisture from the vaginal outlet). The most effective technique in the early stages is a teasing approach in which stimulation is varied and random, from lips to breasts to thighs to labia, interlaced with stroking of nonsexual areas (stomach, back, etc.). The male must concentrate on fulfilling the female's sensual desires, rather than trying to force responsivity.

When success is obtained in manual genital excitation, coitus can be engaged in using the female superior position. The initial focus is again on penile containment, the male lying still. Once vaginal sensations develop, the male may thrust nondemandingly at a pace suggested by the female; throughout this stage there should be a relaxed atmosphere and frequent interruption of coitus for simple love play. Once confidence has been gained using the female superior coital position and the woman enjoys sensate pleasure and intravaginal containment, the couple may employ a lateral coital position. [NOTE: A. H. Kegal, a gynecologist, has reported success in helping woman overcome difficulties in being sexually responsive by a set of exercises involving the muscles of the vaginal introitus. To learn where and how these muscles function, the woman is instructed to stop the flow of urine voluntarily a few times; the exercise itself involves flexing these same muscles rhythmically, beginning with sets of ten and then repeating the exercise five to six times a day (8).]

DISCUSSION

The three therapies above are extremely abbreviated and deal only with the most common sexual dysfunctions. More complete and detailed descriptions are found in Masters and Johnson's work (6) together with instructions for treatment of other types of sexual dysfunction, e.g., ejaculatory incompetence, vaginismus, and dyspareunia (male and female).

Since the appearance of the monumental works of Masters and Johnson, a number of other researchers and therapists have published modifications, innovations, and elaborations of the Masters and Johnson material. In a number of places throughout the country, sexual therapy is done in a way different from that which Masters and Johnson insisted was necessary. For instance, Masters and Johnson required that a couple reside near the Reproductive Biology Research Foundation in St. Louis during a 2-week period for optimal results. In many university centers where sexual therapy is now being done, couples appear at the clinic once a week for several hours over a period of 6 to 10 weeks. Other couples may set aside 1 day a week for sexual therapy after a short, more intensive period of work-up and evaluation. Masters and Johnson also insisted that there be co-therapists, a male and a female, who could offer different perspectives about male and female sexuality as well as be able to obtain different facets of a sexual history from the sexual partners. In contrast, a number of sexual counseling centers have reported success using a single therapist (9).

DESENSITIZING THE PHYSICIAN

Many physicians are reluctant to tackle a thorough job of sexual counseling because of their own discomfort when discussing or describing sexual material. Physicians are like the rest of the population; they have grown up with taboos, values, and assumptions which may make complete comfort in verbal sexual communication difficult. Audiovisual media, "desensitization verbal exercises," audiotapes, slides, etc. can all be a boon to the physician to help desensitize him through repeated exposure to explicit sexual material, so that he can become more comfortable when discussing such material with his patients. A frequent inital response to sexually stimulating material which is "required viewing" is irritation, anger, or shock, often accompanied by discomfort at one's own erotic response to the material. After a while, the material produces less-intense emotions in the viewer and, if the material is poorly made, outright boredom. Many of the materials described in this chapter may, after the physician has seen them several times, still be mildly stimulating to him, but the feelings may be toned down sufficiently that the physician can consider: (1) his own emotional reactions to the material in a somewhat "detached" way (so that this reaction does not interfere with treatment goals); (2) what the media has to teach patients in terms of communication, techniques, expressions of intimacy, etc.; and (3) how he might incorporate such material, if it is appropriate, in the treatment of patients with a sexual problem. The best way to use such materials for desensitization purposes is to view or listen to them with a friend, a colleague, or a discussion group and then discuss the experience and trade personal observations about individual reactions to the materials.

Audio Tape for Explicit Language Desensitization

George Carlin: "Seven Words You Can Never Say on Television," from *Class Clown* (tape). Little David Records, Atlantic Recording Corp., 1841 Broadway, New York, NY 10023; #LID CS 1004 0697.

This is a hilarious takeoff on the "seven bad words" and is excellent not only for desensitizing physicians but as an ice-breaker to begin sexuality conferences for counselors, teachers, etc.

Desensitizing Verbal Exercises

The following two exercises, developed through the Planned Parenthood Center of Seattle (Information and Education Department),* have been extremely useful for helping sexual counselors increase their level of comfort in using the language of some of their clientele. (Many persons who come to counselors or physicians often either do not know or choose not to use words such as "coitus" and "penis.") The second exercise is useful in teaching actual or potential sexual counselors how to share their own sexual value biases while learning about someone else's values.

Exercise 1
Word Games: With at least one other person, translate the following paragraphs from slang terms into "neutral" or "clinical" terms as appropriate:

---

*This exercise was developed and made available to the author, courtesy of Ms. Victoria Campbell, formerly Education Director, Planned Parenthood Center of Seattle, WA. Exercise 2 was developed by Gary Howard, Director of Threshold, Seattle, in conjunction with Ms. Campbell.

1. *Balling* (Translate into neutral terms.) A guy and a chick begin (usually) by making out. The man rubs the woman's tits, sometimes sucking on them. The woman rubs the man's balls and rod, and he gets it up. The man plays with the woman's pussy and clit, separating her lips and turning on her juice. The man's prick goes into the woman's box, and they slide it back and forth until they both come.
2. *Oral Sex (Mutual)* (Translate into slang.) Mutual oral sex is the caressing of the genitals of one partner with the mouth of the other partner. The man separates the labia of the woman's vulva, and his tongue and lips caress the woman's genitals. The woman can hold the shaft of the man's penis in one hand while kissing, caressing with her tongue and lips, and sucking on the glans and shaft of the penis.
3. *Playing With Yourself—Female* (Translate into neutral terms.) A gal plays with herself by rubbing her clit with her fingers or by rubbing her whole pussy with her hand. She lies down and separates her lips and rubs over her cunt until she comes. Sometimes a chick wants to get off with something inside her twat, so she uses her finger or something else shaped like a cock.
4. *Masturbation—Male* (Translate into slang.) The usual way for a man to masturbate is to make a fist, hold the penis in it, and move his hand up and down vigorously until he reaches orgasm and ejaculates. Because the most sensitive part of the penis is where the glans meet the shaft, some men use the tips of their fingers to stroke the glans, increasing the motion until orgasm occurs.

Exercise 2

Practice this exercise (asking the questions and giving answers) with another person. Try to ask the questions as tactfully as possible and to get as much information as your partner feels comfortable in disclosing.
1. What is the earliest sexual experience you can remember from your own childhood? How old were you?
2. When, if ever, did you begin masturbating? What were/are your feelings about this?
3. What are your remembrances/feelings about the sexual behavior you observed between your parents?
4. From whom or what in your past have you learned the most about sex?
5. What sexual feelings or behavior have you experienced toward a person of your own sex?
6. What feelings have you had about your own body as a child? As a teenager? As an adult?
7. What feelings do you remember having about your first experience with intercourse?
8. What have been the sexual high points for you as you look back over your past?
9. What things do you wish could have been different about your sexual development?

Films

A large number of desensitization or "educational" films are now available. Some of these have been designed for desensitization purposes only; many of them—once the physician has been desensitized—are excellent for instructing either the physician or his patients in specific techniques of sexual therapy, sexual counseling, or attitude examination. An annotated listing of recommended films appears below, together with the distributor of the film.

Films can be timesavers in sexual therapy by showing a couple a technique the doctor feels is appropriate for them. For instance, it is rather difficult to tell someone how to do sensate focus exercises; a film, on the other hand, can demonstrate some aspects of the technique, and, especially if shown more than once, may encourage the couple to elaborate on ideas implicit in the movie. Some therapists arrange for patients to see such films by themselves in a room in the physician's office; some lend the film to the couple for use at home; some show the films and then follow them by a discussion with the couple about what each of them got out of the film and what they felt about it. Each of these ways of using the film has advantages, depending on the couple and the circumstances. Discussion after the film is almost always helpful provided the physician is properly desensitized about the sexual material itself and is well informed and sensitive to the feelings of his patients. The therapist can then be sure that the couple really has understood, assimilated, and become comfortable with the message imparted by the film—that they may be ready to put the techniques into operation themselves.

A Quickie 1' 45" 16 mm	Multimedia Resource Center, 540 Powell St., San Francisco, CA. 94105. (415) 421-5035. An excellent speeded-up version of a sexual encounter with Buster Keaton slapstick qualities. Very good for desensitization and for opening meetings (breaking the ice).
Margo 11' 16 mm	Multimedia Resource Center. Sensitive film about female masturbation (instructs how to masturbate). Would be good for nonorgasmic female who is unsure or uninformed about masturbation, as well as for desensitization purpose.
One to One 10' Super-8 with mag. sound	Multimedia Resource Center. Good film showing male masturbation (adolescent boy), including his use of fantasy material. Good for group discussion and to increase level of comfort about male masturbation.
Touching 15' 16 mm	Multimedia Resource Center. A very sensitive film about a male paraplegic and his sexual partner. It is excellent for showing to paraplegic patients to encourage their sexual experimentation and pleasure and give them hope about the possibilities of an active sexual life. Also very good for physical medicine, occupational therapy, and rehabilitation services.
Give to Get 11' 16 mm	Multimedia Resource Center. Shows sexual massage and pleasuring techniques; it also gives the viewer a sense that the relationship is not transient. Shows female caressing man. Should be used with *The Erogenists*.

The Erogenists 11' 16 mm	Multimedia Resource Center. Also shows sexual massage (sensate focus and pleasuring). Male massaging female to orgasm, with a great deal of pleasure and closeness shown.
A Ripple of Time 24' 16 mm	Multimedia Resource Center. This is an excellent film showing a couple, aged 50 and 63, with strong physical and emotional attachment to each other. Their natural, loving, and mature expression of sexuality and affection demonstrate that sexuality is valuable to older persons and not just to the young. This is an excellent film for teaching, therapy, and even inspiration.
Free 12' 16 mm	Multimedia Resource Center. A delightful movie showing a young black couple having sexual relations outdoors, playing sexually, and obviously having a good time. It is useful in raising the issue of "play," openness in sexuality, "looking," and enjoying visual stimuli while having sex.
Vir Amat 15' 16 mm	Multimedia Resource Center. A warm, and, to many people, moving film about a young male homosexual couple, showing their life style and "ongoing relationship" as well as explicit sexual scenes. This film is excellent in desensitization purposes. It is particularly good with groups of physicians or medical students to serve as a basis for discussion of values, judgments, counseling roles, etc. Also useful with homosexual groups as a film which, in effect, says that homosexual relationships are O.K. (Negative comments suggest that the couple appears to have no relationship except the sexual one.)
The Look of Love 40' 16 mm	Dick Kornbackher, Inc., 1525 37th Street, Seattle, WA. Explicit heterosexual movie excellent for desensitization; shows a close relationship, "fun" sexual activity, etc.
Holding 15' 16 mm	Multimedia Resource Center. Female homosexual movie for desensitization, showing life style of two women, as well as explicit scenes. Good, except for bombastic musical soundtrack.
Squeeze Technique 12' 16 mm	Multimedia Resource Center. Shows technique developed by Dr. James Semens for dealing with premature ejaculation. Well done and instructional, with voice-over soundtrack giving instructions. (Revised version.)

About Sex 25' 16 mm	Texture Films, 1600 Broadway, New York, NY 10019. Lively, colorful, and reassuring film for and about teenagers. Starts with a rap session led by a young man answering questions about adult sexual behavior, directly and without embarrassment. The second part of the film explores various myths about sexual fantasies, homosexuality, masturbation, abortion, etc. excellent for use by a physician or health educator, followed by discussion.
Sexuality and Communication 60' 16 mm	Mobius Productions, Ltd., 49 Palmerston Gardens, Toronto, Ontario, Canada. Excellent film that emphasizes talking with a sexual partner about needs and stresses as well as sexual problems. Excellent for educating adults (including physicians) about how to approach potential sexual difficulties or dysfunctions within a relationship. Informative, humorous, and warm.
Like Other People 40' 16 mm	Didactic Films, Perenial Education, Inc., P.O. Box 236, 1825 Willow Road, Northfield, IL 60093. A very moving film about the loving relationship between a man and a woman handicapped by cerebral palsy. The message that they have a right to love and live together can be applied to any handicapped person, especially the mentally retarded. Sound track occasionally difficult because of speech defects and British accents.
Heterosexual Intercourse Super-8 20' 16 mm Sony video casette	EDCOA Productions, Inc., 310 Cedar Lane, Teaneck, NJ 07666. The natural and unrehearsed love-making techniques of an attractive young couple are depicted. This silent color production is an excellent desensitizing and therapeutic presentation. The couple employ a variety of foreplay techniques, including oral-genital stimulation. Several coital positions are depicted.
An Experiment in the Teaching Methodology of Sensate Focus Super-8, 18' 16 mm Sony video casette	EDCOA Productions, Inc. A brief explanation of sensate focus, its purpose and goals, is followed by an unusual experimental presentation. Dr. Neubardt directs an unrehearsed young couple in a series of sensate focus type exercises, culminating in intromission in the female superior position. Didactic material is presented for the student.

Old Enough to Know 22' 16 mm	Planned Parenthood Center of Seattle, 2211 E. Maidson Street, Seattle, WA 98144. A film designed to help parents be more comfortable answering the questions small children (6 and under) ask about sex. The film deals with attitudes rather than imparting information and would be superb as the background for a discussion with parents. A discussion leader should always accompany the film to answer questions; a discussion leader's guide comes with each film.
The Trying Time 20' 16 mm	Planned Parenthood Center of Seattle. Excellent film for the parents of people entering their teens. Intended to stimulate discussion among adults about the physical and emotional uncertainties and discomfort felt by young teenagers. Some emphasis on sexual values. Should be followed by a discussion (discussion leader's guide provided with each film).

NOTE: Multimedia Resource Center has both an 8-mm "package" and a video "package" of a number of their films for sale, which a physician group might consider if they were planning to use the films a great deal.

Films can serve as a springboard for discussion between patients and physicians about sexuality, sexual counseling, or sexual dysfunctions; they can also educate and desensitize. Books are often similarly useful, either to provide information to the physician or to give or lend to patients for a specific reason. The following list contains suggestions for the use of the books. They are paperbacks, unless otherwise noted.

The following pamphlets from the Glide Foundation Publications, 540 Powell St., San Francisco, CA 94105 are excellent and very affirmative about sexual activity and sexuality. They could increase the "comfort level" of readers.

You Can Last Longer: illustrated; shows squeeze technique.

Lesbian Love and Liberation: about female homosexuality; illustrated; for information about life styles and values.

Gay Men Speak: about male homosexuality; illustrated; for information about life styles and values.

When You Don't Make It: about impotence; suggests ways a man can become more comfortable and positive about his own body; illustrated.

Getting In Touch: shows a female caressing herself. It would be useful for instructing a female in masturbation and gaining greater comfort with her own body.

Other paperback books (not from the Glide Foundation) include the following:

Barbach, L.: *For Yourself: The Fulfillment of Female Sexuality*. Doubleday, New York. 1975.

Boston Women's Health Book Collective: *Our Bodies, Ourselves*. Simon and Schuster, New York, 1976. (For women: affirmative about female sexuality; contains a lot of information and resources.)

Braun, P. and Foulder, C.: *Learning to Love: How to Make Bad Sex Good and Good Sex Better*. Universe Books, New York, 1978.

Comfort, Alex: *The Joy of Sex*. Fireside (Simon and Schuster), New York, 1973.

Comfort, Alex: *More Joy of Sex*. Fireside (Simon and Schuster), New York, 1975.

Hansen, Lyn, et al: *How to Have Intercourse Without Getting Screwed*. Associated Students of the University of Washington, Women's Commission, Seattle, 1980. (Excellent and inexpensive, 30¢; includes such topics as anatomy, contraception, pregnancy, abortion, venereal disease, infections, sexual counseling, myths about sex and conception, etc.)

Hastings, Donald W.: *A Doctor Speaks on Sexual Expression in Marriage*. Bantam Books, New York, 1966.

Hymes Jr., James L.: *How to Tell Your Child About Sex*. Public Affairs Pamphlet No. 476, New York, 1972. 25¢.

Johnson, Eric W.: *Sex: Telling It Straight*. Bantam Books, New York, 1970.

Katchadourian, Herant: *Human Sexuality: Sense and Nonsense*. Portable Stanford, Stanford Alumni Association, Stanford, CA, 1972. (An excellent and sophisticated book describing Masters and Johnson data, including information about sexual functioning, techniques, attitudes, values, etc.)

Meilach, Dona, and Mandel, Elias: *A Doctor Talks to 5 to 8 Year Olds*. Budlong Press, Chicago, 1969.

Planned Parenthood/World Population: *Sex Alphabet*. Planned Parenthood/World Population, New York, 1973.

Planned Parenthood/World Population: *How To Talk With Your Teenager About Something That's Not Easy To Talk About*. Planned Parenthood/World Population, New York, 1973.

Planned Parenthood/World Population: *So You Don't Want to be a Sex Object*. Planned Parenthood of Colorado, Denver, 1973.

Pomeroy, Wardell: *Boys and Sex*. Dell, New York, 1968. (Gives pros and cons for different kinds of sexual activity and provides a great deal of information for children, especially adolescents.)

Sexuality and Subnormality, A Swedish View. National Society for Mentally Handicapped Children, Swedish Board of Health and Welfare, Stockholm, 1970. (Has specific instructions about how to provide sex education to retarded children and adults.)

Wilderberg, Sive: *The Kids Own XYZ of Love and Sex*. Stein and Day, New York, 1973. (A superb book using simple, direct, nonclinical language to explain sexual behavior and sexual feelings to young children.)

Yale University: *Student Guide to Sex On Campus*. Signet, New York, 1970.

Several additional hardback books should be on every physician's shelf. These are:

Belliveau, F. and Richter, L.: *Understanding Human Sexual Inadequacy*. Little Brown, Boston, 1970.

Green, R. (ed): *Human Sexuality*. Williams and Wilkins, Baltimore, 1970.

Kaplan, H. S.: *The New Sex Therapy: Active Treatment of Sexual Dysfynction*. Brunner/Mazel, New York, 1974.

Kaplan, H. S.: *The Illustrated Manual of Sex Therapy*. Quadrangle Press, New York, 1975.

Katchadourian, H., and Lunde, D.: *Fundamentals of Human Sexuality*. Holt, Reinhart, and Winston, New York, 1972.

LoPiccolo, J. and LoPiccolo, L. (eds): *Handbook of Sex Therapy*, Plenum Press, New York, 1978.

Vincent, C.: *Sexual and Marital Health: The Physician as a Consultant*. McGraw-Hill, New York, 1973.

REFERENCES

1. Annon, J. S. (1976): *Behavior Treatment of Sexual Problems*. Harper & Row, New York.
2. Lurie, H. J. (1978): Sexual complaints in family practice. *Med. Aspects Hum. Sexuality*.
3. Berman, E. M., and Lief, H. I. (1975): Marital therapy from a psychiatric perspective: an overview. *Am. J. Psychiatry*, 132:583.
4. Hampson, J.: Department of Psychiatry and Behavioral Sciences, University of Washington, Seattle. Personal communication.
5. Group for the Advancement of Psychiatry (1973): *Assessment of Sexual Function: A Guide to Interviewing*, Report 88, pp. 830–831. GAP, New York.
6. Masters, W. H., and Johnson, V. (1970): *Human Sexual Inadequacy*, pp. 34–51, 830–831. Little Brown, Boston.
7. Coffin: *Guidelines to Sexuality and Health*. Planned Parenthood, Seattle.
8. Katchadourian, H. (1975): *Human Sexuality: Sense and Nonsense*. Portable Stanford Press, Stanford, California.
9. Levay, A. N. and Kagle, A. (1978): Recent advances in sex therapy: Integration with dynamic therapies. *Psychiatric Quarterly*, 50:1.

24

Mental Health of the Physician

If one judges by statistics, the mental health of many physicians is in need of heroic resuscitative measures. The suicide rate of doctors is among the highest of comparable professional groups (exceeded only by pharmacists, medical technicians, chemists, and dentists) (1). Among physicians aged 24 to 64, the suicide rate is approximately 2.5 times that of the general population (controlled for sex, social class, etc.), and many of the physicians on the lower end of the age spectrum kill themselves during residency training. Among physicians 65 and older, the suicide rate is four times that of the general population. Drinking too much and drug use are also well known professional hazards among physicians, the latter particularly, as drugs are much more easily available to doctors than to other professional groups.

There have been many studies and much speculation about why doctors are so vulnerable. A number of hypotheses have emerged, although no one factor can be applied uniformly (2–6).

1. Many doctors have compulsive personalities, and their inherent compulsiveness becomes more intensified by the rigor and pace of medical school. Such compulsiveness predisposes the doctor to drive himself too hard, to ignore his emotional needs even when they are pressing, and to become unusually depressed when losses occur during later life.

2. The process of medical education, both during medical school and residency training, is dehumanizing in a very literal way for many physicians (7). Many predictable major stresses face the medical student and resident, and such stresses are usually ignored or minimized by medical faculty, administrators, or program chiefs. Such predictable stresses include: (a) sleep deprivation with a secondary mild dementia, present in many residents one-third to one-half of the time; (b) situational depression, experienced in its most severe form during the first year of residency or internship, where 30% of residents have a significant depressive disorder, 25% have suicidal ideas, and 18% a suicidal plan (14); (c) severe role

transition, where residents are not sure if they are doctors or students; (d) severe marital stress, secondary to medical and time demands: the spouse at home frequently feels trapped, neglected, and depressed, and there is often minimal peer or social support; (e) sensory deprivation—athletic, sexual, gastronomic, social—is often the hallmark of the more rigorous moments in "quality" medical education; (f) sudden and intensive interaction with patients, many of whom are dying, producing feelings of helplessness, failure, or incompetence in many residents and students; (g) confronting demanding patients who do not accept "no" for an answer (and a student's or resident's reaction of feeling guilty if he must say no); (h) brainwashing and modeling by professors and teachers who usually value productivity, stoicism, and efficiency far more than humanistic values such as self-care, relaxation and recreation, and nonmedical interests; (i) assimilation of the medical ethic that one should never complain if one is tired or depressed, or that if one does, one "doesn't have what it takes" to be in medicine. Besides, one should solve one's problems alone and should not need advice or support; (j) assimilation of the medical ethic that being in medicine itself will somehow solve life's problems (personal meaning, intimacy, recreation, a balanced life including work and pleasure, etc.).

3. Many doctors are "loners." The American myth of the "old family doctor" who drives out in the middle of the night in his Model T or horse and buggy to care for his patients persists to some extent. Many physicians feel that they are being self-indulgent or neglectful if they delegate some responsibility to other workers or go into partnerships or group practices rather than "doing it all themselves." With notable exceptions, medical school training does not really prepare a physician to work as a member of a "team." A doctor is usually trained to be autonomous, self-sufficient, and to mistrust the judgment of almost everyone else. Learning to share responsibility with colleagues is difficult for many doctors after such an emphasis on independence. Of course, many physicians in rural areas who are the sole medical resource for a large geographical area have been forced, at least medically, to be loners.

4. Doctors are often put in a god-like position by their patients, who expect medical and psychological miracles from them, and by their communities, to whom they may represent reason, scientific objectivity, and all the positive qualities attributed to education. Doctors, in fact, do have life-and-death powers over people. Hearing about these powers from adoring patients or sensing a sort of dumb worship and gratitude makes one less able to recognize one's own *human* needs, limitations, and isolation. All too often, a doctor is forced into the uncomfortable position of living up to his (unreal) image.

5. Because many doctors have been taught to be healers and not to notice or complain about their own feelings, when they discover that they themselves are depressed or depleted it feels like a betrayal of both themselves and their profession. Self-medication through drinking, amphetamines, or opiates seems to many doctors a better and less embarrassing route to coping with dysphoric feelings than talking with a colleague or (God forbid) a mental health professional. Drugs are more to be trusted than people!

6. The process of medical education and medical practice is, for many physicians, an intense, narrowing, and myopic experience. Hence a doctor may easily lose touch with his original humanistic ideals, a broader concept of living, and a sense of what is really important. Material acquisitions—houses, cars, boats—are seen as supplying both material and spiritual needs. During mid-life, it comes as a shock to discover that these things are "not enough."

7. The social support system of many physicians is inadequate or nonexistent. Many "traditional" medical marriages are similar to movie star marriages: The doctor is surrounded by adoring patients and nymphets for much of the day, his will is law, and almost everyone is grateful for his time and wise words. When he returns home, however, his spouse complains because the dishwasher got plugged up and the children are bringing home poor report cards. The doctor feels abused and unappreciated, and the spouse feels abandoned, patronized, and enraged at the lack of interest and empathy shown by her husband, the physician. The doctor, feeling unloved, leaves and goes to the club, where he feels constrained not to reveal his real concerns to his buddies. Instead, he has a few drinks, jokes a bit, speculates about having an affair with the new office nurse, and staggers home to a frigid house. The pattern, interspersed with occasional committee meetings, repeats itself like a broken record. The doctor feels lonely, depressed, and isolated but concludes that there is no one he dare talk with for fear of jeopardizing his local reputation, hospital affiliation, or his standing with his county or state medical society.

8. The demands of what was formerly called "traditional family practice" (which may be a solo practice, entailing being available much of the time for emergency calls) are extremely wearing and exhausting. Hostile, demanding, dependent, and hysterical patients take their toll. So does the more subtle torment of the demand for paper work from third-party insurance carriers, community gossip that the doctor overhears about "rich doctors" and how they "exploit us poor patients," and pressure from professional societies for peer review, patient audits, more elaborate charting procedures, and problem-oriented records. All of these are bound to be resented to some degree by the overworked physician, even if he understands and agrees with the need for accountability, improving patient care, cutting medical costs, etc.

9. In exchange for giving the doctor a prestigious position in the community, many communities, in turn, believe that the doctor, like the city park, belongs to them and should be available to meet their needs whenever and wherever they arise. The doctor may be asked to serve on the school board, do voluntary physical examinations for high school athletes, serve on community advisory committees, etc. Unfortunately, many doctors are reluctant to educate their communities and their patients about their own private needs for space and time, and can be wheedled and cajoled into doing much more than they should. The community's flattery and pressure conspires with the doctor's inability to set limits and results in the doctor's early coronary occlusion.

The inability to stop, assess the situation, and then set goals accounts for those doctors who realize they are spending too little time with their families but do not arrange to spend more. Doctors work too hard and feel they do not have time for vacations; but then they get drunk at parties or take amphetamines to maintain their energy after a hard day. Many middle-aged physicians drift into casual extramarital affairs, not because of the pleasure they achieve but because they are hunting for something which has meaning. Although many doctor's children wish to emulate their parent and go into medicine, an equally large number feel that being the son or daughter of a doctor is a hardship. They experience semi-isolation from the community, and the physician-parent can often offer only financial—not emotional—support.

WHAT CAN BE DONE?

Recently medical conferences and scholarly articles have begun to study how physicians can avoid the "Four Ds of doctoring": depression, drinking, drugs, and divorce (8). A number of individual doctors have also expressed some ideas.

1. If you are in solo practice, you should recognize that you are considerably more vulnerable than most other physicians to becoming isolated, depressed, and exhausted. Group practice or partnership is by no means a panacea, but it provides considerably greater support for most doctors than solo practice. This statement is made with the full realization that many communities do not have even one physician. Nonetheless, the health of the solo practicing physician is of significant importance to a community and helping support a small clinic with several physicians would be in the interest of both doctor and townspeople. Some physicians in solo practice have hired a physician's assistant or a nurse practitioner to work in collaboration with them. Many physicians feel that even if the work load is not reduced by this move the shared responsibility and sense of having at least one colleague to grumble with is a supportive experience.

2. Periodic life planning and stress reduction sessions with one's spouse, and sometimes with the entire family, are often useful in helping the doctor assess whether he is getting what he wants out of his life and his practice. Professional organizations, such as the American Academy of Family Physicians (through its Mental Health Committee), The American Academy of Pediatrics, and the American Psychiatric Association, as well as "well-being" or "personal problems" committees of various state medical associations (e.g., those in Oregon, Pennsylvania, California, Washington, and Ohio) have all sponsored meetings to look at the well-being of doctors and to give doctors and their families an opportunity to discuss such personal issues in depth. Personal growth centers (e.g., Esalen and the National Training Laboratories of Applied Behavioral Sciences of the National Education Association) have also offered experiences of various kinds leading to life planning and assessment. Life planning methodology is described elsewhere in this book (Chapter 21); it is very hard to do one's life planning alone, and a workshop or course setting is preferable to a "do it yourself" approach at home. Many doctors and their families who have participated in such workshops report improved com-

munication within the family, better use of leisure time, and more meaningful time that the couple spends with each other (15).

3. Preventive educational programs to anticipate the predictable stresses of residency and medical practice are getting under way. Spearheaded by the Mental Health Committee of the American Academy of Family Physicians, a series of stimulus videotaped vignettes together with discussion guides was developed to be used in all Family Practice Residency Programs in the United States and has been incorporated into a number of family residency curricula (7). (Details about this are available from the Academy of Family Physicians Office, Kansas City, MO.) Through the collaboration of Blue Cross and Blue Shield Associations, the Center for Well-Being of Health Professionals (Chapel Hill, NC) has developed an instructional package (9) designed to alert doctors in practice and in training to the current research about physician disability, and telling them where to obtain information about prevention and treatment. The American Medical Association has helped promote national conferences on preventing physician impairment, as well as publishing such books as *Beyond Survival* (10), which is a manual for medical students and residents about coping with the physical and psychological rigors of medical training and practice. All of these are useful first steps. The wheels of institutional medical training move exceedingly slowly. Courses to sensitize students and faculty to these issues and the institutional development of strategies to identify or prevent future psychological disability in doctors will not come easily or quickly.

4. Distance makes the heart grow fonder (and prevents the coronaries). Even in a small community, it has been possible for doctors to make arrangements to take occasional long vacations, with coverage from colleagues or a *locum tenens* physician. If one is in a group practice, an alternative is taking less-frequent half-year or year-long sabbaticals for study, travel, and renewal (11). The reason that such arrangements are not more common seems to reflect the physician's inability to consider that such an option is possible as much as the actual difficulties in arranging the option.

5. Many doctors go to medical society meetings as much for their social and supportive aspects as for their learning component. It is refreshing to see colleagues from other towns, to do some mutual consultation, and to feel free to bitch about common problems (the hospital administrator, problem patients, PSROs, insurance forms, etc.). Seeing people in the medical world may not, however, be as refreshing as seeing nonmedical people. Cultivating a relaxing hobby (e.g., painting, music, or sports), particularly if these interests can be shared to some extent with nonmedical individuals, affords a physician not only support but new perspectives on the world.

6. There is no reason why a doctor cannot change his career or life style; nonphysicians are doing this with increasing frequency. When a doctor is "fed up," he may impulsively decide to get out of medicine altogether or at least to leave a medical position that involves direct patient care. Although this is, of course, a real option, frequently it is not an option that will produce happiness once the career change is made. Like the man who finds himself making a series of bad marriages,

the physician who finds himself fed up and overwhelmed by his practice may have difficulty saying "no" when it is necessary. He probably also has difficulty limiting the hours of his practice and taking time off when he is exhausted. Hence such patterns might continue in a new occupation as well.

The syndrome of self-neglect and guilt in caring for one's self and one's own needs is often the real culprit in the decision to leave medicine. It generally is far better to look at one's personal needs and arrange to have them met while still practicing medicine than to run away from the whole situation (even if it feels good for a while). This, of course, does not mean that a doctor—for reasons of health, the welfare of his family, or his personal satisfaction—may not decide to change his career or his specialty or style of practice through additional training. The issue is whether the urge to leave is dictated by the chance for new growth, enrichment, and an opportunity for additional human satisfaction and service or is simply a push to "get the hell out." If the latter is the motivating force, the doctor would be well advised to stick around and figure out (with outside help) how to improve things in his own life rather than hurl himself into new occupations which will probably offer the same perils as his present life style.

7. Everybody, including doctors, needs a "support system." It is essential to maintain a productive life, especially with heavy demands on time, energy, and talent. A support system can include the person who smiles casually at you in the elevator every morning, a colleague with whom one jokes, one's drinking buddies, one's family, or one's old college roommate with whom one talks on the phone from time to time. Just as the doctor is frequently part of the support system of his patients, relationships with some patients, particularly those that have been maintained for many years, are often supportive to the doctor. Many doctors look forward to the visits of certain patients whom they like and with whom they can have an interesting conversation.

Even a highly individualistic person such as a doctor should recognize the wisdom of asking for and receiving support when it is needed—and should recognize that everyone needs it at one time or another. For intimate matters, a minister, a colleague, or a friend may provide a great deal of support. On the other hand, many personal situations are extremely complex, and professional counseling may be the optimal choice.

For doctors "getting into trouble" because of personal problems, organizations in more enlightened states have been set up to offer formal support or referral. Through this means, a doctor perceiving himself (or perceived by patients and colleagues) to be in trouble has an opportunity for help before considerations of ethics or competence are raised in a formalized "legal" way. For each hospital to have such a small committee which works in collaboration with the appropriate committee of the state medical association makes a lot of sense. Doctors can keep practicing who otherwise might drop out of the medical community because of drug or alcohol abuse, personality disintegration under pressure, or incompetence stemming from being too busy to keep up with new information in their fields. "Institutional" support systems which allow and encourage a physician to get help professionally without jeopardizing his status as a staff member in the hospital have been found to be extremely workable in such diverse places as Oregon, Washington, and Pennsylvania (12).

The upshot of all this is that physicians must learn to treat themselves in a humane way, in the same way they try to treat their patients. Patients need warmth and understanding—someone who has the time to listen and who can encourage the individual to cope and thereby allow him to mobilize his resources to go on with the struggles of his life. Physicians need the same things as their patients, only they often are too proud to ask for it. Hopefully, they can learn to ask, and their friends and colleagues can learn to offer. As one of my family doctor friends said about the needs of doctors: "We all have to learn to reach out and touch (13)."

REFERENCES

1. Rose, K., et al. (1973): Physicians who kill themselves. *Arch. Gen. Psychiatry*, 29:800.
2. Pearson, E. (1973): The Sick Physician. Address given at the Eleventh Annual Colloquium of the American Psychiatric Association on the postgraduate teaching of psychiatry, Charleston, SC.
3. Valliant, G. (1970): Physicians' use of mind-altering drugs. *N. Engl. J. Med.*, 282:365.
4. Valliant, G. (1972): Some psychological vulnerabilities of physicians. *N. Engl. J. Med.*, 287:272–375.
5. Middleton, J. (1970): Drug-abuse—growing occupational hazard for doctors. *Hosp. Physician*, 6:60.
6. Council on Mental Health, American Medical Association (1973): The sick physician. *JAMA*, 233:684.
7. Lurie, H. J., producer/scriptwriter (1979): *Coping: Stress and the Resident Physician* (videotape and discussion leader's guide). American Academy of Family Physicians, Kansas City, MO.
8. American Psychiatric Association: Eleventh Annual Colloquium on Postgraduate Teaching of Psychiatry. Charleston, SC, 1973; "Coping Conferences" (Mental Health Committee of the American Academy of Family Physicians, Sponsor), 1966–1970.
9. Pfifferling, J. H.: *The Impaired Physician: An Overview*. Health Sciences Consortium, Inc., Chapel Hill, NC.
10. Tokarz, J. P., Bremer, W., et al. (1979): *Beyond Survival*. American Medical Association, Chicago.
11. Aller, L.: Personal communication.
12. Personal Problems of Physicians Committee, Washington State Medical Association, Seattle, WA. (Media outlining how such a "personal problems committee" can operate is also available from Washington State Medical Association.)
13. Hazelrigg, J.: Personal communication.
14. Valko, R. J. and Clayton, P. J. (1975): Depression in the internship. Diseases of the Nervous System, 36:26–29.
15. Lurie, H. J. (producer/scriptwriter) (1981): *Coping: Stress and the Practicing Physician* (videotape and discussion leaders guide). American Academy of Family Physicians, Kansas City, Missouri.

Subject Index

A

Abstract thinking, impaired, 161
Abusive elderly patient, 88–89
Acetamenophen, for chronic pain, 95
Acquiescence and deflection, and seductive patient, 37–38
Acting out, 75
Addiction
  to chlordiazepoxide, 133
  and confrontative interviewing style, 17
  to meprobamate, 133
Adolescents and adolescence, 58–70
  anxiety disorders in, 43,59
  Brief Reactive Psychosis in, 64,65–67
  and deescalation, 60–61
  defenses in, male, 75
  depression in, 59,121–122
  family of, 68,69–70,121–122
  friendly and objective counseling in, 61
  identity crisis in, 64–65,165–166
  interviewing, 44–45
  and office team, 3
  and parents, 58,60,61
  and physician's role, 60–62
  preoccupation of, with body, 62,63,219
  rapport with, 60
  reaction of, to physical illness, 62–63
  schizophrenia in, 64,66–70
  schizophreniform disorder in, 65–66
  sexual activity of, 59,63,64
  sexual concerns of, 63–64,219–220
  suicidal, 121–122
  therapy group for, 169
  turmoil in, 58
  values of, 58
  values clarification for, 61

Adult development, 72–79,154,202,203
Adult life
  false assumptions about, 73–74
  sexual concerns in, 221
Adulthood, early, depression in, 122–124
Advice-giving interviewing style, 17–19
Affect, in mental status examination, 160
Affection-seeking, 33
Affective disorders, *see specific disorder*
Aging; *see also* Elderly
  facts about, 80–81
  myths about, 80,81,83,222
Alcohol intoxication, treatment of, 177
Alcohol withdrawal, in differential diagnosis of anxiety, 131
Alcoholics Anonymous, 181,182
Alcoholism, 175–183
  acute treatment of, 177
  behavioral contract in, 177,180,200
  and change in beliefs, 177–178
  and depression, 113–114
  development of, factors correlated with, 177
  diagnosis of, 175–177
  disulfiram in, 179,181
  employer confrontation in, 180–181
  group therapy in, 181–182
  hospital and residential treatment in, 181
  individual therapy for, 179–180, 175
  and physician, 178–179
  among physicians, 237,238
  problems in implementing treatment in, 182–183
Allied health personnel, 4
Alprazolam, for panic attacks, 132
Altruism, in mid-life, 75
Amitriptyline, 114,116
Amoxapine, 114,115

245

Analgesics, for chronic pain, 95
Anger, and advice-giving interviewing style, 18
Anger phase of dying, 92, 94
Anorexia nervosa, in children, 44
Antianxiety drugs
  for acute anxiety, 132
  for chronic anxiety, 132–133,134
  for anxiety with depression, 113
  for delirium tremens, 144
  for physical symptoms, 26–27
  psychiatric side effects of, 149
Anticholinergics, psychiatric side effects of, 149
Anticipation, in mid-life, 75
Anticonvulsants, psychiatric side effects of, 148
Antidepressants, 126; see also Tricyclic antidepressants
Antiemetics, 96
Antihistamines, psychiatric side effects of, 149
Antiparkinsonian drugs, psychiatric side effects of, 149
Antipsychotic drugs
  for acute psychosis in adolescence, 65–66
  for adolescent schizophrenia, 67–68,69,70
  in chronic anxiety, 133
  in depression with anxiety, 116
  long-acting injectable, 68,70,168
  psychiatric side effects of, 149
  for schizophrenia, 68,69–70,166–168
  for schizophrenic patient in relapse, 144
Antisocial personality disorder, 43
Anxiety, 131–138
  acute, management of, 132
  in adolescence, 43,59
  athletics for, 137
  and attention span, 161
  and calculating ability, 161
  catastrophizing in, cognitive approaches to, 136
  in children, 43,133
  and depression, 113,115–116
  desensitization and hypersensitization for, 197
  differential diagnosis of, 131–132
  and judgment, 162
  measures of, 188–189
  medications for, 132–133,134; see also Antianxiety drugs
  reassurance and support in, 135–136
  reciprocal inhibition for, 195
  relaxation rituals for, 138
  saunas, spas, and hot tubs for, 138
  sexual activities for, 137
  stress reduction procedures for, 135
  structured activities for, 135
  therapy groups for, 136–137
  touch for, 137
  vegetative symptoms in, 25
Appearance, in mental status examination, 157
Aspirin, for chronic pain, 95
Assertiveness training, 198
Athletics, for chronic anxiety, 137
Atropine compounds, psychiatric side effects of, 149
Attention deficit disorder, 43,120
  assessment of, 47–51
  differential diagnosis of, 48
  parent education about effects of medication for, 49–50
  treatment of, 48–51
Attention-seeking, 33
Attention span, impaired, 161
Audio tapes, for explicit sexual language desensitization, 229
Auditory hallucinations, 160
Authority, and advice-giving interviewing style, 18–19
Aversion therapy, in alcoholism, 181

B

Barbiturates, 133,144,148
Bargaining phase of dying, 92
Beck Depression Inventory (BDI), 189
Behavior
  adolescent, strange, 59
  in mental status examination, 157,160
Behavior modification, 191,196–197
  in attention deficit disorder, 49
Behavior techniques, 191–201
  for attention deficit disorder, 50–51
  for physical symptoms, 27

SUBJECT INDEX

for sexual dysfunction, 225–228
Behavioral contract, *see* Contract, behavioral
Beliefs, change in, and treatment of alcoholism, 177–178
Bellevue Index of Depression, 103
Bender-Gestalt Test, 185–186
Benton Visual Retention Test, 186
Benzodiazepines, for anxiety, 116,132–133,134
Bereavement, uncomplicated, 103–104,105
Biofeedback, 199
  with relaxation, 135
Bipolar disorder, *see* Manic-depressive disorder
Body, adolescent's preoccupation with, 62,63,219
Body language, 19
Body movement, in mental status examination, 160
Books, for desensitizing physician about sexual material, 234–236
Boundary issues, in marriage, 76,77
Brief Reactive Psychosis, 166
  in adolescent, 64,65–67
  symptoms of, 158,161
  treatment of, 158
Bromides, psychiatric side effects of, 148
Bulimia, in children, 44
Butyrophenones, for schizophrenia, 168

C

Caffeine, overuse of, in differential diagnosis of anxiety, 131
Calculation ability, impaired, 161
California Psychological Inventory (CPI), 186
Catastrophizing, cognitive approaches to, 136
Catatonia, 165
  symptoms of, 158
  treatment of, 158
Chemical restraints, 144–145
Child abuse, 146
  sexual, 52–58
Child abusers, 146
Childbirth and depression, 123–124

Childhood onset pervasive developmental disorder, 43–44
Children
  anxiety in, 43,133
  assertiveness training for, 198
  attention deficit disorder in, 43,47–51,120
  and behavioral contracts with parents, 200
  conduct disorders of, 43
  depression in, 45,100,103–104,119–121,122
  developmental deviations in, 43
  diagnostic issues and treatment implications with, 42–44
  dying, 52,93
  eating disorders of, 44
  external conflict in, 42–43
  functional encopresis in, 44
  functional enuresis in, 44
  healthy responses of, 42
  interviewing, 44–47, 53–57
  mental retardation in, 43
  and office atmosphere, 7
  oppositional disorders in, 43
  phobias in, 133
  psychological tests for, 185,186
  reactions of, to illness and hospitalization, 51–52
  sexual abuse of, 52–57
  sexual concerns of, 218–219
  stereotyped movement disorders in, 44
  stuttering disorders in, 44
  therapy groups for, 169
Chlorazepate, for anxiety, 132,133
Chlordiazepoxide
  for alcohol withdrawal syndrome, 177
  for anxiety, 133
  physical addiction to, 133
Chlorpromazine
  for alcohol withdrawal syndrome, 177
  for schizophrenia, 166–167
Chronic brain syndrome, acute (reversible), 162–166; *see also* Organic brain syndrome
  differential diagnosis of, 138
  symptoms of, 158
  treatment of, 158,163–166

Chronic brain syndrome (irreversible), 162–166; *see also* Organic brain syndrome
 differential diagnosis of, 163
 symptoms of, 158,161
 treatment of, 158,162–166
Cimetidine, psychiatric side effects of, 149
Civil commitment procedures, 145
Clarifying interviewing style, 14–15
Clinical observation, in assessment of attention deficit disorder, 48
Closed relationships, 20,21
Clubs, for chronic anxiety, 137
Codeine, in chronic pain, 95
Cognitive distortion, and depression, 105,109
Combative elderly patient, 88–89
Communication
 of adolescent with parents, 58
 dysfunctional, 210
 in dysfunctional family, 70
 and marriage and family counseling, 209–210
 nonverbal, 19
Community mental health center, for ex-mental patient, 170
Compazine®, in vomiting, 96
Competitive patient, 34–36
Complaint sessions, for hypochrondriasis, 127–128
Compulsive personality, of physician, 237
Conduct disorder, 43
Confidentiality
 and adolescent sexual concerns, 220
 and children, 47
 and psychological tests, 184
Conflict
 in children, 42–43
 counseling for, 23
 marital, 76,77; *see also* Marital counseling
Confrontation, and seductive patient, 37
Confrontative interviewing style, 15–17
Confusion, clarifying interviewing style in, 15
Consciousness, impaired, 161

Contract, behavioral, 199–200
 in alcoholism, 179
 in counseling, 22
 in depression, 109–110
Conversion phenomena, 26
Corticosteroids, psychiatric side effects of, 150
Counseling, 21–24; *see also* Marital and family counseling; Sexual counseling
 of adolescent, 61
 crisis, 22
 education as, 23
 in emotional conflict, 23
 for ex-mental patient, 170
 group, 111–113
 marital, 125
 support, 22–23
Crisis
 and acute depression, 154
 and advice-giving interviewing style, 19
 life, and interviewing style, 15
 mid-life, *see* Mid-life crisis
Crisis counseling, 22
Crisis intervention, 110–111,139,152–155
Culture
 and alcoholism, 177
 and counseling, 122–123
 and marital and family counseling, 209
 and symptoms, 26
Cyclothymic disorder, 101–102

D

Day-treatment programs
 for adolescent schizophrenic, 70
 in depression, 111
 for ex-mental patient, 170
Decadron®, in chronic pain, 95
Defenses, in adult male life cycle, 75–76
Delinquency, and alcoholism, 177
Delirium, 161,162; *see also* Chronic brain syndrome, acute (reversible)
 and hallucinations, 160
 in intoxication, 163,164
Delirium tremens, 177
 antianxiety drugs for, 144, 177
 hallucinations with, 160

SUBJECT INDEX

Dementia, 104,161,162–163; *see also* Chronic brain syndrome, irreversible
Denial phase of dying, 92,94
Dependent patient, 14,18,32–34
Depression, 99–130
  in adolescents, 59,121–122
  and advice-giving interviewing style, 19
  causes of, 104–105
  in children, 45,100,103–104, 119–121,122
  classification of, 99,100–102
  crisis taking form of, 154
  differential diagnosis of, 102–103,137–138
  and dying, 128
  in early adulthood, 122–124
  in elderly, 86–87,127–128,159, 162–163
  measures of, 189
  in men, 99,100,124–125
  in middle age, 124–125
  in physician, 125
  recurrent, 101,117
  secondary, in attention deficit disorder, 50
  after surgery, 139,140–141
  symptoms of, 25,99,100–101,120–121
  treatment of, 105–119,122
  in women, 99,100,124
Depression phase of dying, 92–94
Depressive episode, major, with psychosis
  treatment of, 159
  symptoms of, 159
Depressive equivalents, 125
Desensitization, of physician, to sexual material, 228–236
Desensitization and hypersensitization, 197
Desipramine, 114,116
Development, adult, *see* Adult development
Developmental changes, and crisis, 154
Developmental deviations, in children, 43
Developmental disorders, pervasive, 43–44
Developmental stress, 208

Dexamethasone suppression test, 117
Dextroamphetamine
  abuse of, in differential diagnosis of anxiety, 132
  in attention deficit disorder, 49–50
Diary, patient, 35,109
Diazepam
  for anxiety, 132,133
  for anxious depression, 116
  physical addiction to, 133
  psychological dependence on, 133
Difficult-problem patient, 28–41
Digitalis glycosides, psychiatric side effects of, 150
Dilaudid®, in chronic pain, 95
Disorganized (hebephrenic) psychosis, 165
  symptoms of, 158
  treatment of, 158
Disorientation, 161
  at night, in organic psychosis, 164
Disulfiram, 179,181
  psychiatric side effects of, 149
Doxepin, 114,115
Drawings, children's, 46–47
Droperidol, for nausea, 96
Drug abuse
  adolescent's, 59
  and depression, 113–114
  physician's, 238
Drug-drug interactions, 115
Drug intoxication, 66,104,144–145,163
Drugs
  psychiatric complications of, 103,148–150
  and sexuality, 225
DSM III, 39,43,65,99
Dying
  stages of, 92–93
  teaching about, 93–94
Dying patient, 92–98
  and cautious optimism, 96
  child, 52,93
  and chronic pain, 94–95
  and continuity of care, 97
  and depression, 128
  and hospice movement, 94–96
  interviewing, 94

Dying patient (*contd.*)
  and nausea, 96
  and quiet confidence, 96
Dysfunctional communication styles, 70,210
Dysthymic disorder, 101,102

E

Eating disorders, 44
ECT, 118–119
Education
  limited formal, and impaired thinking, 161
  medical,10,212–213,214,216
  patient, 3,8–9,23
  preventive, 241
Elderly, 80–91; *see also* Aging
  abusive, combative, 88–89
  depression in, 86–87,118,127–128, 137–138,159
  depression mimicking dementia in, 162–163
  diagnostic and treatment issues in nursing
    home care of, 86–90
  ECT in, 118
  forgetfulness of, 88
  and losses, 80,127
  mental status examination of, 83
  and office organization, 2
  and office team, 3
  organic brain syndrome in, 163
  and orientation, 83–85
  and planning and prevention, 85–86
  psychotic, 89–90
  sexual concerns of, 222
  touch for, 137
  treatment techniques with, 81–83
Electroconvulsive therapy (ECT), 118–119
Electroencephalogram,
  in organic psychosis, 164–165
  sleep, 117
Emergencies, psychiatric,
  31–41,139–147; *see also specific emergency*
Empathic style of interviewing, 12–14

Empathy, 18
  versus sympathy, 13
Employer confrontation, in alcoholism, 180–181
Encopresis, functional, in children, 44
Empty nest syndrome, 124
Endocrine disorders, and sexuality, 224
Eneurisis, functional, in children, 44
Environment, in organic psychosis, 163–164
Ex-mental patient, 169–171
Exploration, empathic interviewing as, 14
Extinction phenomenon, 196
Eye contact, 19

F

Facial expression, in mental status examination, 157
Family; *see also* Parents
  of adolescent depressive patient, 121–122
  of adolescent schizophrenic, 68,69–70
  and alcoholism, 180
  assessment of, and children's problems, 47
  communication in, 70, 209–210
  counseling of, *see* Marital and family counseling
  and depression, 107–108
Family therapy, in depression, 107–108,122; *see also* Marital and family counseling
Fantasies, eliciting, in children, 46–47
Feelings
  in mental status examination, 160
  problems with, and empathic interviewing style, 14
Films, for desensitizing physician to sexual material, 230–234
Flooding, 197
Fluphenazine decanoate, for schizophrenia, 168
Fluphenazine enanthate, for schizophrenia, 168
Flurazepam, for anxiety, 133
Forgetfulness, of elderly, 88

G

Generalized anxiety disorder, 131; *see also* Anxiety
Genital diseases, and sexuality, 225
Goldfarb 10-point scale, 83
Grief, normal, *see* Bereavement, uncomplicated
Gross motor coordination, 47
Group therapy
　for alcoholism, 181–182
　for chronic anxiety, 136–137
　for depression, 111–113, 122
　in office, 3
　for physical symptoms, 27
　for posttraumatic stress disorder in Vietnam veterans, 174
　for schizophrenia, 169
Guanethidine, psychiatric side effects of, 150

H

Hallucinations
　auditory, 160
　in mental status examination, 160
　tactile, 160
　visual, 160
Hallucinogen intoxication, 145
Halogenated phenothiazines, 166–167
Haloperidol
　for alcohol intoxication, 177
　for schizophrenia, 168
　for schizophreniform disorder, 66
　for Tourette's syndrome, 44
Hamilton Anxiety Scale, 189
Hamilton Depression Scale, 189
Heredity
　and alcoholism, 177
　and depression, 105
Heroin, for chronic pain, 95
Hierarchy of restraint, 143–145
History
　in diagnosis of attention deficit disorder, 48
　sexual, 199, 222–224
　and somatization, hypochondriasis, and chronic pain complaints, 40
Hobbies, physician's, 241
Holistic medicine, 8–9
Home, structured, in attention deficit disorder, 48–49
Home visits, 3, 33, 107
Homicidal behavior
　causes of, 145
　immediate precipitants of, 145–146
Homicidal patients, 145–146
Homosexual experiences, of adolescent, 63, 64, 220
Hopkins Symptom Checklist (HSCL), 189
Hospice movement, 94–96
Hospitalization
　for adolescent schizophrenia, 67, 70
　for alcoholism, 181
　avoidance of, for adolescent schizophrenia, 68
　reactions of children to, 51–52
　for schizophrenia, 71, 169
Hostile patient, 29–32
　and reasons for anger, 29–30
　strategies and approaches to, 30–32
Hostility, adolescent, 58, 59, 60
Hot tubs, for chronic anxiety, 138
Humor, in mid-life, 75
Hyperthyroidism, in differential diagnosis of anxiety, 132
Hypochondriasis, 39, 40–41
　in adolescent males, 75
　complaint sessions for, 127–128
Hypoglycemia, in differential diagnosis of anxiety, 132
Hysterical personality, and clarifying interviewing style, 15
Hysterical phenomena, 26

I

Identity, women's, 77–78
Identity crisis, adolescent, 64–65, 165–166
　differentiating from schizophrenia, 165–166
Identity disorder, 64
Illness
　and depression, 102–103, 113–114
　reaction of adolescent to, 62–63

Illness *(contd.)*
  reaction of child to, 51–52
  and sexuality, 224–225
Illusions, 160
Imipramine
  for anxiety, 43,133
  for depression, 114
  for phobias, 133
Independence, adolescents, 59
Impotence, 226–227
Indomethacin, psychiatric side effects of, 149
Infantile autism, 43–44
Insight, impaired, 161–162
Insomnia, anxiety about, 132
Institutional support system, for physician, 243
Intellectual functioning, in mental status examination, 161–162
Intellectualizing, in adolescent males, 75
Intelligence tests, 184–185
Interview
  sexual, 223–224
  Structured Family, 212–214
Interviewer, relationship to, in mental status examination, 160
Interviewing, 10–21
  assumptions about, 11–12
  children, 44–47,53–57
  dying patient, 94
  suicidal patient, 141
  victim of child sexual abuse, 53–58
Interviewing styles
  advice-giving, 17–19
  clarifying, 14–15
  confrontative, 15–17
  empathic, 12–14,223–224
Intoxication
  and hallucinations, 160
  and organic psychosis, 163,164
Isoniazid, psychiatric side effects of, 150

J
Judgment, impaired, 161,162

K
Kegal exercises, 228
Kinetic Family Drawing, 46

L
Law suits, 31
Learned helplessness, and depression, 104–105
Levodopa, psychiatric side effects of, 149
Levodromeran®, in chronic pain, 95
Life cycle
  of adult men, 74–76
  and depression, 119–125,127–128
  and developmental stress, 208
  of marriage, 76–77
Life planning, 202–207
  analysis of present situation in, 205
  development of new goals in, 205
  identity questions in, 206
  life roles in, 206
  longitudinal life assessment in, 205–206
  for physician, 240–241
  projection questions in, 206
  values clarification in, 204–205
Lithium, 101,118
Liver diseases, and sexuality, 224
Loose associations, 161
Loss, and depression, 104,127
Lorazepam, for anxiety, 133

M
Male menopause, 125
Manic-depressive disorder, 101,105
  symptoms of, 101,159
  treatment of, 101,118–119,159
MAO inhibitors, 116–117,126
Maprotiline, 114
Marezine®, for vomiting, 96
Marijuana, for chronic pain, 96
Marital assessment test, 215
Marital conflict, 76,77
Marital and family counseling, 208–216
  and communication issues, 209–210
  and cultural issues, 209
  in depression, 125
  and developmental issues, 208
  and diagnostic procedures, 212–214
  and maturational issues, 209
  and personality pathology issues, 210–211
  and referrals, 216
  strategies of, 214–216

and transference and projection issues, 211–212
Marriage
  and depression, 123
  life cycle of, 76–77
  and personality types, 211
  physician's, 239
  and projection, 211–212
  and transference, 211–212
Marriage contract, 215
Masturbation, 63, 219–220
Maturational issues, and marital and family counseling, 209
Media, and patient education, 8, 9
Medical education
  and interviewing and counseling skills, 10
  and stress, 237–238, 239, 241
Meditation, 135
Medrol®, for chronic pain, 95
Memory, impaired, 88, 161–162
Men
  defenses of, 75–76
  depression in, 99–100, 124–125
  and developmental issues, 74–75
  and expression of emotions, 26
Menopause, 124
  male, 124–125
Mental retardation, 19, 43, 161
Mental status examination
  in elderly, 83
  in psychosis, 156–157, 160–162
Methadone, for chronic pain, 95
Meprobamate, physical addiction to, 133
Mercaptophenothiazines, for schizophrenia, 167–168
Methyldopa, psychiatric side effects of, 150
Methylphenidate
  abuse of, in differential diagnosis of anxiety, 132
  for attention deficit disorders, 49
Metoclorpamide, for vomiting, 96
Mid-life
  defenses in, in male, 75
  depression, 124–125
  sexual concerns in, 221–222
Mid-life crisis, 73, 124, 125

Minimal brain dysfunction, test for, 185–186
Minnesota Multiphasic Personality Inventory (MMPI), 187
Monoamine oxidase inhibitors, 116–117, 126
Mood, in mental status examination, 160
Mood fluctuations, in adolescent, 59
Morphine, for chronic pain, 95
Motor performance, test of, 185–186
Motor skills, children's, 47
Motor tic disorder, chronic, in children, 44
Movement disorders, stereotyped, in children, 44
Mutual Story Telling technique, 46

N
Nausea, of dying patient, 96
Navane, for adolescent schizophreniform disorder, 66
Neonatal period, sexual concerns in, 218
Neurologic diseases, and sexuality, 224–225
Neurotransmitters, and depression, 105
No-suicide contract, 109
Nortriptyline, 114, 116
Nurse practitioners, 4
Nursing homes
  diagnosis and treatment issues in, 86–90
  placement in, 33–34

O
Obsessive-compulsive disorders, 131
Office atmosphere, 2, 5–7
  and avoidance of patient hostility, 31
  and elderly, 82–83
Office team, 1–4
  and avoidance of patient hostility, 31
  and crisis intervention, 154, 155
  and therapy group, 169
Open relationship
  advantages of, 19
  disadvantages of, 19–20
  establishing, 19–21
  and personal perceptions, 21

Open relationship (contd.)
  and specific information, 20–21
  and time factor, 20
  and use of feelings, 21
Opiate antagonists, 145
Opiate intoxication, 145
Oppositional disorders, 43
Oral contraceptives, psychiatric side
  effects of, 150
Organic brain syndrome, 19,127,162–165
  differential diagnosis of, 163
  in differential diagnosis of anxiety, 132
  and mental status assessment, 83
  symptoms of, 158,161
  treatment of, 158,163–165
Organic impairment, tests for, 185–186
Orgasmic dysfunction, female, 227–228
Orientation
  of elderly, 83–85
  impaired, 161
Oxazepam, for anxiety, 133
Oxycodone, for chronic pain, 95

P
Pain, chronic, 94–95
Panic, prior to surgery, 140–141
Panic attacks, 132
  in adolescent, 59
  alprazolam for, 132
  tricyclic antidepressants for, 133
Paranoia
  and physical restraints, 144
  symptoms of, 159
  and talking restraints, 143
  treatment of, 159
Paranoid delusions of persecution, 161
Paranoid schizophrenia, 165
Parents; see also Family
  of adolescent, 58,60,61
  and child's illness, 52
  of dying child, 52
  education of, about medications for
    attention deficit disorder, 49–50
  interviewing, 42,44,45
Paroxysmal atrial tachycardia (PAT), in
  differential diagnosis of anxiety, 132
Passive-aggressive adolescent male, 75

Passive-aggressive personality disorder,
  43
Patient
  compliance and noncompliance of,
    26–27,70–71
  dependent, 32–34
  discomfort of, about help, 11–12
  ex-mental, 144–146
  giving information to, 8
  involvement of, 8,35
  and struggles with physician, 15–16
Patient education, 3,8–9,23
PCP intoxication, and chemical restraints,
  144–145
Pemiline, for attention deficit disorders,
  49
Penicillin, psychiatric side effects of, 150
Pentazocine, psychiatric side effects of,
  150
Perceptions, in mental status
  examination, 160
Perceptual-motor problems, tests of,
  185–186
Percodan®, for chronic pain, 95
Perfectionistic patient, 34–36
Perphenazine, 116
Personality disorder
  and confrontative interviewing style,
    17
  explosive, sedatives for, 144
Personality pathology, 210–211
Personality tests, 186–187
Phenacetin, psychiatric side effects of,
  149
Phenelzine, 114
Phenothiazines, 166–168
Phenylephrine, psychiatric side effects of,
  150
Phobias, 131
  in children, 133
  imipramine for, 133
  reciprocal inhibition for, 195
Phone calls, returning, 31–32
Phone contact, 33
Physical restraints, 144
Physician(s)
  and adolescent, 60–62
  alcoholism among, 237,238

beliefs of, 5
career change for, 241–242
with compulsive personality, 237
depression in, 125
desensitizing, about sexual material, 228–236
drug abuse among, 238
education of, 10,237–238,239,241
feelings of, and open relationship, 21
hobbies for, 241
institutional support system for, 243
judging by, 12
level of comfort of, 12
life planning for, 240–241
marriage of, 239
medical society meetings for, 241
mental health of, 125,237–243
patient's struggles with, 15–16
practice of, effect of, 239,240
prestige of, 238,239
preventive education programs for, 241
reactions of, 12
roles of, 12
seductive behavior of, 38–39
social support system of, 239,242,243
suicide rate of, 237
values of, 28
Physician assistants, 4
Physician-patient relationship, 11,12,19–21,28
Pica, in children, 44
Placebos, 27
Play
  structured, 45–46
  unstructured, 45,47
PLISSIT model, 217–218
Posture, in mental status examination, 157
Posttraumatic stress disorder, 131
  in Vietnam veterans, 113,172–174
Practice, solo, 239,240
Prazepam, for anxiety, 133
Pregnancy, and sexual concerns, 218
Premature ejaculation, 226
Prenatal period, sexual concerns in, 218
Prenatal visits, 3
Problem clarification, and seductive patient, 38

Problems, multiple, and clarifying interviewing style, 15
Progressive relaxation, 135
Projection, 75,211–212
Projective tests, 187–188
Propranolol, psychiatric side effects of, 150
Protriptyline, 114,116
Pseudodementia, 127
Psychiatric emergencies, *see* Emergencies, psychiatric
Psychogenic pain disorder, 39,40–41
Psychological intervention, disagreement over value and need for, 10–11
Psychological tests, 184–190
  of anxiety, 188–189
  of depression, 189
  of intelligence, 184–185
  of organic impairment, 164,185–186
  of personality, 186–187
  projective, 187–188
Psychophysiological disorder, adolescent, 59
Psychosis, 156–171
  Brief Reactive, 64,65–67,136,141,161
  in elderly, 89–90
  and mental status examination, 156–157,160–162
  recovering from, and advice-giving interviewing style, 19
  types of, 158–159,162–169
Psychosomatic complaints, as depressive equivalents, 125
Psychotherapy
  for adult schizophrenics, 69
  for alcoholism, 154–155
  in attention deficit disorder, 50
  for depression, 105–106,116
  group, *see* Group therapy

Q
Questionnaire, patient, 8

R
Rationalizing, in adolescent males, 75
Rauwolfia alkaloids, psychiatric side effects of, 103,150

Reaction formation, in adolescent males, 75
Reality orientation, 84, 164
Reassurance
 for acute anxiety, 132
 for chronic anxiety, 135–136
Rebelliousness, of adolescent, 58–59
Recall, tests of, 186
Reciprocal inhibition, 195
Referrals
 for adolescent homosexuality, 63
 for marital and family problems, 216
Regressive behavior, of ill children, 51
Rehabilitation
 and abusive, combative patient, 88–89
 and depression, 86–87
 and disorientation, 84–85
 and forgetfulness, 88
 and psychotic elderly, 89–90
Reinforcement
 in behavior modification, 196
 in depression, 105
Relationship, see Closed relationship; Open relationship; Physician-patient relationship
Relaxation rituals, for chronic anxiety, 138
Relaxation training, 135, 192–195
Resensitization, 198
Reserpine, psychiatric side effects of, 150
Reserved people, and confrontative interviewing style, 17
Residential treatment, for alcoholism, 181
Resistance, confrontative interviewing style for, 17
Restraints
 chemical, 144–145
 physical, 144
 talking, 143–144
Rigid patient, 34–36
Rituals, relaxation, for chronic anxiety, 138
Rorschach Test, 187

S

Sabbaticals, for physician, 241
Salicylates
 for chronic pain, 95

 psychiatric side effects of, 150
Saunas, for chronic anxiety, 138
Scandinavian system, of dealing with depression, 108–109
Schizophrenia, 164–169
 adolescent, 64, 66–70
 depression in, 104
 symptoms of, 66–67, 158, 160–161
 theories of, 68–69
 treatment of, 158, 166–168
Schizophreniform disorder, 166
 in adolescent, 65–66
 and disorientation, 161
School, structured, in attention deficit disorder, 49
School behavior, troublesome, behavior contract in, 200
Sedative-hypnotics, 133, 144, 148, 164
Seductive patient, 36–39
 elderly, 82
 and meaning of behavior, 36–37
 strategies and approaches to, 37–38
Self-esteem, low, in attention deficit disorder, 50
Self-help groups, for alcoholism, 182
Sensate focus exercises, 226, 227
Separation anxiety, 43, 104
 in adolescent, 59
 and hospitalization, 51
Sexual abuse of children, 52–57
Sexual activity
 of adolescent, 59, 63, 64
 for chronic anxiety, 137
Sexual concerns, 217–222
 in adolescence, 63–64, 219–220
 in adult years, 221
 in childhood, 218–219
 in mid-life, 221–222
 in neonatal period, 218
 in old age, 222
 in prenatal period, 218
Sexual counseling, 217–236
Sexual dysfunction, 197, 217–236
Sexual history, 222–224, 227
Sexual therapy, 225–228
Siblings, and death, 52
SIGEP program, 50–51, 199
Situational homosexuality, 64

SUBJECT INDEX

Sleep EEG, 117
Social class, 182
Social contacts, of adolescent schizophrenic, 68
Social factors, and symptoms, 25–27
Social skills training, 199
  in attention deficit disorder, 50–51
Social support system, physician's, 239,242,243
Solu-medrol®, for chronic pain, 95
Somatic symptoms
  and depression, 25,125,127
  and social factors, 25–27
Somatization disorder, 39,40–41
Spas, for chronic anxiety, 138
Spatial perception, tests of, 186
Speech, in mental status examination, 157
State-Trait Anxiety Inventory (STAI), 188
Stereotyped movement disorders, in children, 44
Steroids, for chronic pain, 95
Stimulants
  abuse of, in differential diagnosis of anxiety, 132
  for attention deficit disorder, 49,50
Stranger anxiety, 51
Stress, life, and depression, 104,119
Stress, in medical education, 237–238
Stress reduction procedures, 135
Structured Family Interview, 212–214
Sublimation, in mid-life, 75
Suicidal patient, 19,121–122,141–143
Suicide rates
  and age, 127
  among physicians, 237
Sulfonamides, psychiatric side effects of, 150
Support
  for chronic anxiety, 135–136
  and symptoms, 27
Support counseling, 22–23
Support groups, 136–137
Support system
  in depression, 106–107,108
  of physician, 239,242,243
  in schizophrenia, 168–169

Suppression, in mid-life, 75
Surgery, 139–141
Surgical conditions, and sexuality, 225
Symbolic giving, 82
Sympathy vs. empathy, 13
Symptoms
  counting, 35
  log of, 135
  and social factors, 25–27

T

Tactile hallucinations, 160
Talking down, 144,145
Talking restraints, 143–144
Talking, Thinking, and Feeling Game, 46
Tardive dyskinesia, 68,168
Taylor Manifest Anxiety Scale (TMAS), 188
Teacher rating scale, 48
Teenagers, *see* Adolescents and adolescence
Thematic Apperception Test (TAT), 188
Therapist-patient relationship, 191
Thinking
  in mental status examination, 160–162
  nonlogical, 161
Thioridazine
  for anxious depression, 116
  for schizophrenia, 167–168
Touch, for chronic anxiety, 137
Tourette's syndrome, 44
Tranquilizers
  major, *see* Antipsychotic drugs
  minor, *see* Antianxiety drugs
Transactional analysis, 211,212
Transference, 37,211–212
Transient tic disorder, in children, 44
Tranylcypramine, 114
Traumatic neurosis, 197
Treatment plan, written, 35–36
Tricyclic antidepressants, 113,114–116,117,122,126; *see also* Antidepressants
  for anxiety in children, 133
  prediction of response to, 117
  for prevention of panic attacks, 133
  psychiatric side effects of, 149
Trifluoperazine, for schizophrenia, 167

U

Undifferentiated psychosis
  symptoms of, 159
  treatment of, 159
Unipolar disorder, *see* Depression

V

Values
  adolescent's, 58–59
  physician's, 28
  and sex, 222
Values clarification
  and adolescent, 61
  in life planning, 204–205
Ventilation, and empathic interviewing, 14
Verbal exercises, for sexual language desensitization, 229–230
Veterans, Vietnam, posttraumatic stress disorder in, 113, 172–174
Vietnam Outreach, 173
Violent patient, 143–145
Visiting team, in depression, 107
Visual hallucinations, 160
Visual performance, tests of, 185, 186

W

Wechsler Adult Intelligence Scale (WAIS), 185
Wechsler Intelligence Scale for Children (WISC), 185
Wechsler Preschool and Primary Scale of Intelligence (WPPSI), 185
Women
  depression in, 99, 100, 124
  and developmental issues, 77–79
  and expression of emotion, 26
  orgasmic dysfunction in, 227–228
Work groups, for chronic anxiety, 137